PARALYSIS RESOURCE GUIDE

SECOND EDITION

By Sam Maddox
Knowledge Manager

Christopher and Dana Reeve Foundation/Paralysis Resource Center

Christopher and Dana Reeve Foundation, Short Hills, New Jersey

PARALYSIS RESOURCE GUIDE
SECOND EDITION

by Sam Maddox

This book was produced by the Paralysis Resource Center (PRC) through a cooperative agreement with the Centers for Disease Control and Prevention (award No. 1U59DD000338). The contents of this book are solely the responsibility of the PRC and do not necessarily represent the official views of the Centers for Disease Control and Prevention.

Cover photograph by Timothy Greenfield-Sanders
Book design by Laura Mazy
Production by Sam Maddox

The material contained in this book is presented for the purpose of educating and informing readers about paralysis and its effects. Nothing contained herein should be construed as medical diagnosis or treatment advice. This information should not be used in place of the advice of a physician or other qualified health care provider. If any questions arise while reading this book, the PRC strongly recommends contacting a physician or the appropriate healthcare provider.

Library of Congress Control Number: 2003094719
ISBN 0-9726831-1-9

For information or to get additional copies of this book:
Paralysis Resource Center
636 Morris Turnpike, Suite 3A
Short Hills, New Jersey 07078
toll-free 1-800-539-7309
e-mail c/o *info@paralysis.org*
on the Internet see *http://www.paralysis.org*

ACKNOWLEDGMENTS

Welcome to the revised and updated edition of the PARALYSIS RESOURCE GUIDE. I would like to recognize several individuals who made this book possible. First, thanks to Christopher and Dana Reeve for recognizing the need for the Paralysis Resource Center (PRC), which produced the book.

Thanks also to key personnel at the Christopher and Dana Reeve Foundation (CDRF), including Executive VP/Director of Research Susan Howley and Senior VP, Marketing and Communications Maggie Goldberg. At the Paralysis Resource Center, thanks to Director and VP/Quality of Life Joe Canose and PRC Librarian Sheila Fitzgibbon. The PRC team of Information Specialists helped with the revision. Thanks also to Jesse Hagy and Rose Rossier in the California office.

This book is made possibly by the support of the Department of Health and Human Services (HHS), Centers for Disease Control and Prevention (CDC), National Center on Birth Defects and Developmental Disabilities (NCBDDD).

The PRC's Paralysis Task Force (see page 304) assisted with connections and research. Many other organizations in the disability community provided resources and helped the text approach the highest standard of verisimilitude.

The PARALYSIS RESOURCE GUIDE is dedicated to the memories of Christopher Reeve and Dana Morosini Reeve. They lived life fully and fearlessly, with purpose and passion. The spirit of Chris and Dana is embodied in the pages of this book: Life is dear, choice is good, hope is irrepressible.

SM
Westlake Village, California

Table of Contents

*H*ello, *and welcome* to the Paralysis Resource Guide. This book, created by the Christopher and Dana Reeve Foundation Paralysis Resource Center (PRC), offers comprehensive information and connections. Our goal is to help you find what you need to stay as healthy, as active and as independent as possible. The book serves the full community of people affected by paralysis, including of course loved ones and caregivers – people who know how paralysis can be a family issue.

Our founders, Chris and Dana, understood how frightening it is to suddenly become paralyzed. Being active one day and immobile the next thrusts you suddenly into an entirely new existence. The changes are enormous and often overwhelming.

First, let us assure you that you are not alone. In the U.S. alone, there are 400,000 people living with paralysis caused by spinal cord injury, and hundreds of thousands of others with paralysis caused by other types of trauma or disease. Although it's a club no one would

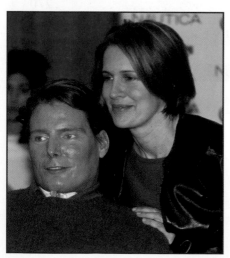

choose to join, there are people who have gone through similar situations who are eager to help you maximize your health and well-being.

The PRC was created to provide information services and resources on the full range of topics related to paralysis, including specific health and clinical information on the various conditions that cause paralysis, whether by stroke, trauma or disease. We have formed partnerships with many national organizations to make sure you get the most relevant and reliable information.

Paralysis is much more than a medical issue, of course. The PRC hopes to encourage you to be active and to participate in your community as much on your own terms as possible. We have resources available on travel and recreation, specialized assistive equipment and automobiles, and key information to help navigate the health care and insurance systems.

You'll also find information on a multitude of organizations around the country that offer programs to promote independent living for children and adults with paralysis. You will find numerous listings in this book devoted to accessibility, health promotion, advocacy, research, and more. We have funded numerous Quality of Life grants through the PRC and the Christopher and Dana Reeve Foundation to support organizations like those around the country.

If you don't find what you need here in the book, be sure and visit the PRC Website, *www.paralysis.org*. If you prefer to speak to a trained information specialist, please contact us by phone (toll-free 1-800-539-7309) or email (*info@paralysis.org*) and we will research your question for you.

Finally, and perhaps most importantly, we want you to know that paralysis is not a hopeless condition. You will know this in more detail after reading Chapter Four in this book, Research. Scientists are making steady progress in deciphering the complexities of diseases and injuries to the brain and spinal cord; we are convinced that they will succeed in developing treatments for acute and chronic paralysis. To learn even more about promising research, and how to support the Foundation's mission, visit the Website *www.ChristopherReeve.org*.

–The PRC Staff

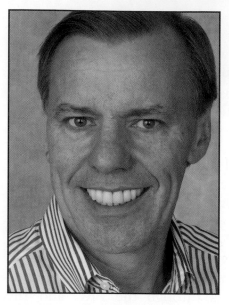

Welcome to the Paralysis Resource Guide, a one-stop handbook to guide you and your loved ones through the often bewildering world of paralysis.

The goals of this book and of the Christopher and Dana Reeve Foundation (CDRF) Paralysis Resource Center are to improve the lives of millions of people living with paralysis. We offer information you can trust in order to make the best choices for a fulfilling and active life.

CDRF has over the years invested millions of dollars to support research to restore function in the damaged spinal cord. While we expect the long-term payoff of treatments and cures, we understand the day-to-day challenges of living with paralysis. That's why we offer tools, services and resources, here and now, through our Quality of Life grants and the Paralysis Resource Center.

We also advocate for the rights of people with disabilities; we want you to be armed with the information and knowledge you need to face the world of paralysis with the fierce determination and courage of our namesakes.

We have a wonderful, dedicated team here at the Foundation carrying on Christopher and Dana's vision and keeping their legacy of hope and perseverance alive. But we all know there is much work ahead of us; we have yet to reach our goal of mobility, full participation and independence for all citizens.

Until that day, we will continue to Go Forward.

Peter Wilderotter, President
Christopher and Dana Reeve Foundation

MESSAGE FROM THE PRC DIRECTOR

The Paralysis Resource Center was created in 2002 to provide a comprehensive, national resource to help people living with paralysis, their caregivers and loved ones promote health, foster community involvement and improve quality of life. What we do is provide a roadmap to help people navigate the chaos of paralysis.

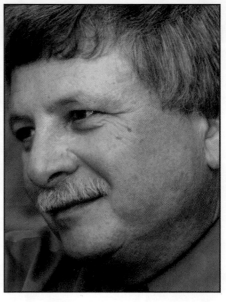

Our message, like that of our namesakes and founders, Chris and Dana, is full of hope. It is consistently upbeat and encouraging, credible and realistic. Paralysis can be a devastating occurrence – for the affected individual, of course, but also for families and friends.

The PRC, formed through a cooperative agreement with the Centers for Disease Control and Prevention, offers information (in English, Spanish and several Asian languages, including Chinese, Vietnamese and Korean) directly by telephone from our team of information specialists (toll-free 1-800-539-7309), by email or online at *www.paralysis.org*, and in print here in the Paralysis Resource Guide.

The PRC is also a large library, open to the public in Short Hills, New Jersey; our books, videos and other materials are available for loan to anyone, at no cost, through the national interlibrary loan program. Click on our homepage for details on the collection, and on the loan procedures. If we can be of further assistance, contact us by phone or email.

Joseph Canose, Director, VP Quality of Life
Christopher and Dana Reeve Foundation/Paralysis Resource Center

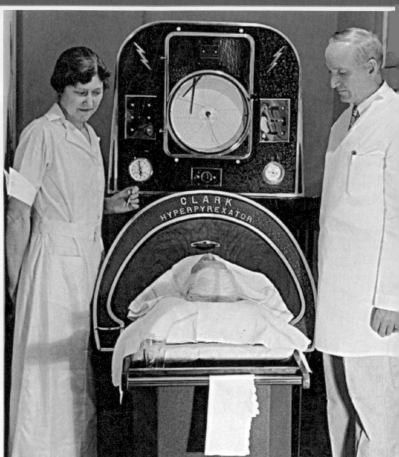

BASICS BY CONDITION

Paralysis is the result of nerve damage in the brain or spinal cord, due to trauma, disease or birth condition. This chapter characterizes the primary causes.

ALS

Amyotrophic lateral sclerosis (ALS), called Lou Gehrig's disease after the New York Yankee baseball player who was stricken by it, is a progressive neurological disease affecting as many as 30,000 Americans with about 5,600 new cases occurring in the United States alone each year.

Amyotrophic lateral sclerosis belongs to a group of disorders known as motor neuron diseases. Motor neurons are nerve cells located in the brain, brainstem and spinal cord that serve as control units and communication links between the nervous system and the voluntary muscles of the body. The loss of these cells causes the muscles under their control to weaken and waste away, leading to paralysis. ALS is often fatal within five years of diagnosis, mainly due to respiratory failure. People who opt for permanent use of a feeding tube and a ventilator after failure of swallowing and respiratory muscles can generally be kept alive for many more years.

Amyotrophic lateral sclerosis manifests itself in different ways, depending on which muscles weaken first. Symptoms may include frequent tripping and falling, loss of control in hands and arms, difficulty speaking, swallowing and/or breathing, persistent fatigue, and twitching and cramping. Typically, ALS strikes in midlife. For reasons unknown, men are about one-and-a-half times more likely to have the disease as women.

Because ALS affects motor neurons, the disease does not usually impair a person's mind, personality, or intelligence. It does not affect the ability to see, smell, taste, hear or recognize touch. People with ALS usually maintain control of eye muscles and bladder and bowel function, although these functions can be affected.

There is no known cure for ALS, nor is there a therapy to prevent or reverse its course. Riluzole is the only FDA approved drug shown to prolong the survival of people with ALS – but only for a few extra months. Riluzole is believed to reduce damage to motor neurons by minimizing damage due to the release of glutamate. The drug may also extend the time before a person needs ventilation support. Riluzole does not reverse the damage already done to motor neurons, and people taking the drug must be monitored for liver damage and other possible side effects. Because of its expense and limited efficacy, riluzole is not always considered by people who could benefit by using it. Aventis Pharmaceuticals offers a patient assistance program that helps qualified patients receive the drug without charge. Many private health plans cover the cost of Riluzole.

ALS experts have identified at least 20 compounds that show promise for treating the disease. Several drugs are currently being tested in patients. See *www.clinicaltrials.gov.*

Physical or occupational therapy and special equipment can enhance independence and safety throughout the course of ALS. Low-impact aerobic exercise such as walking, swimming and stationary bicycling can strengthen unaffected muscles, prevent deconditioning, improve cardiovascular health, and help patients fight fatigue and depression. Range-of-motion and stretching exercises can help prevent painful spasticity and muscle contractures. Occupational therapists can suggest devices such as ramps, braces, walkers and wheelchairs that help people conserve energy and remain mobile, while making it easier to perform activities of daily living.

Respiratory weakness: People with ALS are at risk for pneumonia and pulmonary embolism. Indicators of deteriorating respiratory status can include difficulty breathing, especially when lying down or after meals; lethargy; drowsiness; confusion; anxiety; irritability; loss of appetite; fatigue; morning headaches and depression. When the muscles that assist in breathing weaken, use of ventilatory assistance (intermittent positive pressure ventilation, IPPV; or bi-level positive airway pressure, BiPAP) may be used to aid breathing during sleep. When muscles are no longer able to maintain oxygen and carbon dioxide levels, these devices may be used full-time.

Another problem common to many people with ALS is the inability to cough strongly enough to clear away even normal amounts of mucus. People are advised to make sure their fluid intake is sufficient to keep the secretions thin; some take an over-the-counter cough medicine containing the expectorant guaifenesin, a mucus thinner. A weak cough can be made more effective by quad coughing (assisting a cough by applying a sort of Heimlich-like maneuver as the patient coughs), supplying fuller breaths with an ambu-bag to improve the cough, or using a devise such as a "cofflator" or "In-Exsufflator" (delivers deep breaths through a mask and then quickly reverses to negative pressure to simulate a cough).

Drooling: While people with ALS do not overproduce saliva, their swallowing problems can create sialorrhea, the term for excess salivation and drooling. Sialorrhea can be under-treated—it may take trials of several medications until one provides relief without undesirable side effects.

Muscle problems: Spasticity is present in some people with ALS. It causes a tightening of muscles and a stiffening of the arms, legs, back, abdomen or neck. It can be triggered by a simple touch and can be painful especially if it sets off muscle cramps, common in ALS because of muscle fatigue. Cramps can be very painful but become less severe with time—weakening muscles can't tighten into a cramp anymore. Fasciculation (muscle twitching) is common, too, though they aren't painful so much as annoying.

Loss of communication: While the loss of the ability to communicate is not life-threatening or painful, being "locked-in" is a devastating, extremely frustrating aspect of ALS. Although assistive technology offers many solutions, it may be underutilized because people lack information about what is available. Equipment is available to magnify a weak whisper into audible speech. As long as a person can move nearly any body part there is potential for some basic communication. Numerous communication devices are on the market and can be found in many home health dealers or at Internet shopping sites. See *www.ALSA.org* for a list of products and vendors. These devices range from simple call buttons and sensitive switches to small communication boards that speak pre-recorded words and messages.

In experiments using brain waves, people who are locked in due to ALS have learned to communicate by way of a computer using only their thoughts. Using a headband sensor, Brainfingers is a brain-actuated hands-free mouse that enables a user to steer a cursor, change its speed and resolution, perform left and right mouse button functions, and send keyboard characters and character string commands – all by thought control. Visit *http://brainfingers.com*.

Another more sophisticated device in the clinical testing phase is The BrainGate System, which implants a sensor in the brain to transmit, analyze and, as the company puts it, "apply the language of neurons." Early trials show great promise for the technology. For more detail see *www.Cyberkineticsinc.com*.

There are other ways that computers can be used by people who are almost totally paralyzed. See page 227 for more on hands-free control of cursors for communication, entertainment and even work. Research holds great promise for treatments for ALS, including drugs, cell transplants, gene therapy and immune system modulation. See page 144 for more on the efforts to treat or even cure ALS.

Sources
National Institute on Neurological Disorders and Stroke, ALS Association

ALS RESOURCES

ALS Association (ALSA), a partner with the Christopher and Dana Reeve Foundation Paralysis Resource Center, is rich with news, research support and resources, and it has a national network of connections, support groups, clinics and specialty hospitals. ALSA has awarded more than $30 million to fund research seeking to identify the cause, means of prevention and cure for ALS. ALSA National Office, 27001 Agoura Road, Suite 150, Calabasas Hills, CA 91301; toll-free 1–800–782–4747; or visit the Internet site *http://www.alsa.org*

The ALS Therapy Development Foundation is a nonprofit biotechnology company working to discover treatments for patients alive today. ALS Therapy Development Foundation, 215 First Street, Cambridge, MA 02142; telephone 617-441-7200; on the Internet see *http://www.als.net*

ARTERIOVENOUS MALFORMATIONS

Arteriovenous malformations (AVMs) are defects of the circulatory system that are believed to arise during fetal development or soon after birth. They are comprised of snarled tangles of arteries and veins. Arteries carry oxygen-saturated blood away from the heart to the body's cells; veins return oxygen-depleted blood to the lungs and heart. The presence of an AVM disrupts this vital cycle, reducing oxygen to nervous system tissue and increasing the risk of bleeding.

Arteriovenous malformations can form wherever arteries and veins exist. The ones that form in the brain or spinal cord can be especially problematic. Even in the absence of bleeding or significant oxygen loss, large AVMs can damage the brain or spinal cord by their presence. They can range in size from a fraction of an inch to more than 2.5 inches in diameter. The larger the lesion, the greater the amount of pressure there is on surrounding brain or spinal cord structures.

AVMs of the brain or spinal cord (neurological AVMs) affect approximately 300,000 Americans. They occur in males and females of all racial or ethnic backgrounds at roughly equal rates.

Common symptoms of AVMs are seizures and headaches. Other neurological symptoms may include muscle weakness or paralysis in one part of the body; loss of coordination (ataxia), pain, or disturbances of vision or speech. Mental confusion or hallucination is also possible. There is evidence that AVMs may also cause subtle learning or behavioral disorders during childhood.

Diagnosis of AVM is by either computed axial tomography (CT) or magnetic resonance imaging (MRI) scans. Angiography is an accurate way to get the exact location of the malformation. A thin tube is inserted in a leg artery, threaded toward the brain and then injected with a dye. Pictures reveal the AVM tangle.

Arteriovenous malformations can put veins under great pressure since there are no capillaries to slow blood flow. Over time, the AVM may rupture and cause a hemorrhage. While the risk of hemorrhage is small, the risk increases over time. Therefore, treatment is usually recommended.

Treatment: Advances in technique have made surgical treatment of most cases of AVM safe and effective. Surgery inside the skull may attempt to cut out or burn away the AVM with a laser. Another option for smaller AVMs is stereotactic radiosurgery, which focuses radiation on AVM blood vessels to slowly obliterate them; it may take from one to three years to remove the AVM.

A third treatment option is endovascular embolization, which is similar to an angiogram. A catheter is inserted into a leg artery and threaded through the body toward the affected arteries. A glue-like substance is injected to block key blood vessels leading to the AVM, thus reducing its size so stereotactic radiosurgery or conventional surgery may be used to treat it.

Surgery is a decision that must be made with full understanding of risks. Untreated, AVMs have the potential to hemorrhage, which may lead to serious neurological deficits or death. Surgery on the central nervous system, however, has known risks as well; AVM surgery is invasive and can be quite complex. It carries an estimated 8 percent risk of serious complications or death.

Sources
National Institute of Neurological Disorders and Stroke, Mayo Clinic, National Organization for Rare Disorders

---

AVM RESOURCES

Mayo Clinic offers many educational materials about arteriovenous malformation and provides treatment at three centers. Mayo Clinic, 200 First St. S.W., Rochester, MN 55905; 507-284-2511. See *http://www.mayoclinic.org/arteriovenous-malformation*

The National Institute for Neurological Disorders and Stroke (NINDS) offers clinical detail and resources on AVM. NINDS, 31 Center Drive, Bethesda MD 20892-2540; 301-496-5751, toll-free 800-352-9424; *http://www.ninds.nih.gov/disorders/avms/avms.htm*

National Organization for Rare Disorders (NORD) includes AVM in its materials. NORD, 55 Kenosia Avenue, Danbury, CT 06813-1968. 203-744-0100; 800-999-6673. See *http://www.rarediseases.org,*

BRACHIAL PLEXUS INJURY

Brachial plexus injuries are caused by excessive stretching, tearing, or other trauma to a network of nerves between the spine and the shoulder, arm, and hand. Symptoms may include a limp or paralyzed arm, loss of muscle control or sensation in the arm, hand, or wrist. Chronic pain is often a concern. Injuries often occur due to vehicular accidents, sports mishaps, gunshot wounds, or surgeries; many of these injuries happen during birth if the baby's shoulders become impacted during the birth process, causing the brachial plexus nerves to stretch or tear.

Some brachial plexus injuries may heal without treatment; many children improve or recover by 3 to 4 months of age. Treatment for brachial plexus injuries includes occupational or physical therapy and, in some cases, surgery. For avulsion (tears) and rupture injuries there is no potential for recovery unless surgical reconnection is made in a timely manner. For neuroma (scarring) and neuropraxia (stretching) injuries the potential for recovery is more encouraging. Most people with neuropraxia injuries recover.

Sources
United Brachial Plexus Network, Brachial Plexus Palsy Foundation, National Institute of Neurological Disorders and Stroke

BRACHIAL PLEXUS RESOURCES

Brachial Plexus Palsy Foundation supports research and education. Contact c/o 210 SpringHaven Circle, Royersford, PA 19468; toll-free 1-800-668-2778; see *http://membrane.com/bpp*

United Brachial Plexus Network provides support related to brachial plexus injuries. Contact c/o 1610 Kent Street, Kent, OH 44240; toll-free 1-866-877-7004; see *http://www.ubpn.org*

SUNY at Syracuse provides a course overview of brachial plexus. Contact c/o State University of New York, Upstate Medical University, 750 Adams Street, Syracuse, NY 13210; telephone 315-464-5540; see *http://www.upstate.edu/cdb/grossanat/limbs2.shtml*

BRAIN INJURY

The brain is the control center for all of the body's functions, including conscious activities (walking, talking) and unconscious ones (e.g., breathing, digestion). The brain also controls thought, comprehension, speech and emotion. Injury to the brain, whether the result of severe trauma to the skull or a closed injury in which there is no fracture or penetration, can disrupt some or all of these functions.

Traumatic brain injury (TBI) results mainly from motor vehicle accidents, falls, acts of violence and sports injuries. It is more than twice as likely in males than in females. The estimated incidence rate is 100 out of 100,000 persons. The Centers for Disease Control and Prevention estimates that 5.3 million Americans are living with disabilities from brain trauma, added to more than 50,000 deaths per year. The highest incidence is among persons 15 to 24 years of age and 75 years and older. Alcohol is associated with half of all brain injuries, either in the person causing the injury or in the injured person.

Brain injury can have serious and lifelong effects on physical and mental functioning, including loss of consciousness, altered memory and/or personality, and partial or complete paralysis. Common behavioral problems include verbal and physical aggression, agitation, learning difficulties, poor self-awareness, altered sexual functioning, impulsivity and social disinhibition. Mood disorders, personality changes, altered emotional control, depression and anxiety are also prevalent after TBI.

Social consequences of mild, moderate and severe TBI are numerous, including higher risk of suicide, divorce, chronic unemployment and substance abuse. The annual cost of acute care and rehabilitation in the United States for new cases of TBI is enormous: $9 to $10 billion. Estimates for average lifetime cost of care for a person with severe TBI range from $600,000 to $1,875,000.

Enclosed within the bony framework of the skull, the brain is a gelatinous material that floats in cerebrospinal fluid, which acts as a shock absorber in rapid head movements.

Injury to the brain can be caused by a fracture or penetration of the skull (vehicle accident, fall or gunshot wound), a disease process (neurotoxins, infection, tumors, metabolic abnormalities, etc.), or a closed head injury such as shaken baby syndrome or rapid acceleration/deceleration of the head. The outer surface of the skull is smooth, but the inner surface is jagged – this is the cause of significant damage in closed head injuries as the brain tissue rebounds inside the skull over rough bony structures.

With traumatic injury, brain damage may occur at the time of impact or may develop later due to swelling (cerebral edema) and bleeding into the brain (intracerebral hemorrhage) or bleeding around the brain (epidural or subdural hemorrhage).

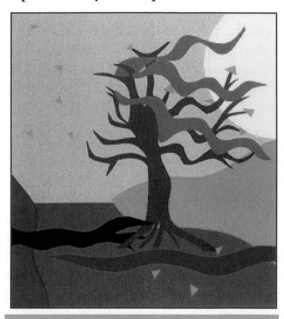

ARTWORK CREATED FOR THE NIH CONSENSUS DEVELOPMENT CONFERENCE ON REHABILITATION OF PERSONS WITH TRAUMATIC BRAIN INJURY, OCTOBER 1998, SPONSORED BY THE NATIONAL INSTITUTE OF CHILD HEALTH AND HUMAN DEVELOPMENT AND THE NIH OFFICE OF MEDICAL APPLICATIONS OF RESEARCH. FOR FULL STATEMENT SEE WWW.CONSENSUS.NIH.GOV

If the head is hit with sufficient force, the brain turns and twists on its axis (the brainstem), interrupting normal nerve pathways and causing a loss of consciousness. If this unconsciousness persists over a long period of time, the injured person is considered to be in a coma, a disruption of nerve messages going from the brainstem to the cortex.

A closed head injury often occurs without leaving obvious external signs, however the difference between closed and penetrating injuries can be significant. A bullet wound to the head, for example, might destroy a large area of the brain but the result may be minor if the area is not a critical one. Closed head injuries often result in more damage and extensive neurologic deficits, including partial to complete paralysis; cognitive, behavioral and memory problems; and persistent vegetative state.

Injured brain tissue can recover over a short period of time. However, once brain tissue is dead or destroyed, there is no evidence that new brain cells can regrow. The process of recovery usually continues even without new cells, perhaps as other parts of the brain take over the function of the destroyed tissue.

The rehabilitation process begins immediately after injury. Once memory begins to be restored, the rate of recovery often increases. However, many problems may persist, including those related to movement, memory, attention, complex thinking, speech and language, and behavioral changes. Beyond the obvious physical effects of brain injury, survivors frequently cope with depression, anxiety, loss of self-esteem, altered personality and, in some cases, a lack of self-awareness by the injury survivor of any existing deficits.

Rehab may include cognitive exercises to improve attention, memory and executive skills. These programs are structured, systematic, goal-directed and individualized; they involve learning, practice and social contact. Sometimes memory books and electronic paging systems are used to improve particular functions and to compensate for deficits. Psychotherapy is an important component of a comprehensive rehabilitation program; it's used to treat depression and loss of self-esteem. Rehab may also include medications for behavioral disturbances associated with TBI. Some of these drugs have significant side effects in persons with TBI and are used only in compelling circumstances.

Behavior modification has been used to reduce personality and behavioral effects of TBI and in retraining social skills. Vocational training is also common to many rehab programs. According to a consensus statement on brain injury from the National Institutes on Health, persons with TBI and their families should play an integral role in the planning and design of their individualized rehabilitation programs.

Sources

National Institute of Neurological Disorders and Stroke, Texas Head Injury Association, Brain Injury Resource Center, National Institute on Deafness and Other Communication Disorders

BRAIN INJURY RESOURCES

Brain Injury Association of America (BIAA) features resources on living with brain injury, treatment, rehabilitation, research, prevention, etc. It also has state-by-state affiliates. BIAA, 8201 Greensboro Dr., Suite 611, McLean, VA 22102; telephone 703-761-0750 or toll-free 1-800-444-6443; or visit the Internet site *http://www.biausa.org*

Brain Injury Resource Center/Head Injury Hotline (BIRC) operates a resource center "to empower you to have your needs met and avoid exploitation." BIRC, P.O. Box 84151, Seattle, WA 98124; 206-621-8558; or visit *http://www.headinjury.com*

Defense and Veterans Brain Injury Center (DVBIC) serves active duty military, their dependents and veterans with traumatic brain injury (TBI) through medical care, clinical research and educational programs. DVBIC, Walter Reed Army Medical Center, 6900 Georgia Avenue NW, Washington DC 20307-5001. Telephone 202-782-6345, toll-free 1-800-870-9244. See *http://www.dvbic.org*

Traumatic Brain Injury (TBI) Model Systems of Care are specialty head injury clinics with federal grants for developing and demonstrating expertise with TBI. See *http://www.tbindc.org*

The following are the current U.S. model systems centers for brain injury:

Spain Rehabilitation Center, Birmingham, AL. *http://www.uab.edu/tbi*

Santa Clara Valley Medical Center, San Jose, CA. *http://www.tbi-sci.org*

Craig Hospital, Englewood, CO. *http://www.craighospital.org*

Spaulding Rehabilitation Hospital, Boston, MA. *http://spauldingrehab.org*

Rehabilitation Institute of Michigan, Detroit, MI. *http://www.semtbis.org*

Mayo Clinic, Rochester, MN. *http://www.mayo.edu/model-system*

Methodist Rehabilitation Hospital, Jackson, MS. *http://www.mmrcrehab.org*

Carolinas Rehabilitation, Charlotte, NC. *http://www.carolinashealthcare.org/services/*

JFK-Johnson Rehabilitation Institute, Edison, NJ. *http://www.njrehab.org/*

Mount Sinai Medical Center, New York, NY. *http://www.mssm.edu/tbicentral/nytbims/*

Ohio State University, Columbus, OH. *http://www.ohiovalley.org*

Moss Rehabilitation Research Institute, Philadelphia, PA. *http://www.einstein.edu*

University of Pittsburgh Medical Center, Pittsburgh, PA. *http://www.rehabmedicine.pitt.edu*

University of Texas Southwestern Medical Center, Dallas, TX. *http://www.utsouthwestern.edu*

The Virginia Commonwealth University, Richmond, VA. *http://www.neuro.pmr.vcu.edu*

University of Washington, Seattle, WA. *http://depts.washington.edu*

CEREBRAL PALSY

Cerebral palsy (CP) refers to a group of conditions that affect control of movement and posture. CP disorders are not caused by problems in the muscles or nerves. Instead, faulty development or damage to areas in the brain cause inadequate control of movement and posture. Symptoms range from mild to severe, including forms of paralysis.

Cerebral palsy does not always cause profound disability. While a child with severe CP might be unable to walk and need extensive care, a child with mild cerebral palsy might only be slightly off-balance and require no special assistance. Cerebral palsy is not contagious nor is it usually inherited. With treatment, most children significantly improve their abilities. While symptoms may change over time, cerebral palsy by definition is not progressive; if impairment does increase, it's usually something other than CP.

Children with cerebral palsy often require treatment for mental retardation, learning disabilities, seizures, plus vision, hearing and speech difficulties.

Cerebral palsy usually is not diagnosed until a child is about two to three years old; it affects about 2 to 3 children out of 1,000 over the age of three and about 500,000 children and adults in the United States have CP. There are three major types:

1. Spastic cerebral palsy: About 70–80 percent of those affected have spastic cerebral palsy, in which muscles are stiff, making movement difficult. When both legs are affected (spastic diplegia), a child may have difficulty walking because tight muscles in the hips and legs cause the legs to turn inward and scissor at the knees. In other cases, only one side of the body is affected (spastic hemiplegia), often with the arm more severely affected than the leg. Most severe is spastic quadriplegia, in which all four limbs and the trunk are affected, often along with the muscles of the mouth and tongue.

2. Dyskinetic (athetoid) cerebral palsy: About 10–20 percent have the dyskinetic form, which affects the entire body. It is characterized by fluctuations in muscle tone from too tight to too loose) and sometimes is associated with uncontrolled movements (which can be slow and writhing or rapid and jerky). Children often have trouble learning to control their bodies well enough to

sit and walk. Because muscles of the face and tongue can be affected, there also can be difficulties with swallowing and speech.

3. Ataxic cerebral palsy: About 5–10 percent have the ataxic form, which affects balance and coordination. They may walk with an unsteady gait and have difficulty with motions that require coordination, such as writing.

In the United States, about 10–20 percent of children who have CP acquire the disorder after birth, the result of brain damage in the first few months or years of life; brain infections, such as bacterial meningitis or viral encephalitis; or head injury. Cerebral palsy present at birth may not be detected for months. In most cases, the cause of congenital cerebral palsy is unknown. Scientists have pinpointed some specific events during pregnancy or around the time of birth that can damage motor centers in the developing brain. Until recently, doctors believed that a lack of oxygen during a difficult delivery was the primary cause of cerebral palsy. Studies show that this causes only about 10 percent of cases.

A child with CP usually begins physical therapy to increase motor skills (sitting and walking), improve muscle strength, and help prevent contractures (shortening of muscles that limit joint movement). Sometimes braces, splints or casts are used to improve function of the hands or legs. If contractures are severe, surgery may be recommended to lengthen affected muscles.

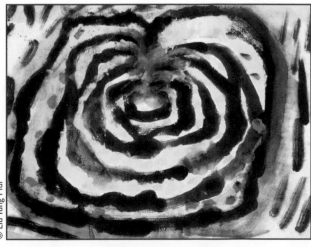

© Liu Tung Mui

BREAKOUT GOUACHE

"PAINTING IS HAPPINESS AS WELL AS SADNESS. IT'S MY PRIVATE CONVERSATION WITH THE UNIVERSE AND THE SYMBOL OF MY EXISTENCE."

- LIU TUNG MUI, A SELF-TAUGHT ARTIST WHO HAS CEREBRAL PALSY

Drugs may ease spasticity or reduce abnormal movement. Injection of the drug directly into spastic muscles is more helpful than oral drugs. In some cases, a small pump is implanted under the skin to continuously deliver the anti-spasm drug baclofen. Some success has been reported using botox to selectively quiet muscles. For younger children with spasticity affecting both legs, dorsal rhizotomy may permanently reduce spasticity and improve the ability to sit, stand and walk. In this procedure, doctors cut some of the nerve fibers that contribute most to spasticity. As a child with cerebral palsy grows older, therapy and other support services will change. Physical therapy is supplemented by vocational training, recreation and leisure programs and special education, when necessary. Counseling for emotional and psychological issues is critical during adolescence.

Sources

United Cerebral Palsy, March of Dimes, National Institute of Neurological Disorders and Stroke

CEREBRAL PALSY RESOURCES

United Cerebral Palsy (UCP), a partner with the Christopher and Dana Reeve Foundation Paralysis Resource Center, offers resources on CP health and wellness, plus lifestyle, education and advocacy resources. A national organization of more than 100 affiliates in most states, UCP advances full inclusion of people with disabilities, through the principles of independence, inclusion and self-determination; two-thirds of people served by UCP have disabilities other than cerebral palsy. UCP National, 1660 L Street, NW, Suite 700, Washington, D.C. 20036; telephone 202–776–0406; or visit the Internet site *http://www.ucp.org*

The March of Dimes Birth Defects Foundation features resources and connections to address four major problems that threaten the health of America's babies: birth defects, infant mortality, low birth weight and lack of prenatal care. March of Dimes, 1275 Mamaroneck Avenue, White Plains, NY 10605; toll-free 1–888–663–4637; on the Internet site *http://www.modimes.org*

FRIEDREICH'S ATAXIA

Friedreich's ataxia is an inherited disease that causes progressive damage to the nervous system. It can result in muscle weakness, speech difficulties or heart disease. The first symptom is usually difficulty in walking.

It is named after the physician Nicholas Friedreich, who first described the condition in the 1860s. "Ataxia" refers to coordination problems and unsteadiness and occurs in many diseases and conditions. Friedreich's ataxia is marked by degeneration of nerve tissue in the spinal cord and of nerves that control arm and leg movement. The spinal cord becomes thinner and nerve cells lose some of the myelin insulation that helps them conduct impulses.

Friedreich's ataxia affects about 1 out of 50,000 people in the United States. Males and females are affected equally. Symptoms usually begin between the ages of 5 and 15, but can appear as early as 18 months or as late as age 30. Early signs may include unsteady posture, frequent falling and progressive difficulty walking due to an impaired ability to coordinate voluntary movements. Rapid, involuntary movements of the eyeball are common. Most people with Friedreich's ataxia develop scoliosis (curving of the spine to one side), which, if severe, can impair breathing.

> **"Although there is no hard proof that they work, many people with Friedreich's ataxia take antioxidant vitamins to limit cell destruction."**

There is currently no effective cure or treatment for Friedreich's ataxia. However, many of the symptoms and accompanying complications can be treated. Many people take antioxidant vitamins to counteract oxidative stress and cell destruction; faulty cellular chemistry causes muscle or nerve cells to release excess free radicals, which wreak havoc on healthy cells. Antioxidants, such as vitamin E and coenzyme Q10, stabilize the free radicals. It is not clear that these supplements can affect the course of the disease.

There is currently a clinical trial in the United States and in Europe sponsored by Swiss drug company Santhera to evaluate Idebenone, a form of coenzyme Q10, on heart function in people with Friedreich's Ataxia. Early results showed improvement of neurological parameters and activities of daily living scores.

Sources

National Institute of Neurological Disorders and Stroke, National Organization for Rare Disorders, Friedreich's Ataxia Research Alliance, Muscular Dystrophy Association

FRIEDREICH'S ATAXIA RESOURCES

Friedreich's Ataxia Research Alliance (FARA) offers information on Friedreich's ataxia and the related ataxias, including current research, ongoing studies, as well as information for researchers, patients, families and caregivers. FARA also offers support and information for the newly diagnosed. FARA, P.O. Box 7537, Springfield, VA 22151; telephone 703–413–4468; or visit the Internet site *http://www.curefa.org*

National Ataxia Foundation (NAF) supports research into hereditary ataxia, with numerous affiliated chapters and support groups in the United States and Canada. The foundation offers information, education and referral. NAF, 2600 Fernbrook Lane Suite 119, Minneapolis, MN 55447; telephone 763–553–0020; or visit the Internet site *http://www.ataxia.org*

National Organization for Rare Disorders (NORD) is committed to the identification and treatment of rare disorders through education, advocacy, research and service. There are more than 6,000 rare disorders, including Friedreich's ataxia, that together affect about 25 million Americans. For more on specific disorders visit the Internet site *http://www.rarediseases.org*

Muscular Dystrophy Association (MDA) offers news and information about neuromuscular diseases, including ataxias. MDA National Headquarters, 3300 E. Sunrise Drive, Tucson, AZ 85718; toll-free 1-800-344-4863; or visit the Internet site *http://www.mdausa.org*

GUILLAIN-BARRÉ SYNDROME

Guillain-Barré (ghee-yan bah-ray) syndrome is a disorder in which the body's immune system attacks part of the peripheral nervous system. The first symptoms include varying degrees of weakness or tingling sensations in the legs. The weakness and abnormal sensations often spread to the arms and upper body and can increase in intensity until a person is totally paralyzed. Many people require intensive care during the early course of their illness, especially if a ventilator is required.

Most people recover from even the most severe cases of Guillain-Barré, although some continue to have some degree of weakness.

Guillain-Barré syndrome is rare. It usually occurs a few days or weeks after a person has had symptoms of a respiratory or gastrointestinal viral infection. Occasionally, surgery or vaccinations will trigger it. The disorder can develop over the course of hours or days, or it may take up to three to four weeks. It is not known why Guillain-Barré strikes some people and not others, or what sets the disease in motion.

There is no known cure for Guillain-Barré syndrome, but therapies can reduce its severity and accelerate recovery. There are a number of ways to treat the complications. Plasmapheresis mechanically removes autoantibodies from the bloodstream. It's also known as plasma exchange. High-dose immunoglobulin therapy is also used to boost the immune system.

Researchers hope to understand the workings of the immune system to identify which cells are responsible for carrying out the attack on the nervous system and to neutralize the attack.

Source
The National Institute of Neurological Disorders and Stroke

GBS/CIDP Foundation International offers information and interactive bulletin boards, research funding and a global chapter organization. Guillain-Barré Syndrome Foundation International, The Holly Building, 104 1/2 Forrest Ave., Narberth PA 19096; telephone 610-667-0131; or see the Internet site *http://www.gbsfi.com*

THE LEUKODYSTROPHIES

The leukodystrophies are progressive, hereditary disorders that affect the brain, spinal cord and peripheral nerves. Specific leukodystrophies include metachromatic leukodystrophy, Krabbe leukodystrophy, adrenoleukodystrophy, Canavan disease, Alexander disease, Zellweger syndrome, Refsum disease, and cerebrotendinous xanthomatosis. Pelizaeus-Merzbacher disease can also lead to paralysis.

Adrenoleukodystrophy (ALD) affected the young boy Lorenzo Odone, whose story is told in the 1993 film "Lorenzo's Oil." In this disease the fatty covering (myelin sheath) on nerve fibers in the brain is lost, and the adrenal gland degenerates, leading to progressive neurological disability. (See *http://www.myelin.org*)

United Leukodystrophy Foundation (ULF) offers resources and clinical detail on the leukodystrophies. ULF, 2304 Highland Drive, Sycamore, IL 60178; toll-free 1-800-728-5483; or visit the Internet site *http://www.ulf.org*

LYME DISEASE

Lyme disease is a bacterial infection transmitted to humans by the bite of certain black-legged ticks. Typical symptoms include fever, headache and fatigue. Lyme disease, which can lead to neurological symptoms, including loss of function in arms and legs, is often misdiagnosed as amyotrophic lateral sclerosis or multiple sclerosis. According to some Lyme disease advocates, standard diagnostic methods fail to discover as many as 40 percent of cases. Most cases of Lyme disease can be treated successfully with a few weeks of antibiotics. While some people with long-term Lyme disease take antibiotics over an extended course of time, most physicians do not consider Lyme to be a chronic infection. There are reports that hyperbaric oxygen and bee venom have been effective in treating symptoms of the disease.

For more information contact the International Lyme and Associated Diseases Society, *http://ilads.org*; American Lyme Disease Foundation, *www.aldf.com*; Lyme Disease Association, *www.lymediseaseassociation.org*

MULTIPLE SCLEROSIS

Multiple sclerosis (MS) is a chronic and often disabling disease of the central nervous system. Symptoms may be mild, such as numbness in a limb, or severe, including paralysis or loss of vision.

Most people with MS are diagnosed between the ages of 20 and 40. MS affects approximately 1 out of 1,000 people. Women are more commonly affected than men. The progress, severity and symptoms of MS in any individual cannot yet be predicted, but advances in research and treatment are giving hope to those affected by the disease.

Multiple sclerosis involves decreased nerve function associated with scar formation on the covering of nerve cells. Repeated episodes of inflammation destroy the myelin sheath that covers nerve fibers, leaving multiple areas of scar tissue (sclerosis) along the covering of the nerve cells. This results in slowing or blockage of nerve impulse transmission in that area. MS often progresses (called exacerbations) with episodes that last days, weeks, or months. Exacerbations often alternate with times of reduced or no symptoms (remission). Recurrence (relapse) is common.

Symptoms of MS include weakness or paralysis of one or more extremities, tremor in the extremities, muscle spasticity (uncontrollable spasms), movement problems, numbness, tingling, pain, loss of vision, loss or coordination and balance, incontinence, loss of memory or judgment, and fatigue.

Fatigue is one of the most common symptoms, occurring in about 80 percent of people with MS. Fatigue can significantly interfere with a person's ability to work and function. It may be the most prominent symptom in a person who otherwise has been minimally affected by the disease. MS-related fatigue generally occurs on a daily basis and tends to worsen as the day progresses. It tends to be aggravated by heat and humidity. MS-related fatigue does not appear to be directly correlated with either depression or the degree of physical impairment. It may occur first thing in the morning even if the person has had a restful full night's sleep.

Symptoms may vary with each attack. Fever can trigger or worsen attacks, as can hot baths, sun exposure and stress.

Multiple sclerosis varies greatly from person to person and in the severity and the course of the disease. A relapsing-remitting course, the most common form of MS, is characterized by partial or total recovery after attacks; 70 to 75 percent of people with MS begin with a relapsing-remitting course.

Relapsing-remitting MS may become steadily progressive. Attacks and partial recoveries may continue to occur. This is called secondary-progressive MS. Of those who start with relapsing-remitting, more than half will develop secondary progressive MS within 10 years; 90 percent within 25 years.

A progressive course from onset of the disease is called primary-progressive MS. In this case, symptoms generally do not remit.

The exact cause of MS is unknown. Studies indicate an environmental factor may be involved. There is a higher incidence in northern Europe, northern United States, southern Australia, and New Zealand than in other areas of the world. There may also be a familial tendency toward the disorder.

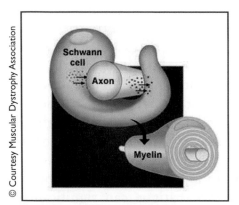

Multiple sclerosis is believed to be an abnormal immune response directed against the central nervous system (CNS). The cells and proteins of the body's immune system, which normally defend the body against infections, leave the blood vessels serving the CNS and pour into the brain and spinal cord where they destroy myelin. The specific triggering mechanism that causes the immune system to attack its own myelin remains unknown, although a viral infection combined with an inherited genetic susceptibility is a leading suspect. Although many different viruses have been thought to cause MS, there has been no definitive evidence linking any one virus to the autoimmune reaction responsible for demyelination.

According to the National Multiple Sclerosis Society, MS was among the first diseases to be described scientifically. The 19th-century doctors did not fully understand what they saw and recorded, but drawings from autopsies done as early as 1838 clearly show what is known today as MS. In 1868, Jean-Martin Charcot, a professor of neurology at the University of Paris, carefully examined a young woman with a tremor of a sort he had never seen before. He noted her other neurological problems, including slurred speech and abnormal eye movements, and compared them to other patients he had seen. When she died, he examined her brain and found the characteristic scars or "plaques" of MS.

> **"The specific triggering mechanism that causes the immune system to attack its own myelin remains unknown; a viral infection combined with genetic susceptibility is a leading suspect."**

Dr. Charcot wrote a complete description of the disease and the changes in the brain that accompany it. He was baffled by its cause and frustrated by its resistance to all of his treatments, including electrical stimulation and strychnine (a poison that is a nerve stimulant). He also tried injections of gold and silver, as they were somewhat helpful in the other major nerve disorder common at that time, syphilis.

One century later, in 1969, the first successful scientific clinical trial was completed for a treatment of MS. A group of patients who were having MS exacerbations were given the steroid ACTH. This treatment proved superior to the placebo (a similar-looking dummy drug) in speeding recovery. This primitive therapy led to the modern steroid therapy in use today for acute exacerbations.

Clinical trials since then have led to approvals of six drugs shown to affect the course of MS. In 1993, Betaseron was approved to reduce the severity and frequency of attacks. In 1996, Avonex was approved to slow the development of disability and reduce the severity and frequency of attacks. The same year Copaxone was approved for treating relapsing-remitting MS. Those with a relapsing-remitting course are now placed on immune modulating therapy that requires injection under the skin or in the muscle once or several times a week. Rebif, a form of interferon beta-1 similar to Betaseron and Avonex, was shown to be more effective than Avonex in reducing the number and frequency of relapses and in slowing the progression of disability. One other drug, Novantrone, has been approved for treating advanced or chronic MS. The drug, also used as an anti-cancer treatment, reduces the number of relapses and in some people decreases the progression of disability.

In 2006 Tysabri was approved for relapsing multiple sclerosis, with very restrictive prescription policies due to a high risk for side effects. The drug is monoclonal antibody that appears to hamper movement of potentially damaging immune cells from the bloodstream, across the "blood-brain barrier" into the brain and spinal cord. In clinical trails, three people taking Tysabri developed a rare disease called PML (progressive multifocal leukoencephalopathy), caused by a common virus. Two of them died.

Other drugs for people with progressive MS — the forms of the disease that do not have a pattern of attack and recovery – are in development. Exciting areas of exploration include laboratory studies on remyelination. In recent years researchers have identified which immune cells mount the attack, how they are activated to attack, and some of the sites, or receptors, on the attacking cells that appear to be attracted to the myelin to begin the destructive process. This research, it is hoped, will lead to therapies. Meanwhile, physicians today know a lot more about the disease but they are also frustrated by the lack of medical tools to fight it.

Other medicines commonly used for MS symptoms include baclofen, tizanidine or diazepam, often used to reduce muscle spas-

MULTIPLE SCLEROSIS RESOURCES

The National Multiple Sclerosis Society, a partner organization with the Christopher and Dana Reeve Foundation Paralysis Resource Center, provides information on living with MS, treatment, scientific progress, MS specialty centers, clinical research, local chapters and an annotated bibliography for healthcare professionals. The National Multiple Sclerosis Society, national office, 733 Third Avenue, New York, NY 10017; toll-free 1-800-344-4867; or visit the Internet site *http://www.nationalmssociety.org*

INTERNET RESOURCES FOR MS

Multiple Sclerosis Complementary and Alternative Medicine (MS-CAM) is an Internet community site run by the Rocky Mountain MS Center. The goal of the center is to provide accurate unbiased reviews regarding complementary and alternative medicine therapies commonly used by people with MS, such as acupuncture, herbal medicine and homeopathy, and to use scientific methods to measure the experiences of the MS community with particular therapies. See *http://www.ms-cam.org*

The Consortium of Multiple Sclerosis Centers/North American Research Committee on MS (CMSC/NARCOMS) is a rich repository of clinical and research information for people with MS. Publishes the International Journal of MS Care. See *http://www.mscare.org*

The Multiple Sclerosis Society of Canada has information about the disease, progress in MS research, services, details about fundraising events and donation opportunities. See *http://www.mssociety.ca*

Multiple Sclerosis Foundation has an interactive, multimedia MS library and online forum. Visit *http://www.msfacts.org*

Multiple Sclerosis Association of America features news, information and community connections. See *http://www.msaa.com*

Computer Literate Advocates for MS (CLAMS) is a Website bringing those with MS out of isolation and into a virtual community for support, companionship and information. See *http://www.clams.org*

Understanding MS features current information on MS, including treatments, lifestyle issues and new research. This site offers Webcasts, which are moderated audio or video discussions between leading health professionals on a particular topic. Visit the Internet site *http://www.understandingms.com*

MSWatch, sponsored by Teva Marion Partners, a drug company, is a Website dedicated to managing MS. Visitors have the ability to keep a diary on the site, ask an expert a question, and communicate via the message boards. Visit the Internet site *http://www.mswatch.com*

ticity. Doctors prescribe anti-cholinergic medications to reduce urinary problems, and antidepressants to improve mood or behavior symptoms. Amantadine (an anti-viral drug) and pemoline (a stimulant usually prescribed to calm hyperactive children) are sometimes used to treat fatigue.

Physical therapy, speech therapy or occupational therapy may improve a person's outlook, reduce depression, maximize function and improve coping skills. Exercise early in the course of MS helps to maintain muscle tone. Try to avoid fatigue, stress, physical deterioration, temperature extremes and illness to reduce factors that could trigger an MS attack.

Although multiple sclerosis is chronic, unpredictable and at this time incurable, life expectancy can be normal or nearly so. See page 148 for an overview of research to treat multiple sclerosis.

Sources:

National Institute of Neurological Disorders and Stroke, National Multiple Sclerosis Society, Consortium of MS Centers, Multiple Sclerosis Complementary and Alternative Medicine at the Rocky Mountain MS Center

ACUPUNCTURE AND MS?

There is some evidence that the ancient Chinese practice of acupuncture might help people with MS. A Canadian study of 217 people with MS found that two-thirds reported some type of beneficial effect, including improvements in fatigue, pain, spasticity, walking, bowel and bladder difficulties, tingling and numbness, weakness, sleep disorders, loss of coordination, optic neuritis, and MS attacks. These results are promising, but since this was a self-assessment survey it lacks the rigorous elements of a formal clinical trial. More research is needed.

For more information on this and many other alternative treatment options, see Multiple Sclerosis Complementary & Alternative Medicine (MS-CAM), http://www.ms-cam.org

See also The American Academy of Medical Acupuncture, 4929 Wilshire Boulevard, Los Angeles, CA 90010; toll-free 800-521-2262; on the Internet see http://www.medicalacupuncture.org

POST-POLIO SYNDROME

Poliomyelitis is a disease caused by a virus that attacks nerves that control motor function. Polio (infantile paralysis) has nearly been eradicated from nearly every country in the world since the approval of the Salk (1955) and Sabin (1962) vaccines.

The World Health Organization (WHO) estimates there are 12 million people worldwide with some degree of disability caused by poliomyelitis. The National Center for Health Statistics estimates there are 1 million polio survivors in the United States. About 433,000 of them reported paralysis resulting in some form of impairment. The last major outbreaks of polio in the United States were in the early 1950s.

For years most polio survivors lived active lives, their memory of polio long forgotten, their health status stable. But by the late 1970s, survivors who were 20 or more years past their original polio began noting new problems, including fatigue, pain, breathing or swallowing problems, and additional weakness—medical professionals called this the "post-polio syndrome" (PPS).

Some people experience PPS-related fatigue as a flu-like exhaustion that worsens as the day progresses. This type of fatigue can also increase during physical activity, and it may cause difficulty with concentration and memory. Others experience muscle weakness that increases with exercise and improves with rest.

Current research indicates that the length of time one has lived with the residuals of polio is as much of a risk factor as age. It also appears that individuals who experienced the most severe original paralysis with the greatest functional recovery have more problems with PPS than others with less severe original involvement.

The current consensus of opinion explaining post-polio symptoms focuses on the nerve cells and their corresponding muscle fibers. When the poliovirus destroyed or injured motor neurons, muscle fibers were orphaned and paralysis resulted. Polio survivors who regained movement did so because nerve cells recovered to a certain extent. Further recovery is attributed to the ability of non-affected neighboring nerve cells to "sprout" and reconnect to the orphaned muscles.

Survivors who have lived for years with this restructured neuromuscular system are now experiencing the consequences including overworked surviving nerve cells, muscles and joints, compounded by the effects of growing older. While the search for a viral cause continues, there is no conclusive evidence to support the concept that post-polio syndrome is a reinfection of the poliovirus.

Polio survivors take care of their health by seeking periodic medical attention, being nutrition-wise, avoiding excessive weight gain, and by stopping smoking or over-indulging in alcohol.

Survivors are advised to listen to their body's warning signals, avoid activities that cause pain, prevent overuse of muscles, and conserve energy by avoiding tasks that are nonessential.

PPS is not typically a life-threatening condition, but it may cause significant discomfort and disability. The most common disability caused by PPS is deterioration of mobility. People with PPS may also experience difficulties performing daily activities such as cooking, cleaning, shopping and driving. Energy-conserving assistive devices such as canes, crutches, walkers, wheelchairs or electric scooters may be necessary for some people.

Many individuals have

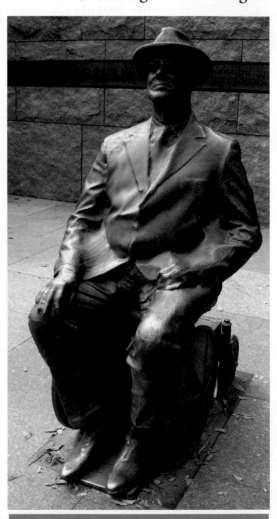

FRANKLIN D. ROOSEVELT, 32ND PRESIDENT OF THE UNITED STATES, HID HIS POLIO FROM THE NATION.

difficulties adjusting to the new disabilities. For some with PPS, reliving childhood experiences of coming to terms with polio can be a traumatic experience. For example, moving from a manual to a power chair can be a difficult transition. Fortunately, PPS is gaining increasing attention in the medical community, and there are many health care professionals who understand PPS and can provide appropriate medical and psychological help. In addition, there are PPS support groups, newsletters and educational networks that provide up-to-date information about PPS while offering individuals the knowledge that they are not alone in their struggle.

Sources

International Polio Network, Montreal Neurological Hospital Post-Polio Clinic

POST-POLIO SYNDROME RESOURCES

Post-Polio Health International offers information for polio survivors and promotes networking among the post-polio community. PPHI publishes numerous useful resources, including the quarterly *Polio Network News*, the annual *Post-Polio Directory*, and *The Handbook on the Late Effects of Poliomyelitis for Physicians and Survivors*. PPHI is the evolution of the GINI organization which was founded as a mimeograph newsletter by Gini Laurie in St. Louis 50 years ago. PPHI, 4207 Lindell Boulevard #110, St. Louis, MO 63108; telephone 314–534–0475; on the Internet see *http://www.post-polio.org*

Montreal Neurological Hospital Post-Polio Clinic offers an online patient handbook on post-polio symptoms and management. See *http://infoneuro.mcgill.ca*, click on Clinics and Programs

Post-Polio Syndrome Central features a massive international list of links related to polio and PPS. Also a repository of international e-mail listservs related to polio, including Post-Polio Med, a forum for PPS researchers, physicians and other medical professionals, polio survivors, families, friends, students, etc. To subscribe (it's free) visit the Internet site *http://www.skally.net/ppsc* and send an email as directed.

SPINA BIFIDA

Spina bifida is the most common permanently disabling birth defect in the United States. One out of 1000 newborns in the United States is born with spina bifida; each year 4000 pregnancies are affected by spina bifida. About 95 percent of babies with spina bifida are born to parents with no family history.

Spina bifida, a type of neural tube defect (NTD), means "cleft spine," or an incomplete closure in the spinal column. This birth defect occurs between the fourth and sixth weeks of pregnancy when the embryo is less than an inch long. Normally, a groove in the middle of the embryo deepens, allowing the sides to meet and enclose the tissue destined to be the spinal cord. In spina bifida, the sides of the embryo do not fully meet resulting in a malformed neural tube, affecting the spinal column and in many cases, forming a spinal cord cleft, or lesion.

The most serious form of spina bifida may include muscle weakness or paralysis below the cleft area, loss of sensation below the cleft, and loss of bowel and bladder control. There are three general types of spina bifida (listed below from mild to severe).

Spina bifida occulta: This is an opening in one or more of the vertebrae (bones) of the spinal column without apparent damage to the spinal cord. Approximately 40 percent of all Americans may have spina bifida occulta, but because they experience little or no symptoms, very few of them ever know that they have it.

Meningocele: The meninges, or the protective covering around the spinal cord, pushes out through the opening in the vertebrae in a sac called the meningocele. The spinal cord remains intact; this can be repaired with little or no damage to the nerve pathways.

Myelomeningocele: This is the most severe form of spina bifida, in which a portion of the spinal cord itself protrudes through the back. In some cases, sacs are covered with skin; in others, tissue and nerves are exposed. A common effect of myelomeningocele is an accumulation of fluid in the brain (hydrocephalus). A large percentage of children born with myelomeningocele have hydrocephalus, which is controlled by a surgical procedure called shunting. This relieves the fluid buildup in the brain and reduces the risk of brain damage, seizures or blindness. Hydrocephalus may occur without spina bifida, but the two conditions often occur together. In some cases, children with spina bifida who also have a history of hydrocephalus experience learning problems. They may have difficulty with paying attention, expressing or understanding language, and grasping reading and math. Early intervention with children who experience learning problems can help considerably to prepare them for school and life.

Examples of secondary conditions associated with spina bifida are orthopedic problems, latex allergy, tendinitis, obesity, skin breakdown, gastrointestinal disorders, learning disabilities, depression and social and sexual issues.

Although spina bifida is relatively common, until recently most children born with a myelomeningocele died shortly after birth. Now that surgery to drain spinal fluid and protect against hydrocephalus can be performed in the first 24 hours of life, children with myelomeningocele are much more likely to live. Quite often, however, they have a series of operations throughout their childhood. Advances in neurosurgery and urology make it possible for 90 percent of infants born with spina bifida to live full and active lives into adulthood. It is estimated that about 70,000 people are living with spina bifida in the United States today.

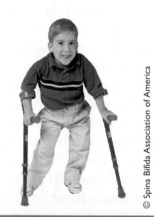

© Spina Bifida Association of America

SPINA BIFIDA MOSTLY OCCURS IN FAMILIES WITH NO HISTORY OF THE DISORDER.

Spina bifida usually is an isolated birth defect. Although scientists believe that genetic and environmental factors may cause this and other neural tube defects, 95 percent of babies with spina bifida are born to parents with no family history of the disorder. While spina bifida appears to run in certain families, it does not follow any particular pattern of inheritance.

Women with certain chronic health problems, including diabetes and seizure disorders (treated with anticonvulsant medications), have an increased risk (approximately 1 out of 100) of having a baby with spina bifida.

Birth defects can happen in any family. Many things can affect a pregnancy, including family genes and things women may come in contact with during pregnancy. Recent studies have shown that folic acid is one factor that may reduce the risk of having an NTD baby. Taking folic acid before and during early pregnancy reduces the risk of spina bifida and other neural tube defects. Folic acid, a common water-soluble B vitamin, is essential for the functioning of the human body. During periods of rapid growth, such as fetal development, the body's requirement for this vitamin increases. The average American diet does not supply the recommended level of folic acid; it can be found in multivitamins, fortified breakfast cereals, dark green leafy vegetables such as broccoli and spinach, egg yolks and some fruits and fruit juices.

According to the Spina Bifida Association of America (SBAA), if all women who could become pregnant were to take a multivitamin with 400 micrograms of folic acid, the risk of neural tube defects could be reduced by up to 75 percent.

There are three prenatal tests that can detect spina bifida: a blood test for alpha-fetoprotein; ultrasound; and amniocentesis. These tests do not identify a child with spina bifida in every case.

Children with spina bifida can achieve independence as they learn mobility skills with the use of crutches, braces or wheelchairs. Many children can independently manage their bowel and bladder problems. According the SBAA, it is important that attention be focused on the psychological and social development of children and young adults with spina bifida. Many recent studies, including the SBAA's Adult Network Survey, clearly indicate the presence of emotional problems that result from factors such as low self-esteem and lack of social skills training.

Research continues to discover the exact cause of spina bifida. Innovative surgical procedures, performed on the developing baby before it is born, show promise to reduce neurological damage caused by the disorder. See page 152 for more information on spina bifida research.

Sources

Spina Bifida Association of America, National Institute of Neurological Disorders and Stroke, March of Dimes Birth Defects Foundation

SPINA BIFIDA RESOURCES

Spina Bifida Association (SBA) promotes the prevention of spina bifida and works to enhance the lives of all affected. SBA, 4590 MacArthur Boulevard, NW, Suite 250, Washington, D.C. 20007-4226; telephone 202-944-3295 or toll-free 1-800-621-3141; or visit *http://www.sbaa.org*

March of Dimes Birth Defects Foundation offers information about the four major problems that threaten the health of America's babies: birth defects, infant mortality, low birthweight, and lack of prenatal care. March of Dimes Birth Defects Foundation, 1275 Mamaroneck Avenue, White Plains, NY 10605; toll-free 1–888–MODIMES (663–4637); or visit *http://www.modimes.com*

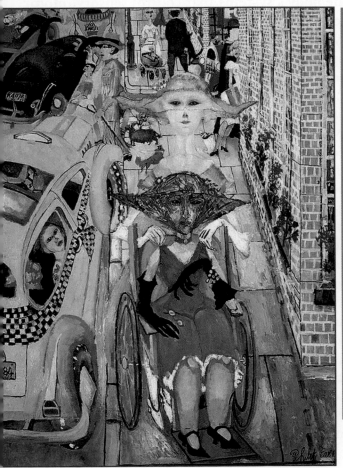

DOWAGER IN A WHEELCHAIR

1952, OIL ON FIBERBOARD, 47 7/8 × 36 IN

PHILIP EVERGOOD, 1901 - 1973, WAS A SOCIAL REALIST PAINTER WHOSE MILITANT SUPPORT OF WORKERS LED TO HIS BEING JAILED SEVERAL TIMES FOR TAKING PART IN STRIKES AND PROTESTS. EVERGOOD OFTEN DEPICTED POLITICAL OPPRESSION AND RACISM, AS WELL AS THE DAILY LIFE OF THE COMMON MAN. HIS STRIDENT EXPRESSIONIST STYLE WAS INFORMED BY A STRONG SENSE OF SOCIAL JUSTICE.

SPINAL CORD INJURY

Spinal cord injury (SCI) commonly leads to paralysis; it involves damage to the nerves within the bony protection of the spinal canal. The most common cause of cord injury is trauma, although damage can occur from various diseases acquired at birth or later in life, from tumors, electric shock, poisoning or loss of oxygen related to surgical or underwater mishaps. The spinal cord does not have to be severed in order for a loss of function to occur. In fact, in most people with SCI, the spinal cord is bruised—and intact.

Since the spinal cord coordinates body movement and sensation, an injured cord loses the ability to send and receive messages from the brain to the body's systems that control sensory, motor and autonomic function below the level of injury.

Spinal cord injury is an age-old problem but it wasn't until the 1940s that the prognosis for long-term survival was very optimistic. Prior to World War II, people routinely died of infections to the urinary tract, lungs or skin; the advent of sulfa drugs changed SCI from a death sentence to a manageable condition. Nowadays, people with spinal cord injury approach the full life span of non-disabled individuals.

Spinal cord trauma is more than a single event. The initial blunt force damages or kills spinal nerve cells. But in the hours and days after injury a cascade of secondary events, including loss of oxygen and the release of toxic chemicals at the site of injury, further damage the cord. Standard acute treatment for SCI trauma includes administration of the steroid drug methylprednisolone, which if given in the first few hours after injury may limit some of the second wave of destruction.

Acute care may involve surgery if the spinal cord appears to be compressed by bone, a herniated disk or a blood clot. Traditionally, surgeons have waited for several days to decompress the spinal cord, since there was some evidence that operating immediately could worsen the outcome. More recently, some surgeons have advocated immediate early surgery.

Generally speaking, after the swelling of the spinal cord begins to go down, most people show some functional improvement after an injury. With many injuries, especially incomplete injuries (some function preserved below the lesion level), a person may recover some motor or sensory function 18 months after the injury. In some cases, people with SCI will regain some function years after the injury.

Nerve cells (neurons) of the peripheral nervous system (PNS), which carry signals to the limbs, torso and other parts of the body, are able to repair themselves after injury. However, nerves in the brain and spinal cord, the central nervous system (CNS), are not able to regenerate.

The spinal cord includes neurons and long nerve fibers called axons that are covered by an insulating substance called myelin, which gives them a whitish appearance; therefore, the region in which they lie is called "white matter." Loss of myelin, which can occur with cord trauma and is the hallmark of such diseases as multiple sclerosis, prevents effective transmission of nerve signals.

The nerve cells themselves, with their tree-like branches called dendrites that receive signals from other nerve cells, make up what is called "gray matter;" this forms a butterfly-shaped region in the center of the spinal cord. As with the brain, the spinal cord is enclosed in three membranes (or meninges): the pia mater, the innermost layer; the arachnoid, the middle layer; and the dura mater, the tough outer layer.

Several types of cells carry out spinal cord functions. Large motor neurons have long axons that control skeletal muscles in the neck, torso and limbs. Sensory neurons called dorsal root ganglion cells, whose axons form the nerves that carry information from the body into the spinal cord, are found immediately outside the spinal cord. Spinal interneurons, which lie completely within the spinal cord, help integrate sensory information and generate coordinated signals that control muscles.

Glia, or supporting cells, far outnumber neurons in the brain and spinal cord and perform many essential functions. One type of glial cell, the oligodendrocyte, creates the myelin sheaths that insulate axons and improve the speed and reliability of nerve signal transmission. Other glia enclose the spinal cord like the rim and spokes of a wheel, providing compartments for the ascending and descending nerve fiber tracts.

DANA REEVE: YOU ARE NOT ALONE

When someone is first injured, it's very disorienting. It's doubly difficult because right after a spinal cord injury there are so many medical problems that crop up. Immediately, the body is bombarded with infection, urinary tract infections, pneumonia, skin breakdown.

It can look very bleak and overwhelming. And yet, if you can focus on one thing at a time, such as the person needing to get well or the person being healthy enough to rehabilitate, a great deal of hope will come from that focus. Once you get to that phase, there will be much forward progress.

There is a tremendous amount of adjustment that needs to go on mentally. And you need to face the new normal, face the adjustments, the loss. You have to grieve for the loss because it's the only way to get through it. The only way for grief to be alleviated is to grieve.

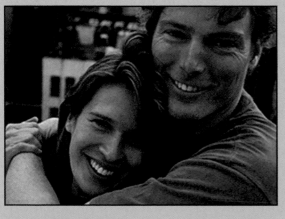

But at the same time, once you do that, you're opening up a whole new area where you can have so much hope. There are resources out there. You don't have to go through it alone. You shouldn't. You have to get the support of other people to get through this.

Our resource center is here for people who are newly injured and for people who have been living with injuries. And for the loved ones and families. Certainly, for the newly injured it's so disorientating and so difficult and you have so many questions. It's great to be able to contact someone who can answer each of your questions or, at least, lead you to answers, lead you to the next step.

Call us. There is no question that is not important. It's toll-free, 1-800-539-7309. If you want to use email, send a question to *info@paralysis.org*

Note: recorded April 2005. Dana Morosini Reeve died less than a year later.

CHRIS REEVE: DO NOT BUY INTO FEAR

I live a fearless life on a daily basis. I'm reminded of that every time I come into New York, because I'm put in the back of a van, strapped down by four straps, and driven around by a bunch of guys who just happen to be firefighters from Yonkers. These guys are used to driving fire trucks — at great speed — so when I get into the van, I have to give it up.

This one-hour van trip is a good metaphor for the journey I'd like to talk about. For so many of us, the source of our fear is the loss of control. But the more we try to control what happens to us, the greater our fear that we're no longer empowered, that there's no safety net, and that dangerous, unexpected things may happen. Ironically, the act of trying to control what happens is what actually robs us of great experiences and diminishes us.

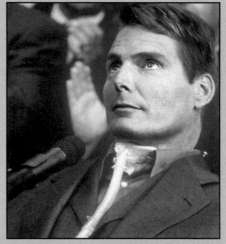

The lesson I had to learn when I had my injury was pretty drastic because my life before that as an actor had been one of self-sufficiency, perseverance, and discipline. I had been extremely self-sufficient from the time I finished high school all the way through college and graduate school, and as I made my way to Off-Broadway, Broadway, television, and film. I had done well and was used to being in charge.

I dealt with [my paralysis] with my wife Dana at my side, thank God. We just decided not to buy into the fear that people tried to instill in us.

This decision was the most important of all. How many people are walking around today three years after they were told that they only had six months to live? How many of us are doing things now that we were told that we could never do? It happens all the time. Our capabilities go way beyond our understanding. Trust in that and go forward.

From Reeve's speech at Omega Institute's Living a Fearless Life conference, 2004.

Astrocytes, large star-shaped glial cells, regulate the composition of the fluids that surround nerve cells. Some of these cells also form scar tissue after injury. Smaller cells called microglia become activated in response to injury and help clean up waste products. All of these glial cells produce substances that support neuron survival and influence axon growth. However, these cells may also impede recovery following injury.

Nerve cells of the brain and spinal cord respond to trauma and damage differently than most other cells of the body, including those in the PNS. The brain and spinal cord are confined within bony cavities that protect them, but this also renders them vulnerable to compression damage caused by swelling or forceful injury. Cells of the CNS have a very high rate of metabolism and rely upon blood glucose for energy—these cells require a full blood supply for healthy functioning. CNS cells are particularly vulnerable to reductions in blood flow (ischemia).

Other unique features of the CNS are the blood-brain barrier and the blood–spinal cord barrier. These barriers, formed by cells lining the blood vessels in the CNS, protect nerve cells by restricting entry of potentially harmful substances and cells of the immune system. Trauma may compromise these barriers, perhaps contributing to further damage in the brain and spinal cord. The blood–spinal cord barrier also prevents entry of some potentially therapeutic drugs.

Finally, in the brain and spinal cord, the glia and the extracellular matrix (the material that surrounds cells) differ from those in peripheral nerves. Each of these differences between the PNS and CNS contributes to their different responses to injury.

Complete vs. incomplete injury. Those with an incomplete injury have some spared sensory or motor function below the level of injury—the spinal cord was not totally damaged or disrupted. In a complete injury, nerve damage obstructs all signals coming from the brain to the body parts below the injury.

Incomplete spinal cord injuries fall into one of several patterns. The anterior cord syndrome results from injury to the motor and sensory pathways in the anterior parts of the spinal cord. Those affected can feel some types of crude sensation via the intact pathways in the posterior part of the spinal cord, but movement and detailed sensation are lost.

The central cord syndrome is caused by injury to nerve cells and pathways located in the center of the cervical spinal cord, which produces weakness, paralysis, and some sensory deficits in the arms. Strength and sensation in the legs are affected much less than in the arms. A so-called "walking quad" fits this category.

Brown-Sequard syndrome results from injury to the right or left half of the spinal cord. Movement and some types of sensation are lost below the level of injury on the injured side, but pain and temperature sensation are lost only on the side of the body opposite the injury—these pathways cross to the opposite side shortly after they enter the spinal cord.

While there's almost always hope of recovering some function after a spinal cord injury, it is generally true that people with incomplete injuries have a better chance of getting more return. In a large study of spinal cord injuries in Colorado reported by Craig Hospital, only 1 out of 7 of those who were completely paralyzed immediately after injury got a significant amount of movement back. But, of those who still had some movement in their legs immediately after injury, 3 out of 4 got significantly better.

About 2 out of 3 of those with neck injuries who can feel the sharpness of a pinprick in their legs eventually get enough muscle strength to be able to walk. Of those with neck injuries who can only feel light touch, about 1 out of 8 may eventually walk.

The sooner muscles start working again, the better the chances are of additional recovery. But when muscles come back later, after the first several weeks, they are more likely to be in the arms than in the legs. As long as there is some improvement and additional muscles recovering function, the chances are better that more improvement is possible. The longer there is no improvement, the lower the odds it will start to happen on its own.

The spinal cord is organized into segments along its length, noted by their position along the 33 vertebrae of the backbone. Nerves from each segment are responsible for motor and sensory functions for specific regions of the body. In general, the higher in the spinal column an injury occurs, the more function a person will lose. The segments in the neck, or cervical region, referred to as C1 through C8, control signals to the neck, arms, hands and, in some cases, the diaphragm. Injuries to this area result in tetraplegia, or as it is more commonly called, quadriplegia.

Injury above the C3 level may require a ventilator for the person to breathe. Injury above the C4 level usually means loss of movement and sensation in all four limbs, although often shoulder and neck movement is available to facilitate sip and puff devices for mobility, environmental control and communication.

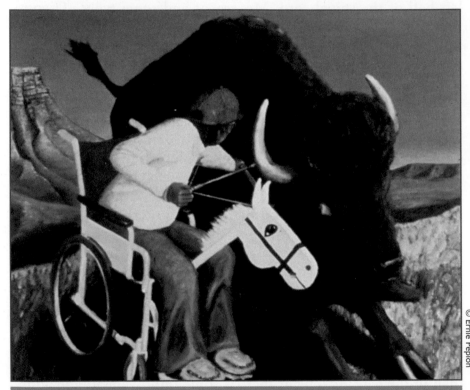

© Ernie Pepion

BUFFALO HUNTER
24 x 30 IN., OIL

"MY PAINTINGS ARE AUTOBIOGRAPHICAL. I USED TO BE A RANCHER UNTIL I WAS 28 AND GOT INJURED [QUADRIPLEGIA]. IN MY MIND I CAN STILL DO THINGS I USED TO DO; SOME OF MY PAINTINGS ARE INSPIRED BY DREAMS. I CAN POW-WOW, HUNT, BUFFALO, LIVE MY PAST LIVES ... PAINTING ALLOWS ME TO BE A PERSON BEYOND THE LIMITS OF RACIAL PREJUDICE AND DISABILITY. ART ENABLES ME TO ADDRESS FEELINGS THAT ARE DIFFICULT FOR ME TO WRITE OR EVEN TALK ABOUT."

- ERNIE PEPION

(UNTIL HIS DEATH IN 2005 PEPION WAS A MEMBER OF THE BLACKFEET TRIBE IN MONTANA)

C5 injuries often spare shoulder and biceps control, but there is not much control at the wrist or hand. Those at C5 can usually feed themselves and independently handle many activities of daily living. C6 injuries generally allow wrist control, enough to be able to drive adaptive vehicles and handle personal hygiene, but those affected at this level often lack fine hand function. Individuals with C7 and T1 injuries can straighten their arms and can typically handle most self-care activities, though they still may have dexterity problems with the hand and fingers.

Nerves in the thoracic, or upper back region (T1 through T12) relay signals to the torso and some parts of the arms. Injuries from T1 to T8 usually affect control of the upper torso, limiting trunk movement as the result of a lack of abdominal muscle control. Lower thoracic injuries (T9 to T12) allow good trunk control and good abdominal muscle control. With great exertion, some paraplegics can use long-leg braces with crutches to get about. Those injured in the lumbar, or mid-back region just below the ribs (L1 through L5), are able to control signals to the hips and legs. A person with an L4 injury can often extend the knees. The sacral segments (S1 through S5) lie just below the lumbar segments in the mid-back and control signals to the groin, toes and some parts of the legs.

Besides a loss of sensation or motor function, injury to the spinal cord leads to other changes, including loss of bowel, bladder and sexual function, low blood pressure, autonomic dysreflexia (for injuries above T8), deep vein thrombosis, spasticity, and chronic pain. See pages 61 - 97 for more on these conditions.

There are a number of conditions secondary to injury that are common to people with SCI and paralysis, including pressure ulcers, respiratory complications, urinary tract infections, pain, obesity, and depression. These secondary conditions are mainly preventable with good health care, diet and physical activity.

Findings from research on aging with disability indicate that respiratory illnesses, diabetes and thyroid disease occur more often in people with SCI than in the rest of the population. For example, people with SCI often have severe lower-respiratory infections, resulting in lost productivity, increased healthcare costs, and increased risk of early death. These problems are common not only in those with high cervical injuries, who have loss of respiratory muscle function, but also in those with paraplegia.

Spinal cord injuries are most commonly caused by motor vehicle accidents, followed by falls and acts of violence. Sports-related spinal cord injuries occur more commonly in children and teenagers, while work-related injuries (mainly construction work) occur with adults. People who sustain a spinal cord injury are mostly in their teens or twenties although as the population ages, the percentage of older persons is increasing. About 4 out of 5 people with spinal cord injuries are male. More than half of all spinal cord injuries occur in the cervical area, a third occur in the thoracic area, and the remainder occur in the lumbar region.

Currently, there is no cure for spinal cord injury. However, ongoing research to test surgical and drug therapies is progressing rapidly. Drugs to limit injury progression, decompression surgery, nerve cell transplantation and nerve regeneration, as well as complex nerve rejuvenation therapies are being examined as a means to treat the effects of spinal cord injury.

Rehabilitation techniques have evolved to the point that exercise and physical activity are believed to be essential to recovery. Seven years after his C2 injury Christopher Reeve gained a modest amount of motor control but a significant amount of sensory function. One of his doctors thinks this was due an aggressive program of physical therapy and exercise. Many people, especially in Europe, have gained function after participating in locomotor or treadmill training. The theory is that movement itself activates neural patterns in the spinal cord.

For the person with a spinal cord injury, it's best to stay active; disregard what you have heard is possible and strive for the maximum outcome. For more on activity based recovery, see page 162. To learn about the Christopher and Dana Reeve Foundation Neural Recovery Network, see page 138.

Sources

American Association of Neurological Surgeons, Craig Hospital, Christopher and Dana Reeve Paralysis Foundation, The National Institute of Neurological Disorders and Stroke

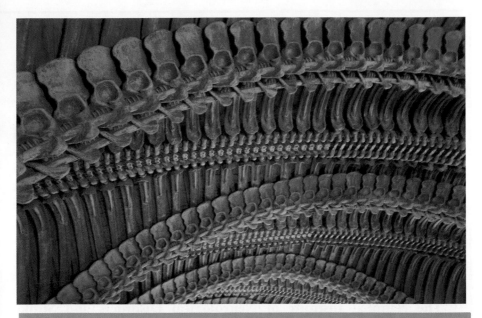

SCI MODEL SYSTEMS CENTERS

University of Alabama, Birmingham, *http://main.uab.edu*

Craig Hospital, Denver, *http://www.craighospital.org*

Shepherd Center, Atlanta, *http://www.shepherd.org*

Boston Medical Center, *http://www.bumc.bu.edu*, click on "Centers and Institutes,"
then New England SCI Center

University of Michigan, Ann Arbor, *http://www.med.umich.edu*

Kessler Institute, New Jersey, *http://www.kmrrec.org*

Mount Sinai School of Medicine, New York, *http://www.mssm.edu/rehab/spinal*

Thomas Jefferson University, Philadelphia, *http://www.jeffersonhospital.org/rehabmed*

University of Pittsburgh, *http://www.upmc-sci.org*

The Institute for Rehabilitation and Research, Houston, *http://www.tirr.org*

University of Washington, Seattle, *http://depts.washington.edu/rehab/sci*

National Rehabilitation Hospital, Washington, DC

Rehabilitation Institute of Chicago,

MetroHealth Spinal Cord Services, Cleveland, *http://www.metrohealth.org*

SPINAL CORD INJURY RESOURCES

The Christopher & Dana Reeve Foundation (CDRF) is committed to funding research that develops treatments and cures for paralysis caused by spinal cord injury and other central nervous system disor-

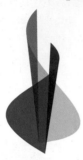

ders. The Foundation also works to improve the quality of life for people living with disabilities through its grants program, Paralysis Resource Center (*http://www.paralysis.org*), and advocacy efforts. For an overview of CDRF's research and advocacy efforts, details on the Quality of Life Program, or to make a contribution, visit *www.ChristopherReeve.org* or write c/o 636 Morris Turnpike, Suite 3A Short Hills, NJ 07078; toll-free telephone 1-800-225-0292.

The National Institute of Neurological Disorders and Stroke (NINDS) offers current and reliable fact sheets on all medical issues related to paralysis. On the Internet: *http://www.ninds.nih.gov*

United Spinal Association provides expertise and access to resources so people with spinal cord injuries and disorders can fulfill their potential as active members of their communities. USA, 75-20 Astoria Boulevard, Jackson Heights, NY 11370, telephone 718-803-3782. On the Internet, *http://www.unitedspinal.org*

National Spinal Cord Injury Association (NSCIA) offers a toll-free help-line, nationwide chapters and support groups. NSCIA, 6701 Democracy Boulevard, Suite 300-9, Bethesda, MD 20817; toll-free 1-800-962-9629; or visit *http://www.spinalcord.org*

The National Spinal Cord Injury Statistical Center (NSCISC) supervises and directs the collection, management and analysis of the world's largest spinal cord injury database, derived from the Model Systems SCI centers. The center is headquartered at the University of Alabama, Birmingham. *http://main.uab.edu,* click on "Information and Statistics." Also the site of the SCI Information Network. Search for details on any topic in paralysis.

Paralyzed Veterans of America (PVA) works toward quality health care, rehabilitation and civil rights for veterans and all citizens with spinal cord injuries and diseases. PVA offers numerous publications, fact sheets and authoritative clinical guidelines for SCI, and supports research by way of its Spinal Cord Research Foundation. The organization sponsors the magazines *PN/Paraplegia News* and *Sports 'N Spokes*. PVA, 801 Eighteenth Street, NW, Washington, D.C. 20006–3517; toll-free 1-800-424-8200; on the Internet see *http://www.pva.org*

The University of Miami School of Medicine offers an easy-to-use online manual on spinal cord injury health and wellness. *http://calder.med.miami.edu/pointis/sciman.html*

The University of Washington School of Medicine, Department of Rehabilitation maintains a useful Website with information on skin care, bowel and bladder management and other topics of concern to people with spinal cord injuries. See the Internet site *http://depts.washington.edu/rehab/sci/index.html*

New York Online Access to Health (N.O.A.H.) offers information and comprehensive links related to spinal cord and head injury treatment, rehabilitation and topics related to children. Many materials are available in Spanish. On the Internet please visit *http://www.noah-health.org*, search under Health Topics

CareCure Community Website offers bulletin boards on SCI and other neuroscience research, caregiving, travel, sex and relationships, sports, equipment, legislation and many other topics. Home of the Spinal Nurses (in the Care section) and of MobileWomen. A lively, helpful, hopeful community. See *http://sci.rutgers.edu*

Craig Hospital, located near Denver, specializes in the rehabilitation of spinal cord injury and traumatic brain injury. Educational materials are available online to help survivors maintain health and wellness. Emphasis on issues related to aging with a disability. See *http://craighospital.org;* click on "Health and Wellness."

SPINAL MUSCULAR ATROPHY

Spinal muscular atrophy (SMA) refers to a group of inherited neuromuscular diseases that affect the nerve cells (motor neurons) and the control of voluntary muscles. SMA causes lower motor neurons in the base of the brain and the spinal cord to disintegrate, preventing them from delivering the necessary signals for normal muscle function.

Involuntary muscles, such as those that control bladder and bowel function, are not affected in SMA. Hearing and vision are not affected, and intelligence is normal or above average.

The three major childhood-onset forms of SMA are now usually called Type 1, Type 2 and Type 3. All three types are also known as autosomal recessive SMA—both parents must pass on the defective gene in order for their children to inherit the disease.

All forms of SMA affect the skeletal muscles of the trunk and limbs. In general, those muscles closer to the center of the body are more affected than those farther away. SMA Type 1, the most severe form, mostly affects the neurons controlling the mouth and throat muscles and therefore involves more problems with chewing and swallowing. Respiratory muscles are involved to varying degrees in all forms of the disease. In SMA Type 1, the onset of the disease is noted within the first six months of the child's life. Children with SMA Type 1 are unable to sit without support, and death usually occurs before age two.

SMA Type 2 is an intermediate form of the disease. Onset is between 7 and 18 months. Children with SMA Type 2 usually learn to sit without support, but they don't learn to stand or walk without aid. The child's survival depends in large part on the degree of respiratory and swallowing difficulties.

SMA Type 3 is a milder form of this condition. Onset occurs after the age of 18 months and most often between the ages of 5 and 15. Weakness of the muscles of chewing and swallowing is rare, and respiratory effects are generally not as severe as in the first two forms. These children may live into adulthood. Respiratory complications, if they occur, pose the most serious threat to life.

At present, there is no known treatment that will stop or

reverse SMA. Physical therapy and orthopedic devices can help preserve walking function. Braces or surgery may also help to counteract scoliosis, or curvature of the spine.

Researchers around the world have collaborated to find the causes of SMA Types 1, 2 and 3. They all seem to result from genetic defects in the same small area of chromosome 5. Scientists hope to characterize the genes, study gene function and disease course, and find ways to prevent, treat and, ultimately, cure these diseases.

Sources

Muscular Dystrophy Association, National Institute of Neurological Disorders and Stroke

SPINAL MUSCULAR ATROPHY RESOURCES

Spinal Muscular Atrophy Foundation hopes to accelerate the development of a treatment or cure for SMA, the number one genetic killer of infants and toddlers. SMA Foundation, 119 West 72nd St. #187, New York, NY 10023l, toll free 1-877-FUND-SMA. See *http://www.smafoundation.org*

Families of Spinal Muscular Atrophy (FSMA) raises funds to promote research into the causes and treatment of the spinal muscular atrophies, and supports families affected by SMA. According to FSMA, SMA is the number one genetic killer of children under the age of two. One in every 6,000 babies is born with SMA. Of children diagnosed before age two, 50 percent will die before their second birthday. For more information contact FSMA, Post Office Box 196, Libertyville, IL 60048–0196; toll-free 1-800-886-1762; or visit the Internet site *http://www.fsma.org*

Muscular Dystrophy Association (MDA) provides services and supports research for a group of hereditary muscle-destroying disorders, including spinal muscular atrophies, metabolic diseases, peripheral nerve problems and immune system related disorders. Contact MDA, 3300 East Sunrise Drive, Tucson, AZ 85718–3208, toll-free 1–800–572–1717; on the Internet search under "Diseases" at *http://www.mda.org*

SPINAL TUMORS

Brain and spinal cord tumors feature abnormal tissue growth inside the skull or the bony spinal column. Tumors are classed as benign (non-cancerous) if the cells that make up the growth are similar to normal cells, grow slowly, and are confined to one location. Tumors are malignant (cancerous) when the cells are different from normal cells, grow quickly, and can spread easily to other locations.

Because the central nervous system (CNS) is housed within rigid, bony quarters (the skull and spinal column), any abnormal growth can place pressure on sensitive nerve tissues and impair function. While malignant cells elsewhere in the body can easily seed tumors inside the brain and spinal cord, malignant CNS tumors rarely spread out to other body parts.

Most spinal cord cancers are metastatic, meaning that they arise from a wide variety of primary cancers. These include lung, breast, prostate, head and neck, gynecologic, gastrointestinal, thyroid, melanoma and renal cell carcinoma.

When new tumors begin within the brain or spinal cord, they are called primary tumors. Primary CNS tumors rarely grow from neurons—nerve cells that perform the nervous system's important functions—because once neurons are mature they no longer divide and multiply. Instead, most tumors are caused by out-of-control growth among cells that surround and support neurons. Primary CNS tumors—such as gliomas and meningiomas—are named by the types of cells comprising them, their location or both.

The cause of most primary brain and spinal cord tumors remains a mystery. Scientists don't know exactly why and how cells in the nervous system or elsewhere in the body lose their normal identity and grow uncontrollably. Some of the possible causes under investigation include viruses, defective genes and chemicals. Brain and spinal cord tumors are not contagious or, at this time, preventable.

Spinal cord tumors are less common than brain tumors. About 10,000 Americans develop primary or metastatic spinal cord tumors each year. Although spinal cord tumors affect people of all ages, they are most common in young and middle-aged adults.

Brain tumors affect about 40,000 Americans each year. About

half of these tumors are primary, and the remainder are metastatic.

Brain and spinal cord tumors cause many diverse symptoms, which generally develop slowly and worsen over time. Some of the more common symptoms of a brain tumor include headaches; seizures (a disruption of the normal flow of brain cell electricity that can lead to convulsions, loss of consciousness or loss of bladder control); nausea and vomiting; and vision or hearing problems. Increased intracranial pressure can also decrease blood flow in the eye and trigger swelling of the optic nerve, which in turn causes blurred vision, double vision or partial visual loss.

Other symptoms of a CNS tumor may include the following:
- Behavioral and cognitive symptoms. Because they strike at the core of the individual's identity, changes in behavior and personality can be the most frightening and devastating symptoms of a brain tumor.
- Motor or balance problems. When tumors affect brain areas responsible for command of body movement, they can produce motor problem symptoms, including weakness or paralysis, lack of coordination or trouble with walking. Motor problems can also include muscle weakness, spasticity in which the muscles stay stiffly contracted, and impaired bladder and/or bowel control. Symptoms may worsen to include muscle wasting and paralysis. Often, muscle weakness or paralysis affects only one side of the body.
- Pain. By putting pressure on the spinal cord, a tumor can trigger pain circuits. This pain is often constant, sometimes severe, and can have a burning or aching quality.
- Sensory changes. This loss of sensation usually takes the form of numbness and decreased skin sensitivity to temperature.

Diagnosis: Special imaging techniques, especially computed tomography (CT) and magnetic resonance imaging (MRI), have dramatically improved the diagnosis of CNS tumors. In many cases, these scans can detect the presence of a tumor even if it is less than half an inch across.

Treatment: The three most commonly used treatments are surgery, radiation and chemotherapy. When a tumor compresses the spinal cord or its surrounding structures, corticosteroids may be given to reduce the swelling and preserve nerve function until the tumor can be removed.

Surgical attempts to remove as much tumor as possible is usually the first step in treating an accessible tumor—as long as the tumor is one that can be removed without unacceptable risk of neurological damage. Fortunately, research has led to advances in neurosurgery that make it possible for doctors to reach many tumors that were previously considered inaccessible. These include:

Microsurgery, a widely used technique where the surgeon looks through a high-powered microscope to get a magnified view of the operating area.

Stereotaxic procedures, which utilize computer information from CT or MRI images to create a three-dimensional map of the operation site. Ultrasonic aspirators use sound waves to vibrate tumors and break them up. Then, like a vacuum, the aspirator sucks up the tumor fragments.

Evoked potentials, a technique in which small electrodes are used to stimulate a nerve so its electrical response, or evoked potential, can be measured. Shunts are flexible tubes used to reroute and drain cerebrospinal fluid and relieve headaches, nausea and other symptoms caused by too much pressure inside the skull.

Doctors treat most malignant, inaccessible or inoperable CNS tumors with radiation and/or chemotherapy. For those who have metastatic CNS tumors, doctors usually focus on treating the original cancer first. However, when a metastatic tumor causes serious disability or pain, doctors may recommend surgery or other treatments to reduce symptoms even if the original cancer has not been controlled. Radiation therapy bombards tumor cells with lethal beams of energy. Most people with primary spinal cord tumors will not require radiation therapy. However, radiation is used for spinal cord compression due to metastatic cancer.

Chemotherapy uses tumor-killing drugs that are given orally or injected into the bloodstream. Because not all tumors are vulnerable to the same anti-cancer drugs, doctors often use a combination of drugs for chemotherapy.

Although most primary tumors of the spinal cord are not life threatening, they can cause significant disability. Goals of rehabilitation include functional improvement in mobility, self-care and pain management.

Sources
    National Institute for Neurological Disorders and Stroke, American Brain Tumor Association, National Cancer Institute

SPINAL TUMORS RESOURCES

The American Brain Tumor Association (ABTA) hopes to eliminate brain tumors through research and works to meet the needs of people with tumors and their families. Offers information, connections and a bibliography. ABTA, 2720 River Road, Des Plaines, IL 60018; toll-free 1–800–886–2282; or visit the Internet site *http://www.abta.org*

The Brain Tumor Society (TBTS) raises funds to find a cure and improve clinical care for brain and spinal cord tumors. It disseminates educational information and provides access to quality of life and psychosocial support. TBTS, 124 Watertown Street, Suite 3-H, Watertown, MA 02472; toll-free 1–800–770–TBTS (8287); or visit the Internet site *http://www.tbts.org*

Musella Foundation for Brain Tumor Research is dedicated to improving the quality of life and survival times for brain tumor survivors. The foundation features detailed information on clinical trials and treatment outcomes. Contact the Musella Foundation for Brain Tumor Research, 1100 Peninsula Boulevard, Hewlett, NY 11557; telephone 516–295–4740; or visit the Internet site *http://www.virtualtrials.com*

Spinal Cord Tumor Support is a Web community that sponsors discussion boards, personal stories and resource materials. *http://spinalcordtumor.homestead.com*

American Cancer Institute, with an annual research budget of over $1.5 billion, is the lead agency in the United States to fight cancer of all kinds. Includes resources and information on brain and spinal cord cancers. On the Internet see *http://cancer.gov*

STROKE

A stroke occurs when the blood supply to the brain is suddenly blocked or when a blood vessel in the brain bursts. Deprived of oxygen, nerve cells in the affected area of the brain can't function and die within minutes. A person with loss of blood flow to the heart is said to be having a heart attack; similarly, a person with loss of blood flow to the brain or sudden bleeding in the brain can be said to be having a "brain attack."

"Stroke is a leading cause of long-term disability in the United States. About 4,500,000 stroke survivors are alive today."

Although stroke is a disease of the brain, it can affect the entire body, including cognitive and memory deficits, speech problems, emotional difficulties, daily living problems and pain. Paralysis is a common outcome of stroke, often on one side of the body (hemiplegia). The paralysis or weakness may affect only the face, an arm or a leg, or it may affect one entire side of the body and face.

A person who suffers a stroke in the left hemisphere of the brain will show right-sided paralysis, or paresis. Likewise, a person with a stroke in the right hemisphere will show deficits on the left side of the body.

There are four main types of stroke. Cerebral thrombosis and cerebral embolism are the most common, accounting for about 70–80 percent of all strokes. They're caused by clots that plug an artery. Cerebral and subarachnoid hemorrhages are caused by ruptured blood vessels. They have a much higher fatality rate than strokes caused by clots.

Ischemia is the term used to describe the loss of oxygen and nutrients for brain cells when there is inadequate blood flow. Ischemia ultimately leads to infarction, the death of brain cells, which are eventually replaced by a fluid-filled cavity (or infarct) in the injured brain.

According to the American Stroke Association, someone in America has a stroke every 45 seconds. It is the nation's third leading cause of death, ranking behind diseases of the heart and all forms of cancer. Stroke is a leading cause of serious, long-term disability in the United States. About 4,500,000 stroke survivors are alive today.

Risk factors: The most important risks for stroke are hypertension, heart disease, diabetes and cigarette smoking. Others include heavy alcohol consumption, high blood cholesterol levels, illicit drug use and genetic or congenital conditions, particularly vascular abnormalities. An increase in the red blood cell count is another risk factor for stroke—excess red blood cells thicken the blood and make clots more likely.

Symptoms: The symptoms of a stroke include sudden numbness or weakness, especially on one side of the body; confusion or trouble speaking or understanding speech; trouble seeing in one or both eyes; sudden trouble walking, dizziness, or loss of balance or coordination; or severe headache with no known cause.

Treatment: Ischemic stroke is treated by removing the obstruction and restoring blood flow to the brain. In hemorrhagic stroke, doctors attempt to prevent the rupture and bleeding of aneurysms and arteriovenous malformations.

When blood flow to the brain is interrupted, some brain cells die immediately; others remain at risk. The damaged cells can often be saved by early intervention with a clot-dissolving drug called tissue plasminogen activator (t-PA) within three hours of the onset of the stroke. Unfortunately, only 3–5 percent of those who suffer a stroke reach the hospital in time to receive treatment.

The appropriate response to a brain attack is emergency action—every minute lost, from the onset of symptoms to the time of emergency contact, cuts into the limited window of opportunity for intervention. Meanwhile, other neuroprotective drugs are being developed to prevent the wave of damage after the initial attack.

Early recovery: The brain often compensates for the damage caused by stroke. Some brain cells that do not die may resume functioning. Sometimes, one region of the brain takes over for a region damaged by the stroke. Stroke survivors can experience remarkable and unanticipated recoveries that can't be explained.

General recovery guidelines show that 10 percent of stroke survivors recover almost completely; 25 percent recover with minor impairments; 40 percent experience moderate to severe impairments requiring special care; 10 percent require care in a nursing home or other long-term care facility; 15 percent die shortly after the stroke

Rehabilitation: This doesn't reverse the effects of a stroke but rehab builds strength, capability and confidence so a person can continue daily activities despite the effects of stroke. Activities may include the following: self-care skills such as feeding, grooming, bathing and dressing; mobility skills such as transferring, walking or moving a wheelchair; communication skills; cognitive skills such as memory or problem-solving; social skills for interacting with other people.

Rehabilitation starts in the hospital, and as soon as possible. For those who are stable, rehab may begin within two days after the stroke has occurred and continue as necessary after release from the hospital. Rehabilitation options may include the rehab unit of a hospital, a subacute care unit, a specialty rehab hospital, home therapy, outpatient care or long-term care in a nursing facility.

Stroke may cause problems with thinking, awareness, attention, learning, judgment and memory. A stroke survivor may be unaware of his or her surroundings. Language problems are common, usually the result from damage to the left lobes of the brain. Also, stroke survivors may experience pain, uncomfortable numbness or strange sensations, due to many factors including damage to the sensory regions of the brain, stiff joints or a disabled limb.

Many people who have had strokes are affected by spasticity, causing stiff, tight muscles. Muscle tightness prevents people from doing everyday things such as holding a spoon or tying a shoe. A combination of medication and physical therapy can loosen the muscles. Some stroke survivors may be candidates for intrathecal baclofen, which places a pump into the abdominal wall to deliver small doses of liquid baclofen into the fluid surrounding the spinal cord. This relaxes the muscles without the mind-numbing side effects often associated with the drug.

A stroke can also lead to emotional problems. Stroke patients may have difficulty controlling their emotions or may express inappropriate emotions in certain situations. One common disability that occurs with many stroke patients is depression. A depressed person may refuse or neglect to take medications, may not be motivated to perform exercises which will improve mobility, or may be irritable.

Depression can create a vicious cycle—it deprives the stroke survivor of social contacts, which could in turn help dispel depression. Family can help by stimulating interest in other people or by encouraging leisure activities. Chronic depression can be treated with counseling, group therapy or antidepressant medications.

Stroke survivors often find that once simple tasks around the house become extremely difficult or impossible. Many adaptive devices and techniques are available to help people retain their independence and function safely and easily. The home usually can be modified so the stroke survivor can manage personal needs. See page 231 for more on home modification and adaptive equipment.

There are numerous research projects related to preventing and treating stroke. See page 166 for more.

Sources
American Stroke Association, National Stroke Association, National Institute of Neurological Disorders and Stroke

STROKE RESOURCES

American Stroke Association (ASA), a partner with the Christopher and Dana Reeve Foundation Paralysis Resource Center, is affiliated with the National Heart Association. ASA covers the full spectrum, including medical, rehabilitation, recovery, caregiving, prevention and research. ASA features a Stroke Family Support Network, providing information and support to stroke families at any stage of recovery. For more information contact ASA, 7272 Greenville Avenue, Dallas, TX 75231; toll-free 1-888-4-STROKE; *http://www.strokeassociation.org*

National Stroke Association (NSA) offers information and support, including publications. NSA, 9707 E. Easter Lane, Englewood, CO 80112; toll-free 1-800-STROKES; or visit the Internet site *http://www.stroke.org*

TRANSVERSE MYELITIS

Transverse myelitis (TM) is a neurological disorder caused by inflammation of the spinal cord. The term "myelitis" refers to inflammation of the spinal cord; "transverse" describes the position of the inflammation across the width of one spinal cord segment. Attacks of inflammation can damage or destroy myelin, the fatty insulating substance that covers nerve cell fibers. This causes scars that interrupt communication between the nerves in the spinal cord and the rest of the body.

Symptoms of TM include a loss of spinal cord function over several hours to several weeks. What usually begins as a sudden onset of lower back pain, muscle weakness or abnormal sensations in the toes and feet can rapidly progress to more severe symptoms, including paralysis. Demyelination (loss of nerve fiber conductivity) usually occurs at the thoracic level, causing problems with leg movement and bowel and bladder control.

> **"In TM, a sudden onset of back pain or muscle weakness can rapidly progress to more severe symptoms, including paralysis."**

Some people recover from TM with minor or no lasting problems, while others have permanent impairments that affect their ability to perform ordinary tasks of daily living.

Transverse myelitis occurs in adults and children, in men and women, and in all races. No familial predisposition is apparent. The peak number of new cases per year appears to occur in people between 10 and 19 years and 30 and 39 years. About 1,400 new cases of transverse myelitis are diagnosed annually in the United States, and approximately 33,000 Americans have some type of disability resulting from TM.

The exact causes of transverse myelitis are not known. The inflammation that damages the spinal cord may result from viral infections, abnormal immune reactions or insufficient blood flow through the blood vessels located in the spinal cord. Transverse myelitis may also occur as a complication of syphilis, measles,

Lyme disease and some vaccinations, including those for chickenpox and rabies. Transverse myelitis often develops following viral infections due to varicella zoster (the virus that causes chickenpox and shingles), herpes simplex, Epstein-Barr, influenza, human immunodeficiency virus (HIV), hepatitis A, or rubella. Bacterial skin infections, middle-ear infections and bacterial pneumonia have also been linked with TM.

Some experts believe that infection causes a derangement of the immune system, which leads to an indirect autoimmune attack on the spinal cord. The immune system, which normally protects the body from foreign organisms, mistakenly attacks the body's own tissue, causing inflammation and, in some cases, damage to the spinal cord myelin.

Treatment: As with many disorders of the spinal cord, no effective cure exists for people with transverse myelitis. The best medicine has to offer is symptom management.

Therapy generally begins when the patient first experiences symptoms. Physicians may prescribe steroids during the first few weeks of illness to decrease inflammation. The goal is to keep the body functioning, hoping for complete or partial spontaneous recovery of the nervous system.

People with acute symptoms, such as paralysis, are most often treated in a hospital or in a rehabilitation facility under the care of a specialized medical team. Later, if patients begin to recover limb control, physical therapy begins to help improve muscle strength, coordination and range of motion.

Transverse myelitis usually includes the following symptoms: (1) weakness of the legs and arms, (2) pain, (3) sensory alteration and (4) bowel and bladder dysfunction. Most patients will experience weakness of varying degrees in their legs; some also experience it in their arms. Progression of the disease over several weeks often leads to full paralysis of the legs, requiring the use of a wheelchair. Some people may require the use of a respirator.

Pain is the primary symptom of transverse myelitis in about half of all patients. The pain may be localized in the lower back or may consist of sharp sensations that shoot down the legs or arms or around the torso. Most people with transverse myelitis report heightened sensitivity to heat, cold or touch; for some a light touch with a finger may cause significant pain (called allodynia).

The prognosis: Recovery from transverse myelitis usually begins within 2 to 12 weeks of the onset of symptoms and may continue for up to two years. However, if there is no improvement within the first three to six months, significant recovery is unlikely. About one-third of people affected with TM experience good or full recovery. Another one-third show fair recovery and are left with

CODY UNSER DRIVING TOWARD CURE

In February 1999, Cody Unser, daughter of racecar driver Al Unser, Jr., was at 6th grade basketball practice in Albuquerque when she began to feel extra tired. She had difficulty catching her breath and got a pounding headache. Her legs felt heavy, numb and "tingly." She was taken to the emergency room and sent home after evaluation. The next morning, Cody was unable to walk and returned to the hospital, paralyzed below her chest. The mysterious symptoms were finally diagnosed: she had Transverse Myelitis.

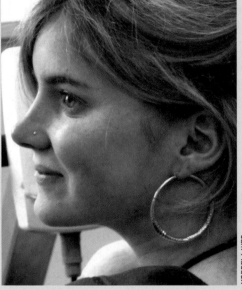

Sam Maddox

Two months later Cody returned home in a wheelchair but energized in her quest to build awareness of TM, promote research and cure paralysis. "The best antidote for my fears is helping other people overcome theirs," says Cody.

The Cody Unser First Step Foundation raises money and spreads the word that treatments for paralysis are within reach. See box on facing page.

deficits such as spastic gait, sensory dysfunction and urinary urgency or incontinence. The remaining one-third show no recovery, using wheelchairs, perhaps with marked dependence on others for basic functions of daily living.

Research: The National Institute of Neurological Disorders and Stroke (NINDS) supports research to clarify the role of the immune system in TM and other autoimmune diseases or disorders. Other work focuses on strategies to repair demyelinated spinal cords, including approaches using cell transplantation. The ultimate goals of these studies are to encourage regeneration in humans and to restore function to paralyzed patients.

Sources

National Institute of Neurological Disorders and Stroke (NINDS), Transverse Myelitis Association

TRANSVERSE MYELITIS RESOURCES

The Transverse Myelitis Association features news and information for the TM community and facilitates support and networking. The association functions as a clearinghouse for articles and research literature about the TM diagnosis. TMA, 1787 Sutter Parkway, Powell, OH 43065–8806; telephone 614–766–1806; or visit the Internet site *http://www.myelitis.org*

The Johns Hopkins Hospital Department of Neurology has established a center of excellence in Baltimore to care for people with non-surgical spinal cord dysfunction, including myelopathy and transverse myelitis. The Center has gathered physicians and health care experts in a variety of disciplines, including neurology, urology, rheumatology, orthopedic surgery, neuroradiology, rehabilitation medicine and physical and occupational therapy. Johns Hopkins Transverse Myelitis Center, toll-free 1-888-JHU-REHAB; or visit the Internet site *http://www.hopkinsneuro.org/tm*

The Cody Unser First Step Foundation is a nonprofit corporation raising research funds to fight paralysis and to build awareness of transverse myelitis. The Cody Unser First Step Foundation, Post Office Box 56696, Albuquerque, NM 87187; telephone 505–890–0086; or visit *http://www.codysfirststep.org*

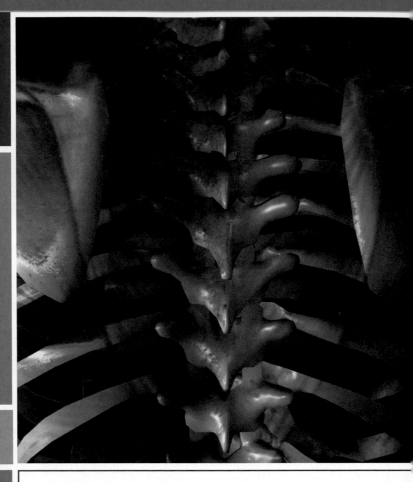

HEALTH MANAGEMENT & WELLNESS

A secondary condition is any medical, social, emotional, mental, family, or community problem that a person with a primary disabling condition (stroke, MS, SCI, etc) likely experiences.

Secondary Conditions
AUTONOMIC DYSREFLEXIA

Autonomic dysreflexia (AD) is a potentially life-threatening medical emergency that affects people with spinal cord injuries at the T5 level or higher.

Autonomic dysreflexia requires quick and correct action. Serious AD can lead to stroke. Because many health professionals are not familiar with this condition, it is important for people who are at risk for AD, including the people close to them, to know all about it.

What to do: If AD is suspected, the first thing to do is sit up or raise your head to 90 degrees. If you can lower your legs, do so. Next, loosen or remove anything tight. Most importantly, locate and remove the offending stimulus, if possible. The signs of AD include high blood pressure, pounding headache, flushed face, sweating above the level of injury, goose bumps below the level of injury, nasal stuffiness, nausea and a slow pulse (slower than 60 beats per minute).

Autonomic dysreflexia is caused by an irritant below the level of injury, usually related to the bladder or bowel. Among the causes are an irritation of the bladder wall, urinary tract infection, blocked catheter or overfilled collection bag, over-distended or irritated bowel, constipation or impaction, hemorrhoids or anal infections, skin infection or irritation, cuts, bruises, abrasions or pressure sores, ingrown toenails, burns (including sunburn and burns from hot water) and tight or restrictive clothing.

Autonomic dysreflexia can also be triggered by sexual activity, menstrual cramps, labor and delivery, abdominal conditions (gastric ulcer, colitis, peritonitis) or bone fractures.

What happens during an episode of AD? Autonomic dysreflexia means an over-activity of the autonomic nervous system — the part of the system that controls things you don't have to think about, such as heart rate, breathing and digestion. A stimulus below the injury level sends nerve impulses to the spinal cord; and they travel upward until they are blocked at the level of injury. Since the impulses cannot reach the brain, a reflex is activated that increases activity of the sympathetic portion of the autonomic nervous system. This results in spasms and a narrowing of the blood vessels, which causes a rise in blood pressure. Nerve receptors in the heart and blood vessels detect this rise in blood pressure and send a message to the brain. The brain then sends a message to the heart, causing the heartbeat to slow down and the blood vessels above the level of injury to dilate. However, the brain cannot send messages below the level of injury, due to the spinal cord lesion, and therefore blood pressure cannot be regulated.

Generally speaking, medications are used only if the offending stimulus cannot be identified and removed or when an episode of AD persists even after the suspected cause has been removed. Potentially useful agents include nitroglycerine, clonidine, hydralazine, minipress and catapres. For most people, autonomic dysreflexia can be prevented. It's important to relieve pressure while in bed or chair – frequently. Use sunscreen, watch water temperatures. Don't wear clothes that are too tight. Adhere faithfully to one's bowel program. Keep catheters clean and stick to your catheterization schedule.

Sources
Spinal Cord Injury Information Network, Paralyzed Veterans of America, Spinal Injuries Association/London, Miami Project to Cure Paralysis/University of Miami School of Medicine

AUTONOMIC DYSREFLEXIA RESOURCES

Paralyzed Veterans of America, in support of The Consortium for Spinal Cord Medicine, offers authoritative clinical practice guidelines for autonomic dysreflexia. PVA, 801 Eighteenth Street, NW, Washington, D.C. 20006; toll-free 1–800–424–8200; or visit the Internet site *http://www.pva.org* and click on Publications, then Medical Guidelines. A consumer guide to AD, co-sponsored by the Paralysis Resource Center, is available.

Spinal Cord Injury Information Network features articles and references for autonomic dysreflexia and all other SCI conditions. Spain Rehabilitation Center, 619 19th Street South SRC 529, Birmingham, AL 35249–7330; or visit the Internet site *http://www.spinalcord.uab.edu* and perform a search under Autonomic Dysreflexia.

BLADDER MANAGEMENT

Paralysis at any level almost always affects control over bladder and bowel function. This is because the nerves controlling these organs attach to the very base of the spinal cord (levels S2–S4) and are therefore cut off from brain input by all but the very lowest of sacral dysfunction.

Although it may not be possible to regain the same control one had before paralysis, a wide range of techniques and tools are available to manage bladder and bowel function. (See page 67 for information on bowel management.)

Here's how the bladder works: Urine consists of excess water and salts that are extracted from the bloodstream by the kidneys. From the kidneys, the urine is pumped down thin tubes called ureters, which normally allow urine to flow only in one direction. The ureters connect to the bladder, a storage bag. When the bag is full, nerves send a message via the spinal cord to the brain.

When one is ready to empty the bladder, the brain sends a message back down the spinal cord to the bladder, telling the detrusor muscle (the bladder wall) to contract and the sphincter muscle (a valve around the top of the urethra) to relax and open. Urine then passes down the urethra to exit the body. It takes a rather elegant process of muscle coordination just to go pee.

After paralysis, however, the body's normal system of bladder control goes haywire; messages can no longer pass between the bladder muscles and the brain. The bladder is usually affected in one of two ways:

1. Spastic (reflex) bladder is when your bladder fills with urine and a reflex automatically triggers the bladder to empty; this usually occurs when the injury is above the T12 level. With a spastic bladder you do not know when, or if, the bladder will empty.

2. Flaccid (non-reflex) bladder is when the reflexes of the bladder muscles are sluggish or absent. If you do not feel when the bladder is full, it can become over-distended, or stretched. The urine can back up through the ureters into the kidneys (called reflux). Stretching also affects the muscle tone of the bladder. Dyssynergia occurs when the sphincter muscles do not relax as when the bladder contracts. The urine cannot flow through the

urethra, which can also result in the urine backing up into the kidneys. The bladder may also not empty completely. Treatments include medications or surgery to open the sphincter.

The most common methods of bladder emptying are with intermittent catheterization (ICP), indwelling catheter (foley), and an external condom catheter (draining to a legbag) for men.

It is quite common for people with multiple sclerosis to have some problems with bladder control. This can involve a little leaking after a sneeze or laugh, or it can involve loss of all control. For many people, appropriate clothing and padding can compensate for lack of control. Some women benefit from strengthening the

CLEAN VS. STERILE

One time use or wash it out? A federal panel reported a few years back on reusable vs. single use intermittent sterile catheters: You run no greater risk for getting a urinary tract infection using either method. Solid medical literature to back this up has yet to be conducted, but it is the basis of current Medicare policy; the feds won't pay for sterile caths until you get really sick from a bladder infection (twice) and can get a doctor to prescribe.

The policy toward re-using caths, the so-called "clean" technique, has mainly been based on cost: it is enormously cheaper to wash them than to toss them.

Things have changed a bit for the better. In 2008, appeals by consumers convinced Medicare to change the way catheters are covered. Many people who used to get four caths a month can now get 200 – they aren't the sterile kind but you don't have to use each one more than once.

If you continue to use the clean method, be sure to wash hands and catheter with mild soap after use. Rinse with water; soaking in bleach or vinegar isn't necessary. After drying the catheter completely, keep it in a container that is not airtight. Some boil or microwave them; there's no proof that's necessary.

pelvic diaphragm (Kegel exercises) to improve retention of urine.

There are several surgical alternatives for bladder dysfunction. A Mitrofanoff procedure constructs a new passageway for urine using the appendix. This allows catheterization to be done through the abdomen directly to the bladder, a great advantage for women and for people with limited hand function. Bladder augmentation is a procedure that surgically enlarges the bladder to reduce the need for frequent catheterization.

Sphincterotomy reduces pressure on the sphincter and thus allows urine to flow out of the bladder easier. There is a chance that the operation will affect a man's ability to obtain a reflex erection. This operation is not normally carried out on women.

Urinary tract infection: People who are paralyzed are at a high risk for urinary tract infection (UTI), which until the 1950s was the leading cause of death after paralysis. The source of infection is bacteria — a group or colony of tiny, microscopic, single-celled life forms that live in the body and are capable of causing disease. Bacteria from the skin and urethra are easily brought into the bladder with ICP, foley and suprapubic methods of bladder management. Also, many people are not able to completely empty their bladder; bacteria are more likely to grow in urine that stays in the bladder.

Some of the symptoms of UTI are fever, chills, nausea, headache, increased spasms and autonomic dysreflexia (AD). You may also feel burning while urinating, and/or discomfort in the lower pelvic area, abdomen or lower back.

The key to preventing UTI is to halt the spread of bacteria into the bladder. Proper cleaning of urinary care supplies can help prevent infection. Sediment in the urine can collect in tubing and connectors. This can make it harder for your urine to drain and can make it easier for bacteria to spread. Clean skin is also an important step in preventing infection.

Drinking the proper amount of fluids can help to "wash out" bacteria and other waste materials from the bladder. This helps prevent UTI and lessens the chance of other problems of the urinary system. Cranberry juice, or cranberry extract in pill form, can be an effective preventative for bladder infections. It works by making it hard for bacteria to stick to the wall of the bladder and colonize. Another way to keep the bacteria from colonizing the bladder wall is the use of D-mannose, a type of sugar available at health food stores. It appears to stick to the bacteria so the bacteria can't stick to anything else.

A complete medical check-up is recommended at least once a year. This should include a urologic exam, including a renal scan or ultrasound to know that the kidneys are working properly. The exam may also include a KUB (kidneys, ureters, bladder), an X-ray of the abdomen that can detect kidney or bladder stones.

Even with a regular bladder management program and proper prevention methods, the risk remains for urinary tract infection. Treatment for a UTI almost always includes an antibiotic medication. Indeed, people prone to UTIs can become resistant to the arsenal of antibiotics.

Bladder cancer is another concern for some individuals with spinal cord injury. Research shows a moderate increase in the risk of bladder cancer among those who have been using indwelling catheters for a long period of time. Smoking also increases the risk for developing bladder cancer.

Sources

National MS Society, Spinal Cord Injury Information Network, University of Washington School of Medicine Department of Rehabilitation Medicine

BLADDER MANAGEMENT RESOURCES

Spinal Cord Injury Information Network links to several articles and fact sheets related to bladder function. Simply search under "Bladder" at *http://www.spinalcord.uab.edu/*

The University of Miami School of Medicine offers clinical information on bladder, bowel and other paralysis-related conditions. See *http://calder.med.miami.edu/pointis/urinary.html*

University of Washington School of Medicine/Department of Rehabilitation Medicine, offers details on bladder management. *http://depts.washington.edu/rehab/sci/bladder-manage.html*

BOWEL MANAGEMENT

The digestive tract in its entirety is a hollow tube beginning at the mouth and ending at the anus. The bowel, the final portion of the tract, is where waste products, digested food, are stored until they are emptied from the body in the form of stool, or feces.

After food is swallowed, it moves through the esophagus to the stomach, which is basically a storage bag, and then on to the intestines or bowels. The absorption of nutrients occurs in the small intestines, the duodenum, the jejunum and the ileum.

Next is the colon, which encircles the abdomen, starting on the right with the ascending colon, passing across the top with the transverse colon, and down the "s"-shaped sigmoid colon to the rectum, which opens at the anus.

"Bowel accidents happen. The best way to prevent them is to follow a regular schedule, to teach the bowel to have a movement when it is most appropriate."

Feces move through the bowel by coordinated muscular contractions of the colon walls called peristalsis. This motion is managed by a network of nerve cells at several different levels. The myenteric plexus nerves direct local intestinal movement, seemingly without input from the brain or spinal cord. More than 100 years ago it was discovered that the intestines, even when removed from the body, have an inherent tendency to produce peristalsis. If the intestine wall is stretched, the myenteric plexus triggers the muscles above the stretch to constrict and those below to relax, propelling material down the tube.

The next level of organization comes from autonomic nerves from the brain and spinal cord to the colon, which receives messages through the vagus nerve. The highest level of control comes from the brain. Conscious perception of a full rectum permits discrimination between solid material and gas, and the decision to eliminate fecal contents when appropriate. Messages relayed via the spinal cord produce voluntary relaxation of the pelvic floor and anal sphincter muscles, allowing the defecation process to occur.

Paralysis often damages the nerves that control the bowel, though injury at the lumbar or sacral areas doesn't affect the digestive system. If the injury is above the T12 level, peristalsis in the large intestine is affected, slowing the movement of fecal matter. The ability to sense a full rectum may also be lost. The anal sphincter will remain tight, however, so bowel movements will occur on a reflex basis. This means that when the rectum is full, the defecation reflex will occur. This is called an upper motor neuron or reflex bowel. It is managed by triggering the defecation reflex at socially appropriate times and places.

Spinal cord dysfunction below T12 may damage the defecation reflex and relax the anal sphincter muscle. This is known as a lower motor neuron or flaccid bowel. Management of this type of bowel problem may require more frequent attempts to empty the bowel and manual removal of stool.

Not being able to control the sphincter can result in an inability to have a bowel movement. This can cause stool to be impacted and the solid waste to be retained. Impaction can be serious if it occurs high up in the bowel.

Bowel Accidents Happen. The best way to prevent them is to follow a schedule, to teach the bowel when to have a movement. Most people perform their bowel program at a time of day that fits in with their prior bowel habits and current lifestyle. The program usually begins with insertion of either a suppository or a mini-enema, followed by a waiting period of approximately 15–20 minutes to allow the stimulant to work. Preferably, this part of the program should be done on the commode.

After the waiting period, digital stimulation is performed every 10–15 minutes until the rectum is empty. Those with a flaccid bowel frequently start their programs with digital stimulation or manual removal. Bowel programs typically require 30–60 minutes to complete.

Antegrade continence enema is another option for some people with difficult bowel problems. This technique involves surgery to create stoma, which allows introduction of liquid above the rectum, thus causing an effective flushing of fecal material from the bowel. In one study, this method was successful in decreasing bowel care time from two hours to 50 minutes daily; allowing for the discontinuation of six bowel medications and eliminating fecal incontinence with no surgical or medical side effects noted.

Some medications common for people with paralysis can affect the bowel. For example, any anti-cholinergic medication has the potential to slow bowel motility, resulting in constipation or even bowel obstruction. This includes drugs commonly used to manage a neurogenic bladder, such as oxybutynin and propantheline; some antidepressant drugs, such as amitryptyline; narcotic pain medications; and some drugs used for the treatment of spasticity, such as dantrolene sodium.

Constipation is a problem for many people with neuromuscular-related paralysis. Anything that changes the speed with which foods move through the large intestine interferes with the absorption of water and causes problems. In amyotrophic lateral sclerosis (ALS), for example, swallowing problems make getting a good diet and sufficient fluids difficult. Breathing problems may make it difficult to take a deep breath and bear down.

There are three main types of laxatives that help with constipation. Bulk or fiber laxatives such as Metamucil supply the fiber necessary to add bulk, which holds water and makes it easier to move the stool through the bowels. Stool softeners, such as Colace, also keep the water content of the stool higher, which keeps it softer and thus easier to move. Stimulants such as bisacodyl increase the muscle contractions (peristalsis) of the bowel, which moves the stool along. Frequent use of stimulants can actually aggravate constipation — the bowels become dependent on them for even normal peristalsis.

Faster than a Speeding ... There are two main types of suppositories, both based on the active ingredient bisacodyl: those with a vegetable base (e.g. Dulcolax) and those with a polyethylene glycol base (e.g. Magic Bullet). Bullets are said to be almost twice as fast as the alternative (see *www.conceptsinconfidence.com* for information on Bullets).

Here are some bowel facts for better digestive management:

- For good health it is generally not necessary to have a bowel movement every day. Every other day is okay.
- Bowels move more readily after a meal.
- Fluid intake of two quarts daily aids in maintaining a soft stool; warm liquid will also aid bowel movement.
- A healthy diet including fiber in the form of bran cereals, vegetables and fruits helps keep the digestive process working.
- Activity and exercise promote good bowel health.

Some people report significant improvements in quality of life after colostomy. This surgical option creates a permanent opening between the colon and the surface of the abdomen to which a stool collection bag is attached. Colostomies sometimes become necessary because of fecal soiling or pressure sores, continual stool incontinence, or excessively long bowel programs. Colostomy enables many people to manage their bowels independently, plus, colostomy management usually takes less time than bowel programs. Studies have shown that people who get colostomies are pleased and would not reverse the procedure; while many may not have embraced the idea of a colostomy at the outset, the procedure can make a huge difference in quality of life, cutting bowel time from as much as eight hours a day to no more than 15 minutes.

Sources

Spinal Cord Injury Information Center/University of Alabama at Birmingham, University of Washington School of Medicine/Rehabilitation Medicine Department, ALS Association of America, National Multiple Sclerosis Society

BOWEL MANAGEMENT RESOURCES

Clinical Practice Guidelines sponsored by the Paralyzed Veterans of America offer reliable information on the management of the neurogenic bowel. Download free from *http://www.pva.org* (click on Publications, then Medical Guidelines).

Spinal Cord Injury Information Center at the University of Alabama, Birmingham, features clinical information about bowel management and all other medical issues of paralysis. Use the search function at *http://www.spinalcord.uab.edu/*

DEPRESSION

Depression is common among people who are paralyzed, but it's not normal – becoming discouraged, grief-stricken or sad is normal, but depression represents a condition that is a health problem unto itself. Most depressions, however, can be treated.

While about 11 percent of the U.S. non-disabled population is said to be moderately or severely depressed, research shows that about 20 - 30 percent of people with long-term disabilities have a depressive condition.

Depression affects a person in many ways. It involves major changes in mood, outlook, ambition, problem solving, activity level and bodily processes (sleep, energy and appetite). It affects health and wellness: People with a disability who are depressed may not look after themselves; they may not drink enough water, take care of their skin, manage their diet. It affects one's social world: Friends and families are tuned out. Depressed people can't find pleasure, success or meaning. Substance abuse may develop. Thoughts of suicide often occur when things look most hopeless.

Many factors contribute to depression. These may include the effects of disability including pain, fatigue, changes in body image, shame, and loss of independence. Other life events, such as divorce, loss of a loved one, loss of a job or financial problems can also lead to or magnify depression.

"Depression is common after paralysis but not normal. It is a health problem unto itself. But depression is highly treatable with therapy and antidepressants."

There are effective ways for helping people cope with the stresses of paralysis. Depression is highly treatable using psychotherapy, pharmacotherapy (antidepressants), or a combination of both. Tricyclic drugs (e.g., imipramine) are often effective for depression but may have intolerable side effects. SSRIs (Selective Serotonin Reuptake Inhibitors, e.g., Prozac) have fewer side effects and are usually as effective as tricyclics. SSRIs may exacerbate spasticity in some persons.

Among the newest antidepressants, venlafaxine (e.g., Effexor) is chemically similar to tricyclics and has fewer side effects. In theory, it may also alleviate some forms of neurogenic pain, a huge contributor to depression. In fact, aggressive treatment of pain problems is crucial to the prevention of depression.

Among those with MS, some experience mood swings and/or uncontrollable laughing or crying (called emotional lability). These result from damaged areas in emotional pathways in the brain. It is important for family members and caregivers to know this and realize that people with MS may not always be able to control their emotions. Mood stabilizing medications such as amitriptyline (e.g., Elavil) and valproic acid (e.g., Depakote) are used to treat these emotional changes. It is also important to recognize that depression is very common in MS – even more so than in other, equally disabling chronic illnesses.

People with major depression may be at risk for suicide. In spinal cord injury, for example, risk is highest in the first five years after the injury. Other risk factors include dependence on alcohol or drugs, lack of a spouse or close support network, or a previous suicide attempt. People who've tried to kill themselves before are likely to try again. The most important factors in preventing suicide are spotting depression early and getting the right treatments for it.

Life is worth living, despite what health professionals are sometimes prone to judge: According to a Colorado survey, 86 percent of SCI high-level quadriplegics rated their quality of life as average or better than average while only 17 percent of their ER doctors, nurses, and technicians thought they would have an average or better quality of life if they acquired quadriplegia.

If you are depressed, get help, including professional counseling or participation in a support group. An active lifestyle can also help to break through depression.

Sources
Rancho Los Amigos National Rehabilitation Center; Paralyzed Veterans of America; National Multiple Sclerosis Society, University of Washington/Department of Rehabilitation Medicine

DEPRESSION RESOURCES

Paralyzed Veterans of America, in support of The Consortium for Spinal Cord Medicine, offers authoritative clinical practice guidelines for depression as a secondary condition of paralysis. PVA, 801 Eighteenth Street, NW, Washington, DC 20006, toll-free 1-800-424-8200, or visit the Internet site, *http://www.pva.org* — click on Publications, then Medical Guidelines.

Spinal Cord Injury Information Network features articles and references related to spinal cord paralysis. Contact Spain Rehabilitation Center, 619 19th Street South - SRC 529, Birmingham, AL 35249-7330. See the Internet site: *http://www.spinalcord.uab.edu*, search under "depression."

National Institute of Mental Health provides free information on depression and other mental illnesses in both English and Spanish. Call toll-free 1-800-421-4211; or see *http://www.nimh.nih.gov*

The National Mental Health Association (NMHA) is the nation's oldest organization dedicated to addressing all aspects of mental health and mental illness, including depression. Contact NMHA toll-free at 1-800-969-6642; visit *http://www.nmha.org*. For an on-line depression screening test, sponsored by NMHA, see the Internet site *http://www.depression-screening.org*

The National Strategy for Suicide Prevention (NSSP) represents the combined work of advocates, clinicians, researchers and survivors to prevent suicide. It is designed to be a catalyst for social change with the power to transform attitudes, policies, and services. Contemplating Suicide? Call toll-free 1-800-SUICIDE. Or see the Internet site *http://www.mentalhealth.org/suicideprevention*

Not Dead Yet was founded 1996 to oppose legalized assisted suicide and euthanasia. The advocacy group opposes a public policy that singles out individuals for legalized killing based on their health status, including physical disability. NDY notes that the duration of disability almost always correlates with acceptance of disability in persons with spinal cord injury paralysis. Not Dead Yet, c/o Progress CIL, 7521 Madison Street, Forest Park, IL 60130; telephone 708-209-1500 or see *http://www.notdeadyet.org*

FATIGUE

Fatigue is a very common symptom of many conditions related to paralysis. About 80 percent of people with multiple sclerosis report that fatigue significantly interferes with their ability to function. It gets worse as the day progresses; it's aggravated by heat and humidity and may be the most prominent complaint in many MSers who otherwise have few other symptoms.

Fatigue is also a prominent symptom of post-polio syndrome. People who had polio long ago, even those who made complete recoveries from their original polio, sometimes begin years later to feel a lack of energy — tiring much faster than in the past, feeling that once simple things now take a huge effort. These symptoms may be caused by the gradual wearing out of already weakened and damaged nerve cells. Some believe chronic fatigue syndrome, which affects about 500,000 people in the United States, may be related to undiagnosed post-polio syndrome.

According to recent research in spinal cord injury, more than 60 percent of people who experience changes in function identified fatigue as a major problem.

Underlying medical problems such as anemia, thyroid deficiency, diabetes, depression, respiratory problems or heart disease may be factors in a person's fatigue. Also, medications such as muscle relaxants, pain drugs and sedatives can contribute to fatigue. Low fitness levels may result in too little energy reserves to meet the physical demands of daily life. People should consult a physician if fatigue becomes a problem.

Disrupted sleep is reported in up to 35 percent of people with MS. The resulting daytime fatigue may be caused by sleep apnea, periodic leg movements, neurogenic bladder problems, spasticity, pain, anxiety or depression. Better sleep starts with better symptom management. Consult your doctor about options for treating pain, depression, sleep apnea, etc. There isn't a single remedy for fatigue. Listen to your body and use your energy wisely.

Sources

National Multiple Sclerosis Society, Rancho Los Amigos Hospital, Paralyzed Veterans of America, Centers for Disease Control and Prevention

DEALING WITH FATIGUE:

- BETTER NUTRITION. Caffeine, alcohol, smoking and a diet high in refined carbohydrates, sugar and hydrogenated fats rob your energy. Lack of protein can also lead to fatigue.

- REST. Take it easy on yourself. Give yourself down time as needed. Reach for the best-feeling thoughts, enjoy a laugh whenever you can, and structure relaxation time at least twice a day using yoga, meditation or prayer.

- STAY COOL. People with MS are less fatigued when they avoid heat and/or use cooling devices (vests, ice packs, etc.).

- FIND NEW WAYS, including the resources of occupational therapy, to simplify work tasks and implement energy saving strategies.

- USE AVAILABLE TOOLS. Adaptive equipment can help preserve the energy you do have. There is a wonderful array of gadgets and timesavers on the market (see page 223 for more). For a person with post-polio, this could mean using a wheelchair instead of a walker. Wheelchair users might add a power assist or move up to a full-power unit.

- CUT STRESS. Some people benefit from stress management, relaxation training, membership in a support group or psychotherapy. Although the link between fatigue and depression is not fully understood, psychotherapy has been shown to lessen fatigue in people with MS who are depressed.

- BUILD STAMINA THROUGH EXERCISE. Physical activity was once thought to worsen fatigue, but aerobic exercise may benefit those with mild disabilities.

- VITAMINS, HERBS, ETC. Some people say their fatigue is improved after taking supplements such as adenosine monophosphate, coenzyme Q-10, germanium, glutathione, iron, magnesium sulfate, melatonin, NADH, selenium, l-tryptophan, vitamins B12, C and A, and zinc. Others include astralagus, borage seed oil, bromelain, comfrey, echinacea, garlic, Ginkgo biloba, ginseng, primrose oil, quercetin, St. John's wort and Shiitake mushroom extract.

- For MS, doctors often prescribe AMANTADINE AND PEMOLINE to relieve fatigue. Since one of the side effects of both drugs is insomnia, they work best if taken in the morning and at noon.

OTHER COMPLICATIONS

Heart Disease: People with spinal cord dysfunction have an increased risk of developing heart disease at an earlier age than those in the rest of the population. Cardiovascular diseases are reportedly the leading cause of death for persons who have had a spinal cord injury for more than 30 years. People with SCI are prone to certain metabolic risk factors. They are generally more insulin resistant, which affects the body's ability to transform blood sugar into energy, and can lead to heart disease, diabetes and other conditions. Contributing to the abnormalities are loss of muscle mass (atrophy), increase in body fat, and a harder time maintaining cardiovascular fitness. Prevention strategies: screening for blood sugar problems, healthy diet, no smoking, moderation with alcohol, regular physical exercise.

Orthostatic hypotension is a condition that results in a decrease in blood pressure when sitting or standing up, causing light-headedness or fainting. It occurs more commonly after spinal cord injury at T-6 or above, in response to lowered blood pressure. Elastic hose and abdominal support help prevent it. It is also helpful to come to a sitting or standing position gradually.

Cyst, or syrinx, is a fluid-filled cavity that develops in the spinal cord and can lead to loss of motor function and sensation. Those who notice significant changes are advised to contact their physician. Treatment may involve cyst drainage or untethering of the spinal cord (freeing the flow of spinal fluid).

Heterotopic ossification (HO) is the development of bone deposits in soft (non-skeletal) tissue, primarily around the hip and knee joints. It occurs in many spinal cord injured individuals and may develop within days following the injury. In most cases, HO causes no significant additional physical limitations but may limit joint motion, cause swelling or increase spasticity in the leg. Drugs are prescribed to treat HO; surgery is sometimes necessary.

Hypo/hyperthermia: Paralysis can cause the temperature of the body to fluctuate according to the temperature of the environment. Being in a hot room may increase temperature (hyperthermia); a cold room may decrease temperature (hypothermia). Temperature management is essential for some people.

CHRONIC PAIN

Pain is a signal triggered in the nervous system to alert us to possible injury. Acute pain results from sudden disease, inflammation or trauma to tissues. Acute pain can usually be diagnosed and treated; the discomfort can be confined to a given period of time and severity.

Chronic pain is the kind that doesn't go away and it's resistant to most medical treatments. There may be an ongoing cause of pain — arthritis, cancer, infection — but some people have chronic pain for weeks, months, even years in the absence of any past injury or evidence of body damage. A type of chronic pain called neurogenic or nerve pain often accompanies paralysis.

The problem with chronic pain is not just the hurting. Pain leads to inactivity, which leads to anger and frustration, which leads to isolation, depression, sleeplessness, sadness, then to more pain. It's a spin cycle of misery with no easy exit.

Treatment options for chronic pain include drugs, acupuncture, local electrical stimulation, brain stimulation and surgery. Psychotherapy, relaxation, biofeedback and behavior modification may also be employed. The goal of pain management is to improve function and allow people to participate in day-to-day activities. These are among the most common treatments:

Acupuncture dates back 2,500 years to China and involves the application of needles to precise points on the body. While some research suggests this technique boosts levels of the body's natural painkillers (endorphins) in cerebrospinal fluid following treatment, acupuncture is not fully accepted in the medical community. Still, it is very popular, noninvasive and inexpensive compared to many other pain treatments.

Anticonvulsants were developed to treat seizure disorders, but are also sometimes prescribed for pain. Carbamazepine is used to treat a number of painful conditions, including trigeminal neuralgia. Gabapentin (sold as Neurontin) is commonly prescribed "off label" (unapproved by the FDA) for neuropathic pain.

Antidepressants can be helpful for the treatment of pain. In addition, antianxiety drugs called benzodiazepines also act as muscle relaxants and are sometimes used as pain relievers.

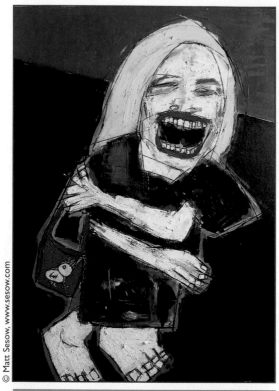

© Matt Sesow, www.sesow.com

ALLEGED

I WANTED TO PORTRAY THE PAIN A PERSON FEELS
WHEN THEIR EXPERIENCE IS REFERRED TO AS
'ALLEGED.' IT IS A COMMON MYTH THAT PAIN IS IN
ONE'S HEAD.

—— MATT SESOW

Biofeedback trains people to become aware of and to gain control over certain bodily functions, including muscle tension, heart rate and skin temperature. One can also learn to effect a change in his or her responses to pain, for example, by using relaxation techniques. With feedback and reinforcement one can consciously self-modify out-of-balance brain rhythms, which can improve body processes and brain physiology. There are many claims made for treating chronic pain with biofeedback, especially using brain wave information (EEG).

Capsaicin is a chemical that puts the heat in chili peppers; it is also a primary ingredient in topical pain-relieving creams and may have other pain-relieving properties.

COX-2 inhibitors ("superaspirins") are nonsteroidal anti-inflammatory drugs (NSAIDs) that work by limiting the production of hormones called prostaglandins, which in turn cause inflammation, fever and pain. COX-2 inhibitors such as rofecoxib (Vioxx) and celecoxib (Celebrex) primarily block cyclooxygenase-2. Due to heightened risk for cardiovascular and liver problems Vioxx was withdrawn from the worldwide market.

Electrical stimulation requires specialized equipment and personnel trained in the procedure being used.

TENS uses tiny electrical pulses, delivered through the skin to nerve fibers, to cause changes in muscles, such as numbness or contractions. This in turn produces temporary pain relief.

In spinal cord stimulation, electrodes are surgically inserted within the epidural space of the spinal cord. The patient delivers a pulse of electricity to the spinal cord using a small box-like receiver and an antenna taped to the skin. This is most commonly used for lower back pain but some people with MS or paralysis can benefit.

Deep brain stimulation is considered an extreme treatment and involves surgical stimulation of the brain, usually the thalamus. It is used for a limited number of conditions, including central pain syndrome, cancer pain, phantom limb pain and other neuropathic pains.

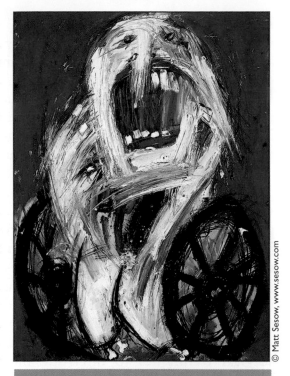

© Matt Sesow, www.sesow.com

THE BODY GETS USED TO THE PAIN
I PAINTED THIS IN RESPONSE TO AN ARTICLE ABOUT OUR TROOPS RETURNING FROM IRAQ AND HAVING DISABILITIES. A DOCTOR WAS QUOTED AS SAYING 'THE BODY GETS USED TO THE PAIN' OR SOMETHING LIKE THAT ... I MAY RETITLE THE PIECE 'THE BODY GETS USED TO THE PAIN (BUT WHAT ABOUT THE MIND?)'
—— MATT SESOW

Exercise is a known link between many types of chronic pain and stress. Even light to moderate walking or swimming can contribute to an overall sense of well-being by improving blood and oxygen flow to tense, weak muscles. Less stress equals less pain.

Hypnosis is commonly used, especially as an adjunct to pain medication. In general, hypnosis is used to control physical function or response — the amount of pain a person can stand. Hypnosis may cause a relief of pain by acting on chemicals in the nervous system, which slows impulses.

Low-power lasers have been used by some physical therapists as a treatment for pain, but like many other treatments, this method is not without controversy.

Magnets are often dismissed as quackery and pseudoscience, but proponents offer the theory that magnets may effect changes in cells or body chemistry, thus producing pain relief. Magnets are usually worn as a collar or wristwatch.

Marijuana is illegal, of course, but its proponents rightfully place pot alongside other pain remedies. In fact, for many years, it was sold in cigarette form by the U.S. government for just that purpose. Twelve states have at least partially decriminalized marijuana for medical reasons but that does not exempt users from federal prohibition laws, nor does it allow doctors to prescribe marijuana. There is evidence, however, to support further study; marijuana appears to bind to receptors found in many brain regions that process pain information.

Nerve blocks employ the use of drugs, chemical agents or surgical techniques to interrupt the relay of pain messages between specific areas of the body and the brain. Types of surgical nerve blocks include neurectomy; spinal dorsal, cranial, and trigeminal rhizotomy; and sympathetic blockade.

Nonsteroidal anti-inflammatory drugs (including aspirin and ibuprofen) are sometimes called non-narcotic or non-opioid analgesics. They work by reducing inflammatory responses in tissues. Many of these drugs irritate the stomach and for that reason are usually taken with food.

Opioids are derived from the poppy plant and are among the oldest drugs known to humankind. They include codeine and the king of opiates, morphine, named for Morpheus, the god of dreams. While morphine is still the go-to therapy at the top of the treatment ladder, it depresses breathing, causes constipation and fogs the brain. And people develop a tolerance for it. Moreover, it isn't effective against many types of neuropathic pain. Scientists hope to develop a morphine-like drug that will have the pain-deadening qualities of morphine but without the drug's debilitating side effects.

Physical therapy and rehabilitation are often utilized to increase function, control pain and speed a person toward full recovery.

Surgeries for pain include rhizotomy, in which a nerve close to the spinal cord is cut, and cordotomy, where bundles of nerves within the spinal cord are severed. Cordotomy is generally used only for the pain of terminal cancer that does not respond to other therapies. The dorsal root entry zone operation, or DREZ, destroys spinal neurons corresponding to the patient's pain. This surgery can be done with electrodes that selectively damage neurons in a targeted area of the brain.

Research in neuroscience will lead to more and better treatments for chronic pain in the years to come. Blocking or interrupting pain signals, especially when there is no injury or trauma to tissue, is a key goal in the development of new medications.

A better understanding of the basic mechanisms of pain is needed for the development of future medicines. As pain is experienced, perhaps as a prick, tingle, sting, burn or ache, receptors on the skin trigger an electrical impulse that travels from the skin to the spinal cord. The spinal cord acts as a relay center where the pain signal can be blocked, enhanced or otherwise modified before it is forwarded to the brain. One area of the spinal cord in particular, the dorsal horn, is important in the reception of pain signals. The most common destination in the brain for pain signals is the thalamus and secondly the cortex, the headquarters for complex thoughts.

Pain is a complicated process that involves an intricate interplay between a number of important chemicals found naturally in the brain and spinal cord. These chemicals, called neurotransmitters, transmit nerve impulses from one cell to another.

There is a critical lack of the essential inhibitory neurotransmitter GABA (gamma-aminobutyric acid) in the injured spinal cord. This may "disinhibit" spinal neurons that are responsible for pain sensations, causing them to fire more than normal. This disinhibition is believed to be the root of spasticity, too. Recent data also suggest that there may be a shortage of the neurotransmitter norepinephrine, as well as an overabundance of the neurotransmitter glutamate. During experiments, mice with blocked glutamate receptors show a reduction in their responses to pain. Other important receptors in pain transmission are opiate-like receptors. Morphine and other opioid drugs work by locking on to these opioid receptors, switching on pain-inhibiting pathways or circuits, and thereby blocking pain.

The body's natural painkillers are promising pain relievers. The brain may signal the release of painkillers found in the spinal cord, including serotonin, norepinephrine and opioid-like chemicals. Endorphins and enkephalins are other natural painkillers. Endorphins may be responsible for the "feel good" effects experienced by people after rigorous exercise; they are also implicated in the pleasurable effects of smoking.

Scientists are working to develop potent pain-killing drugs that act on receptors for the chemical acetylcholine. For example, a type of frog native to Ecuador has been found to have a chemical in its skin called epibatidine. Even though it's highly toxic, epibatidine is a potent pain reliever (200 times the strength of morphine) with a structure akin to nicotine found in cigarettes.

Another promising area of research using the body's natural pain-killing abilities involves cellular transplantation of human neuronal cells. These cells, such as chromaffin cells, derived from the adrenal gland, can be placed into the subarachnoid space in the lumbar cord; they appear to act as little pumps, providing a renewable supply of therapeutic or inhibitory substances. A team from the Miami Project to Cure Paralysis has been working to treat paralysis-related pain, though there are many details to work out, including the source of the chromaffin cells themselves. Researchers are considering non-human cells and engineered cell lines that dampen nerve signals related to pain.

Cytokines, a type of protein found in the nervous system, are also part of the body's immune system — the body's shield for fighting off disease. Cytokines can trigger pain by promoting inflammation, even in the absence of injury or damage. Certain types of cytokines have been linked to nervous system injury. After trauma, cytokine levels rise in the brain and spinal cord and at the site in the peripheral nervous system where the injury occurred. It is hoped that understanding the precise role of cytokines in producing pain may lead to new classes of drugs that can block the action of these substances.

Another frontier in the search for new drug targets is represented by channels — gate-like passages found along the membranes of cells that allow electrically charged chemical particles called ions to pass into the cells. Ion channels are important for transmitting signals through the nerve's membrane. The possibility now exists for developing new classes of drugs, including pain cocktails that would act at the site of channel activity.

Following injury, the nervous system undergoes a tremendous reorganization. The dramatic changes that occur with injury and persistent pain underscore that chronic pain should be considered a disease of the nervous system, not just prolonged acute pain or a symptom of an injury.

Sources
National Institute of Neurological Disorders and Stoke (NINDS), National Multiple Sclerosis Society

CHRONIC PAIN RESOURCES

American Chronic Pain Association (ACPA) offers peer support and education for individuals with chronic pain and their families. ACPA raises awareness among the health care community, policy makers and the public at large about issues of living with chronic pain. ACPA, P.O. Box 850, Rocklin, CA 95677; toll-free 1–800–533–3231; or visit *http://www.theacpa.org*

National Foundation for the Treatment of Pain (NFTP) provides support for people with intractable pain, their families, friends and the physicians who treat them. NFTP, P.O. Box 70045, Houston, Texas 77270; telephone 713-862-9332; or visit the Internet site *http://www.paincare.org*

Spinal Cord Injury Information Center features information on chronic pain and treatment alternatives, plus details on all other medical aspects of spinal cord injury and paralysis. See *http://www.spinalcord.uab.edu*, search under Pain.

Chronic Pain Support Group (CPSG) provides a safe, supportive online environment where people can meet others who live in chronic pain through a message board and chat rooms. The CPSG also offers a newsletter. Subscribe or chat by visiting their website. *See http://www.chronicpainsupport.org/index.html*

RESPIRATORY HEALTH

As we breathe, air is brought into the lungs and into close contact with tiny blood vessels that absorb the oxygen and carry it to all parts of the body. At the same time, the blood releases carbon dioxide, which is carried out of the lungs with exhaled air.

Lungs themselves are not affected by paralysis, but the muscles of the chest, abdomen and diaphragm can be. As the various breathing muscles contract, they allow the lungs to expand, which changes the pressure inside the chest so that air rushes into the lungs. This is the process of inhaling – which requires muscle strength. As those muscles relax, the air flows back out of the lungs.

If paralysis occurs in C-3 or higher, the phrenic nerve is no longer stimulated and therefore the diaphragm does not function. This means mechanical assistance – usually a ventilator – will be needed to breathe.

People with paralysis at the mid-thoracic level and higher may have trouble taking a deep breath and exhaling forcefully. Because they don't have use of abdominal or intercostal muscles, these people also lose the ability to force a strong cough. This can lead to lung congestion and respiratory infections.

Moreover, mucous secretions are like glue, causing the sides of

---

"Pneumonia is the leading cause of death for all persons with spinal cord injury, regardless of the level of injury or time since the injury. "

---

airways to stick together and not inflate properly. This is called atelectasis, or a collapse of part of the lung. Many people with paralysis are at risk for this. Some people have a harder time getting rid of colds or respiratory infections and have what feels like a constant chest cold. Pneumonia is a possibility if secretions become the breeding ground for various bacteria. Symptoms of pneumonia include shortness of breath, pale skin, fever and an increase in congestion.

Be aggressive with pulmonary infections: Pneumonia is one of the

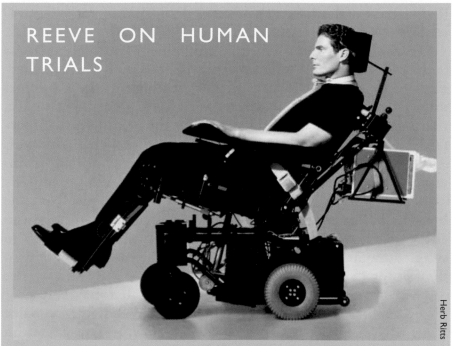

REEVE ON HUMAN TRIALS

Herb Ritts

I was the second patient in the world to have diaphragm pacing implanted into my body. It's like a cardiac pacemaker, but it stimulates the diaphragm to create normal breathing and replace the ventilator. I felt that it was safe and that there was a good chance it would work. It didn't. It failed.

For over a year now, I've had infections and all kinds of signs of rejection by my body, and the site of implantation is still not closed. That's why I am still on this ventilator, why I can't go into the swimming pool anymore, and why I haven't moved beyond my initial level of recovery, where I plateaued. And yet I'm telling you this because it is important to know that living a fearless life means that you might go through an experience that doesn't actually work out for you.

The way to stay positive, to avoid being bitter or feeling like a failure, is to look at the fact that it might help somebody else. For example, this failure of the diaphragm pacing has led to modifications in how doctors perform the procedure, and the set of patients who followed me have all gotten off the ventilator.

Christopher Reeve, from a 2004 speech at Omega Institute's Living a Fearless Life conference, six months before his death.

leading cause of death for all persons with spinal cord injury, regardless of the level of injury or the amount of time since the injury.

Clearing Secretions: A useful technique for clearing secretions is the assisted cough: An assistant firmly pushes against the outside of the stomach and upward, substituting for the abdominal muscle action that usually makes for a strong cough. This is a much gentler push than the Heimlich maneuver; it's also important to coordinate pushes with natural breathing rhythms. Another technique is percussion: this is basically a light drumming on the ribcage to help loosen up congestion in the lungs.

Postural drainage uses gravity to drain secretions from the bottoms of the lungs up higher into the chest where one can either cough them up and out or get them up high enough to swallow them. This usually works when the head is lower than the feet for 15–20 minutes.

There are several machines on the market that may help people on ventilators cough. The Vest (Advanced Respiratory, Saint Paul, MN; 1-800-426-4224; *www.thevest.com*), consists of an inflatable vest connected by air hoses to an air pulse generator, which can rapidly inflate and deflate the vest, thus applying gentle pressure to the chest wall to loosen and thin mucus and move it to the central airways to be cleared by coughing or suctioning.

The CoughAssist (J.H. Emerson; Cambridge, MA; 1-800-252-1414; *www.coughassist.com*) is designed to boost cough function by mechanically simulating the cough maneuver. This device blows in an inspiratory pressure breath followed rapidly by an expiratory flow. This generates enough peak air flow to clear secretions. The CoughAssist has been approved by Medicare for reimbursement if it is determined to be a medical necessity.

Ventilators: There are two basic types of mechanical ventilators. Negative pressure ventilators, such as the iron lung, create a vacuum around the outside of the chest, causing the chest to expand and suck air into the lungs. Positive pressure ventilators, which have been available since the 1940s, work on the opposite principle, by blowing air directly into the lungs.

Ventilators are invasive – an air passage is made in the throat area, fitted with a device most people call a "trach." Some people, including high-level quadriplegics, have had success using a noninvasive breathing system. Positive pressure air is supplied to a mouthpiece from the same type of ventilator used with a trach. The user takes puffs of air as needed. A primary advantage reported for noninvasive ventilation is that there may be fewer respiratory infections because there is less chance of bacterial entry. Also, some patients on non-invasive systems attest to a better, more independent quality of life because they don't have a trach in their neck and they don't have to have suction the trachea as frequently. Clearly, noninvasive ventilation is not for everyone. Candidates must have good swallowing function; they also need a full support network of pulmonary specialists. There are not many clinicians with expertise in the method, thus its availability is limited.

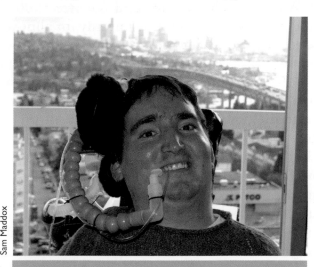

Sam Maddox

JAKE ETCHART'S NON-INVASIVE SYSTEM, WHICH FEATURES A MOUTHPIECE THAT CYCLES AIR FROM A STANDARD VENT INTO HIS LUNGS. JAKE'S MOM SWORE HE'D NEVER USE A TRACH AFTER HIS SISTER, WHO HAD A SIMILAR NEURO-MUSCULAR DISEASE, DIED WHEN HER TRACH MALFUNC-TIONED. ALAS, JAKE WAS ALSO A VICTIM OF TECHNOLOGI-CAL FAILURE. HE DIED IN 2006 WHEN HIS NIGHTTIME BREATHING SYSTEM (A TYPE OF CUIRASS) FAILED.

Some people use a device called a pnuemobelt. This motorized, inflatable bladder alternately expands and contracts, which compresses the abdomen and causes the diaphragm to move upward and take in air. The device has the main advantage of being noninvasive.

Another breathing technique involves implantation of an electronic device in the chest to stimulate the phrenic nerve and send a regular signal to the diaphragm, causing it to contract and fill the lungs with air. Phrenic nerve pacers have been available since the late 1950s. Two companies make diaphragm pacing systems;

both are commercially available. The Avery pacemaker has been in use since before the FDA approved medical devices, going back to the mid-1960s. The Avery has been implanted in over 2,000 patients, with about 600 in use now, some continuously for almost 40 years. The procedure involves surgery through the body or neck to locate the phrenic nerve on both sides of the body. The nerves are exposed and sutured to electrodes. A small radio receiver is also implanted in the chest cavity; this is activated by an external antenna taped to the body. See *www.averylabs.com*

The Synapse system, pioneered in Cleveland, was used by Christopher Reeve in 2003. The Cleveland system, approved by the FDA in 2008, is more simply installed, using an outpatient laparoscopic technique. Two electrodes are placed on each side of diaphragm muscle, with wires attached through the skin to a battery powered stimulator. There are no reported side effects related

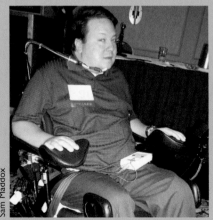

LAZLO NAGY BECAME A C4 QUAD ON A VENT AFTER HE CRASHED HIS MOTOR-CYCLE A FEW YEARS AGO. EVENTUALLY, HE WOUND UP IN A NURSING HOME WITH AROUND-THE-CLOCK CARE, AND QUITE UNSETTLED. "I USED TO CRY MYSELF TO SLEEP EVERY NIGHT BECAUSE OF THE ANXIETY. I WAS CONSTANTLY WORRIED, WOULD MY BATTERY GO DEAD, WOULD THE MACHINE GO ALL NIGHT?"

AFTER NAGY HEARD ABOUT CHRISTOPHER REEVE'S EXPERIENCE IN A DIAPHRAGM PACING CLINICAL TRIAL IN CLEVELAND, HE JOINED THE TRIAL. "THE CHANGE IN MY LIFE HAS BEEN TRULY REMARKABLE," SAYS NAGY. "THE NURS-ING FACILITY WAS BILLING OHIO MEDICAID $16,000 A MONTH. AFTER GETTING THE [PACING] SURGERY, IT WENT TO $3000 — A SAVINGS OF $13,000 A MONTH. EVENTUALLY I RETURNED TO WORK, I'M GETTING MARRIED, I FEEL CONFIDENT I CAN GO OUT IN THE WORLD BY MYSELF, WITHOUT AN ATTENDANT. IT'S GIVEN ME A LOT MORE FREE-DOM. I FEEL SAFE AND COMFORTABLE. I DON'T WORRY THAT I'M GOING TO SUDDENLY DIE."

Sam Maddox

to the exposed wiring; Reeve, however, had chronic infections at the wire site. Synapse expects to get approval to implant the devices in people with ALS, a much bigger market than SCI. See *www.synapsebiomedical.com*

Morning headaches are often the first sign that a person needs help with breathing. Breathing is shallower during sleep, but for people with neuromuscular disease such as amyotrophic lateral sclerosis (ALS), any drop in volume can lead to trouble since they are already breathing shallowly. As the disease progresses, people find themselves waking up with headaches — the shallow breathing causes them to retain carbon dioxide, which gives them a headache. After they wake up and begin breathing more deeply, the headache goes away.

Others may wake up repeatedly during the night as the shallow breathing causes a sudden awakening jolt. Broken sleep causes daytime sleepiness, lethargy, anxiety, irritability, confusion and physical problems such as poor appetite, nausea, increased heart rate and fatigue. At this time, BiPAP (Bi-level Positive Airway Pressure), noninvasive ventilation, is often called for. The devise uses a removable mask over the nose.

BiPAP is not a life-support machine — it cannot completely take over breathing. It delivers a pressurized breath of air into the lungs, then drops the pressure to allow an exhale. The most common use is for people with sleep apnea, characterized by snoring and lack of oxygen during sleep. Sleep apnea is linked to high blood pressure, stroke and cardiovascular disease, memory problems, weight gain, impotency and headaches.

For reasons that are not completely clear, sleep apnea is significantly more common to people with spinal cord injuries, especially quads, among whom an estimated 25–40 percent have the condition. Obesity is a risk factor for sleep apnea, and this is common in the SCI population. Many people with SCI can't change sleep positions and may remain on their backs, which often leads to breathing obstruction. Respiratory muscle weakness is very likely involved. It may also be that certain medications (baclofen, for example, is known to slow down breathing) affect sleep patterns. Quads who rely upon neck and upper chest muscles to help with breathing may be susceptible to sleep apnea because these muscles are inactive during deep sleep.

For people with neuromuscular disease, BiPAP can improve the quality of life while delaying the need for invasive ventilation by months or years. Some people use BiPAP as an intermediary step before going on a ventilator.

Ventilator users with tracheostomies need to have secretions suctioned from their lungs on a regular basis; this may be anywhere from every half hour to only once a day.

Tracheostomy care: There are many potential complications related to tracheostomy tubes, including the inability to speak or swallow normally. Certain tracheostomy tubes are designed to direct air upward during exhalation and thus permit speech during regular, periodic intervals. Another tracheostomy-associated complication is infection. The tube is a foreign body in the neck,

PREVENTING RESPIRATORY COMPLICATIONS:

- MAINTAIN PROPER POSTURE AND MOBILITY. Sit up every day and turn regularly in bed to prevent the buildup of congestion.

- COUGH REGULARLY. Have someone perform manual assist coughs, or perform self-assist coughs; use a machine to help.

- WEAR AN ABDOMINAL BINDER to assist intercostal and abdominal muscles.

- FOLLOW A HEALTHY DIET AND MANAGE YOUR WEIGHT — problems are more likely to occur if you are too heavy or too light.

- DRINK PLENTY OF WATER. Water helps keep congestion from becoming thick and difficult to cough up.

- DO NOT SMOKE OR BE AROUND SMOKERS: Smoking not only causes cancer, but also decreases oxygen in the blood, increases congestion in the chest and windpipe, reduces the ability to clear secretions from lungs, destroys lung tissue, and increases the risk for respiratory infections.

- EXERCISE. Every person with paralysis can benefit from some type of exercise. For those with a high level of paralysis, it may be helpful to do breathing exercises.

- GET VACCINATIONS for both influenza and pneumonia.

and it has the potential of introducing organisms that would ordinarily be stopped by natural defense mechanisms in the nose and mouth. Cleaning and dressing of the tracheostomy site on a daily basis is an important preventive measure.

Sources

Medical RRTC on Secondary Conditions of SCI Research Services/UAB-Spain Rehabilitation Center, Craig Hospital, University of Miami School of Medicine, University of Washington School of Medicine/Department of Rehabilitation Medicine, ALS Association of America

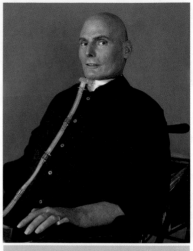

CHRISTOPHER REEVE

DON FLOOD

RESPIRATORY HEALTH RESOURCES

International Ventilator Users Network (IVUN), a resource for people who use ventilators, pulmonologists, pediatricians, respiratory therapists, and ventilator manufacturers and vendors to discuss home ventilation. Features a newsletter, articles from health care professionals and venturesome vent users. Contact Post-Polio Health International, 4207 Lindell Boulevard #110, Saint Louis, MO 63108–2915; telephone 314–534–0475; or visit the Internet site *http://www.post-polio.org/ivun/*

The Center for Noninvasive Mechanical Ventilation Alternatives and Pulmonary Rehabilitation. The New Jersey–based center, under the direction of Dr. John Bach, says it has removed dozens of tracheostomy tubes from ventilator users with no ability to breathe and taught many of them how to breathe without ventilators. *http://www.doctorbach.com/center.htm*

Ventilator Users Support includes links to articles on respiratory management, product manufacturers, etc. See Website to join the vent users mailing list. *http://www.makoa.org/vent/index.html*

SKIN CARE

People with paralysis are at high risk of developing skin problems. Limited mobility coupled with impaired sensation can lead to pressure sores or ulcers, which can be a devastating complication.

The skin, the largest organ system in the body, is tough and pliable. It protects the underlying cells against air, water, foreign substances and bacteria. It is sensitive to injury and has remarkable self-repair capabilities. But skin just can't take prolonged pressure. A pressure ulcer involves damage to the skin and underlying tissue. Pressure ulcers, also called bed sores, decubiti or decubitus ulcers, range in severity from mild (minor skin reddening) to severe (deep craters that can infect all the way to muscle and bone). Unrelieved pressure on the skin squeezes tiny blood vessels, which supply the skin with nutrients and oxygen. When skin is starved of blood for too long, tissue dies and a pressure ulcer forms.

Other factors cause pressure ulcers, too. Sliding around in a bed or chair can cause blood vessels to stretch or bend, leading to pressure ulcers. An abrasion can occur when a person's skin is pulled across a surface instead of lifted. A bump or fall may cause damage to the skin that may not show up right away. Other causes of pressure sores are clothing, braces or hard objects that put pressure on your skin. Also, people with limited sensation are prone to skin injuries from burns.

> **"Take good care or your skin: A serious skin sore can mean several weeks or even months of hospitalization or bed rest in order for the sore to heal."**

Skin damage from pressure usually begins on the body where the bones are close to the skin surface, such as the hip. These bony prominences apply pressure on the skin from within. If there is a hard surface on the outside, too, the skin is pinched off from circulation. Because the rate of circulation is reduced by paralysis to begin with, less oxygen is available to the skin, lowering the skin's resistance. The body tries to compensate by sending more blood to the area. This may result in swelling, putting still more pressure on the blood vessels.

A skin sore begins as a red area on the skin. This reddened area may feel hard and/or hot. For those with black skin, the area may appear shiny. At this stage, the progression is reversible: The skin will return to its normal color if the pressure is removed.

If the pressure is not removed, a blister or scab may form — this means that the tissue underneath is dying. Remove all pressure over the area immediately.

In the next stage, a hole (ulcer) forms in the dead tissue. Frequently, this dead tissue is small on the skin surface, but damaged tissue may extend deep to the bone.

A skin sore can mean several weeks or even months of hospitalization or bed rest in order for the sore to heal. Complex pressure sores may require surgery or skin grafting. All of this can cost thousands of dollars and mean valuable time away from work, school or family.

Skin wound treatment by any means is complicated by hard to treat infections, spasticity, additional pressure and even the psychological makeup of the person (pressure sores have been linked to low self esteem and impulsive behavior). It's too easy to say pressure sores are always preventable. In spinal cord injury, for example, they usually come with the territory.

A wide variety of pressure-relieving support surfaces, including special beds, mattresses, mattress overlays or seat cushions are available to support your body in bed or in a chair. Work with your therapists to know all the options. See page 219 for more on cushions. Search *http://www.abledata.com* for specific products.

Remember that the first line of defense is to be responsible for your own skin care.

Skin stays healthy with good diet, good hygiene and regular pressure relief. Keep the skin clean and dry. Skin that is moist from sweat or bodily discharges is more likely to break down.

Drink plenty of fluids. A healing wound or sore can lose more than a quart of water each day. Drinking 8 to 12 cups of water a day might not be too much. Note: Beer and wine do not count.

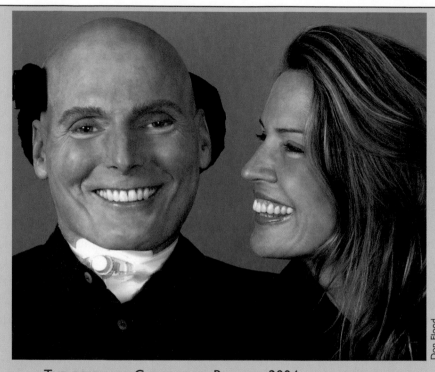

Don Flood

THE DEATH OF CHRISTOPHER REEVE IN 2004 WAS ATTRIBUTED TO HEART FAILURE DUE TO SEPSIS (ALSO KNOWN AS SEPTICEMIA), AN INFECTION THAT SPREADS FROM A SPECIFIC LOCATION (SUCH AS A SKIN SORE OR BLADDER INFECTION) TO THE BLOOD AND OTHER ORGANS. WHAT EXACTLY HAPPENED TO REEVE ISN'T KNOWN. CLEARLY, HIS DEATH WAS RELATED TO PRESSURE SORES; TO BE SURE, REEVE HAD BEEN BATTLING MORE THAN ONE SKIN SORE AND HAD EVEN EXPERIENCED LIFE-THREATENING SEPSIS JUST WEEKS BEFORE HE DIED. BUT ACCORDING TO PEOPLE WHO WERE WITH HIM ON HIS LAST DAY, REEVE DID NOT APPEAR TO HAVE SYMPTOMS THAT WOULD RED-FLAG RECURRENT SEPSIS (HE DID NOT EXHIBIT FEVER, CHILLS, FATIGUE, MALAISE, ANXIETY, CONFUSION).

THE CAUSE OF DEATH WAS NOT DIRECTLY RELATED TO REEVE'S PRESSURE SORES. ACCORDING TO DANA REEVE, THE MORE LIKELY CAUSE OF DEATH WAS A REACTION TO AN ANTIBIOTIC REEVE WAS GIVEN FOR A DEVELOPING INFECTION (HE HAD A HISTORY OF DRUG SENSITIVITY.) REEVE'S BODY IMMEDIATELY WENT INTO SHOCK (ANAPHYLACTIC) BUT NOT SEPTIC.

REEVE CHOSE TO LIVE HIS LIFE FULLY AND WELL, AND AS MUCH AS POSSIBLE ON HIS OWN TERMS. THAT IS HIS MOST LASTING LEGACY.

PRESSURE SORE 101

Stage One

Skin is not broken but is red and color does not fade 30 minutes after pressure is removed. What to do: stay off the sore, practice good hygiene. Explore causes: check out mattress, seat cushion, transfer procedures and turning techniques.

Stage Two

The top layer of skin, the epidermis, is broken. The sore is shallow but open; drainage may be present. What to do: Follow steps in Stage One but cleanse wound with water or saline solution and dry carefully. Apply either a transparent dressing (e.g. Tegraderm) or a hydrocolloid dressing (e.g. DuoDERM). If there are signs of trouble (see below) see your health care provider.

Stage Three

Skin has broken down further, into the second layer of skin, through the dermis into the subcutaneous fat tissue. You must see a care provider at this point as this is getting serious and may need special cleaning or debriding agents to treat. Don't wait.

Stage Four

The skin has broken down all the way to the bone. A lot of dead tissue is present and there is also a lot of drainage. This can be life threatening. You may be looking at surgery.

Healing

Healing occurs when the sore gets smaller, when pinkish skin forms along the edges of the sore. Bleeding might occur but take this as a good sign: circulation is back and that helps healing. Be patient. Skin repair isn't always speedy.

Signs of trouble

The sore is getting bigger; the sore starts to smell bad or the drainage becomes greenish in color. Fever is a bad sign.

When is it safe to put pressure on the affected area again? Only when the sore is completely healed, that is, when the top layer of skin is unbroken and normal looking. The first time pressure is applied, start with 15 minute intervals. Build up gradually over period of a few days to allow skin pressure tolerance to build. If redness occurs, keep pressure off the area.

Alcohol actually causes you to lose water or become dehydrated.

Watch your weight, too. Being too thin causes you to lose the padding between your bones and your skin and makes it possible for even small amounts of pressure to break down the skin. Getting too heavy is risky, too. More weight may mean more padding, but it also means more pressure on skin folds.

Don't smoke. Research has shown that heavy smokers are more prone to skin sores.

Sources

Spinal Cord Injury Information Network, Paralyzed Veterans of America, Craig Hospital, National Library of Medicine, University of Washington School of Medicine/Rehabilitation

SKIN CARE RESOURCES

Paralyzed Veterans of America, in support of The Consortium for Spinal Cord Medicine, offers authoritative clinical practice guidelines for skin care. PVT, 801 Eighteenth Street, NW, Washington, DC 20006, toll-free 1-800-424-8200, or visit the Internet site, *http://www.pva.org*, click on Publications, then Medical Guidelines.

Craig Hospital, with funding from the National Institute on Disability and Rehabilitation Research, has developed educational materials to help people with spinal cord injuries maintain their health. See *http://www.craighospital.org* and click on "Spinal Cord Injury," then on "Health and Wellness."

The Spinal Cord Injury Information Network at the University of Alabama at Birmingham is funded through federal grants to the UAB Rehabilitation Research and Training Center on Secondary Conditions of Spinal Cord Injury and the UAB Model SCI Center. See *http://www.spinalcord.uab.edu* and do a search for "Skin Care" or any other topic in paralysis medicine, lifestyle or resource.

The University of Washington School of Medicine, Department of Rehabilitation maintains a useful, authoritative Website with information on skin care, bowel and bladder management and other topics of concern to people with spinal cord injuries and paralysis. *http://depts.washington.edu/rehab*

SPASTICITY

Spasticity is a side effect of paralysis that varies from mild muscle stiffness to severe, uncontrollable leg movements. Generally, doctors now call conditions of extreme muscle tension spastic hypertonia (SH). It may occur in association with spinal cord injury, multiple sclerosis, cerebral palsy, anoxic brain damage, brain trauma, severe head injury, some metabolic diseases such as adrenoleukodystrophy, and phenylketonuria. Symptoms may include increased muscle tone, rapid muscle contractions, exaggerated deep tendon reflexes, muscle spasms, scissoring (involuntary crossing of the legs) and fixed joints.

When individuals are first injured, their muscles are weak and flexible because of what's called spinal shock: The body's reflexes are absent below the level of injury; this condition usually lasts for a few weeks or several months. Once the spinal shock is over, reflex activity returns.

Spasticity is usually caused by damage to the portion of the brain or spinal cord that controls voluntary movement. Since the normal flow of nerve messages to below the level of injury is interrupted, those messages may not reach the reflex center of the brain. The spinal cord then attempts to moderate the body's response. Because the spinal cord is not as efficient as the brain, the signals that are sent back to the site of the sensation are often over-exaggerated in an overactive muscle response or spastic hypertonia: an uncontrollable "jerking" movement, stiffening or straightening of muscles, shock-like contractions of a muscle or group of muscles, and abnormal tone in the muscles.

Most individuals with SCI have some spasms. Persons with cervical injuries and those with incomplete injuries are more likely than those with paraplegia and/or complete injuries to experience SH. The most common muscles that spasm are those that bend the elbow (flexor) or extend the leg (extensor). These reflexes usually occur as a result of an automatic response to painful sensations.

While spasticity can interfere with rehabilitation or daily living activities, it is not always a bad thing. Some people use their spasms for function, to empty their bladders, to transfer or to dress. Others use SH to keep their muscles toned and improve circulation. It may also help maintain bone strength. In a Swedish study of 353 persons with SCI, 68 percent had spasticity. Of those that did, 41 percent said that their spasticity was a significant problem that reduced activities of daily living or caused pain.

Changing spasticity: A change in a person's spasticity is a symptom to pay attention to. For example, a cyst or cavity in the spinal cord (post-traumatic syringomyelia) could lead to more spasticity. Also, decreasing or disappearing spasticity can also be a sign of a cyst. Untreated, cysts can lead to further loss of function.

Problems outside your nervous system, such as bladder infections or skin sores, can make spasticity increase.

Treatment for spasticity usually includes medications such as baclofen, diazepam or zanaflex. Some people with severe spasms utilize baclofen pumps, which are small, surgically implanted reservoirs that apply the drug directly to the area of spinal cord dysfunction. This allows for a higher concentration of drug without the mind-dulling side effects of a high oral dosage. In recent years some doctors have treated spasticity in children with botox, the muscle-relaxing agent used cosmetically for wrinkles.

Physical therapy, including muscle stretching, range of motion exercises, and other physical therapy regimens, can help prevent joint contractures (shrinkage or shortening of a muscle) and reduce the severity of symptoms. Proper posture and positioning are important for people in wheelchairs and those at bed rest to reduce spasms. Orthotics, such as ankle-foot braces, are sometimes used to limit spasticity. Application of cold (cryotherapy) to an affected area can also calm muscle activity.

For many years doctors have used phenol nerve blocks to deaden nerves that cause spasticity. Lately, a good but more expensive nerve block, botulinum toxin (botox), has become a popular treatment for spasms. An application of botox lasts about three to six months; the body builds antibodies to the drug, reducing its effectiveness over time.

Sometimes, surgery is recommended for tendon release or to sever the nerve-muscle pathway in children with cerebral palsy. Selective dorsal rhizotomy may be considered if spasms interfere with sitting, bathing or general caretaking.

Spasticity comes with the territory for many people who are

paralyzed. Treatment strategy should be based on your function: Is the spasticity keeping you from certain activities? Are there safety risks—losing control while driving your power chair or car? Are spasticity drugs worse than the symptom, affecting concentration or energy? Check with your physician to discuss your options.

Sources

National Multiple Sclerosis Society, United Cerebral Palsy Associations, The National Spinal Cord Injury Statistical Center, Craig Hospital, The University of Alabama at Birmingham/Spain Rehabilitation Center.

SPASTICITY RESOURCES

The Medical Rehabilitation Research and Training Center on Secondary Conditions of Spinal Cord Injury at UAB-Spain Rehabilitation Center has a series of information sheets on topics related to SCI. Visit *http://www.spinalcord.uab.edu* and search under "spasticity."

Medtronic manufactures the implantable pumps for delivery (intrathecal) of drugs such as baclofen to control spasticity. *http://www.medtronic.com*

The National Institute of Neurological Disorders and Stroke (NINDS) offers fact sheets on all medical issues related to paralysis, including spasticity. See *http://www.ninds.nih.gov*

National Multiple Sclerosis Society offers information and resources on spasticity. Call toll-free 1-800-344-4867 or visit *http://www.nationalmssociety.org*; search under "spasticity."

United Cerebral Palsy has resources on spasticity and its treatment options. Call toll tree 1-800-872-5827 to locate the chapter nearest you, or use the search feature at http://www.ucp.org

We Move covers management and treatment of major movement disorders (excessive movement, as in spasticity and restless legs syndrome; also lack of movement, as in bradykinesia). On the Internet see *http://www.wemove.org*

SYRINGOMYELIA | TETHERED CORD

Post-traumatic syringomyelia and tethered spinal cord can occur following spinal cord injury. It can occur from two months to many decades after injury. The results can be devastating, causing new levels of disability long after a person has had a successful rehabilitation. The clinical symptoms for syringomyelia and tethered spinal cord are the same and can include progressive deterioration of the spinal cord, progressive loss of sensation or strength, profuse sweating, spasticity, pain and autonomic dysreflexia (AD).

In post-traumatic syringomyelia (sear-IN-go-my-EE-lia) a cyst or fluid-filled cavity forms within the cord. This cavity can expand over time, extending two or more spinal segments from the level of SCI.

Tethered spinal cord is a condition where scar tissue forms and tethers, or holds, the spinal cord to the dura, the soft tissue membrane that surrounds it. This scar tissue prevents the normal flow of spinal fluid around the spinal cord and impedes the normal motion of the spinal cord within the membrane. Tethering causes cyst formation. Tethered cord can occur without evidence of syringomyelia, but post-traumatic cystic formation does not occur without some degree of cord tethering.

Magnetic resonance imaging (MRI) easily detects cysts in the spinal cord, unless rods, plates or bullet fragments are present.

Post-traumatic tethered cords and syringomyelia are treated surgically. Untethering involves a delicate surgery to release the scar tissue around the spinal cord to restore spinal-fluid flow and the motion of the spinal cord. In addition, a small graft is placed at the tethering site to fortify the dural space and decrease the risk of re-scarring. If a cyst is present, a tube, or shunt, is placed inside the cavity to drain the fluid from the cyst. Surgery usually leads to improved strength and reduced pain; it does not always bring back lost sensory function.

In experiments at the University of Florida, people with spinal cord cysts were treated with injections of fetal tissue. It is unlikely this technique will find its way to the clinic any time soon, but the tissue grew, filled the cavities and prevented further loss of function.

Syringomyelia also occurs in people who have a congenital abnormality of the brain called a Chiari malformation — during development of the fetus the lower part of the cerebellum protrudes from the back of the head into the cervical portion of the spinal canal. Symptoms usually include vomiting, muscle weakness in the head and face, difficulty swallowing, and varying degrees of mental impairment. Paralysis of the arms and legs may also occur. Adults and adolescents with Chiari malformation who previously showed no symptoms may show signs of progressive impairment, such as involuntary, rapid, downward eye movements. Other symptoms may include dizziness, headache, double vision, deafness, an impaired ability to coordinate movement and episodes of acute pain in and around the eyes.

Syringomyelia can also be associated with spina bifida, spinal cord tumors, arachnoiditis and idiopathic (cause unknown) syringomyelia. MRI has significantly increased the number of diagnoses in the beginning stages of syringomyelia. Signs of the disorder tend to develop slowly, although sudden onset may occur with coughing or straining.

Surgery results in stabilization or modest improvement in symptoms for most people. Delay in treatment may result in irreversible spinal cord injury. Recurrence of syringomyelia after surgery may make additional operations necessary; these operations may not be completely successful over the long-term. Up to one half of those treated for syringomyelia have symptoms return within five years.

Source

National Institute of Neurological Disorders and Stroke, American Syringomyelia Alliance Project

SYRINGOMYELIA RESOURCES

American Syringomyelia Alliance Project (ASAP) offers news on syringomyelia, tethered cord and Chiari malformation, sponsors research; supports an e-mail listserv. ASAP, P.O. Box 1586, Longview, TX 75606–1586; toll-free 1-800-ASAP-282; or visit the Internet site *http://www.asap4sm.org*

Syringomyelia Information Page offers general information and links. Spanish version available. See *http://www.syringo.org*

Healthy Living
COPING AND ADJUSTMENT

Individuals who are new to paralysis, whether from a sudden accident or the progression of a disease, will most likely experience grief. Families, too, enter this strange, new why-me world with its hallmarks of mourning, helplessness, second-guessing and regret. While everyone deals with loss and change in their own way, there are aspects of the adjustment process that many people share.

At first, many react to paralysis as if nothing happened, refusing to accept that changes in their body and in their ability to move are not going to get better or heal in ways they always have. Some may see the injury as an annoyance similar to getting the flu that will pass with time. Psychologists call this denial. Elisabeth Kübler-Ross, who has outlined the stages of grieving, notes that denial has a beneficial function as a "buffer" after unexpected shocking news.

Some people find refuge in the denial stage for a long time, using it as an excuse to do nothing, or to do too much to overcome limitations and act "normal." Most, however, will begin to gain knowledge about their condition and have some perspective on what has happened. As denial fades, hope emerges. Thus begins the process of adjustment.

When denial can no longer be maintained, it is often replaced with other dark feelings: anger, rage, envy and resentment. These can be seen as defense mechanisms that allow a person time to mobilize other defenses. Guilt may be part of the mix, too, especially in people whose poor judgment or self-destructive behavior may have contributed to their disability. Self-loathing may also appear when one's notion of "normal" is turned upside down.

Many people within the universe of disability – including those who experience paralysis first hand as well as family members – can become extremely frustrated. They may see themselves as victims whose lives are ruined because they can never live the happy life they always knew they would; they see no way out. These people may react with hostility to others. This, of course, adds stress to caregivers and loved ones. There's nothing wrong with anger — unless you hold on to it and let it smolder. The best advice, easier said than done, is to let anger run its course, and let it go. How? Some find relief in religion, others by quieting the mind using meditation.

Fear is another common feeling: Where is all this chaos leading? Will it get worse? Will my spouse stay with me? Will I ever love or work or be taken seriously again? For many people, the greatest fear is losing control over their lives. These thoughts are common for individuals who are newly paralyzed; many persons continue to hold on to them, even the irrational ones, long after their injury.

Extreme sadness is natural after paralysis — there has, of course, been great loss. Sadness passes. It's important not to confuse the blues we all experience when something bad happens with depression. Depression is a medical condition that can lead to inactivity, difficulty concentrating, a significant change in appetite or sleep time, and feelings of dejection, hopelessness or worthlessness. A depressed person may have thoughts about suicide.

❝There's nothing wrong with anger — unless you hold on to it and let it smolder. The best advice, easier said than done, is to let anger run its course, and let it go.❞

Suicide is two to six times greater for people with spinal cord injuries compared to the nondisabled population. It is the leading cause of death for people with SCI younger than 55.

To be sure, paralysis ignites many emotions and feelings, most of them negative. A person's reactions to all this baggage may result in behavior that is bad for health and happiness. For example, a person who feels worthless may not take proper care of their bladder or skin or nutrition. Also, people with a history of alcohol and/or substance abuse may return to old patterns of self-destruction. Others may start drinking or taking drugs to quiet their anxieties. Unhealthy behavior leads to unhealthy results. Neglect of personal care (which has been called "existential suicide") risks a wide range of health problems such as respiratory complications, urinary tract infection, and pressure sores.

In time, one processes the toxic feelings. Another phase of adjustment begins. Generally, at some point following paralysis, people may begin to admit that they have a serious condition, though they may hold on to the belief that the situation is not a long-term problem.

As the process continues, it is important for people to contact others who share similar experiences. There are peer support groups for every sort of condition related to paralysis in most communities, and the Internet is a great tool for connecting with paralysis survivors who have been down the same path and can testify that there is still a future ahead full of life and rewarding experience.

Given time, a person will eventually come to terms with their loss and reach the final stage of the grieving process: acceptance. Most people come to accept a realistic view of their condition, find meaning in life, and begin to make plans for the life ahead of them.

Adjustment may ultimately depend on motivation. Early on, people may be motivated to work hard at therapy to gain strength and function, still believing, perhaps, that paralysis can be beaten by sheer will power. Many people with spinal cord injuries continue to hope that they will walk again. While treatments for paralysis are coming, the best approach is to move forward and live a full life now. Hope for restoring function is fine and not unrealistic, but if it means waiting on the sidelines until medical research delivers the cure, it's an aspect of denial.

People who adjust well to life after paralysis are motivated by personal goals – getting through college, getting a good job, raising a family. People who set these kinds of goals report greater life satisfaction, and they feel less shameful about their condition. How do you get motivated? It may help to think about what you always wanted out of your life before. Most people have the same personality, the same sense of style and humor as they did before being paralyzed; there is no reason not to strive for the same things.

Of course getting things done after losing function to paralysis is a challenge. It may mean learning lots of new ways to solve problems. It may be necessary to ask others for help, even when doing everything on your own becomes a stubborn way to assert your independence. Asking for help is okay – it's one of the ways to get what you need and get things done.

Adjustment to paralysis is a process; changing one's thoughts, feelings, and behavior doesn't happen overnight. It takes time to know what is true, what is realistic, what is rational. It takes time to rebuild one's identity, to find a new balance in relationships, to discover that what is important is what is happening now. Negative emotions are self-limiting, but they can be transformed. Keep your options as open as you can. Don't ignore the support and problem-solving experiences of others in similar circumstances. Figure out what's next and how to get there.

Sources

University of Alabama at Birmingham Research and Training Center on Secondary Conditions of Spinal Cord Injury/UAB Spain Rehabilitation Center; National Multiple Sclerosis Society; Quebec Paraplegic Association; Paralyzed Veterans of America; American Stroke Association

ANGER MANAGEMENT

You can't eliminate anger, and it wouldn't be a good idea if you could. Life will always bring you your share of frustration, pain, loss, and the unpredictable actions of others. You can't change that; but you can change the way you let such events affect you, especially if anger is an issue.

Simple relaxation techniques, such as deep breathing and pleasing imagery, can help calm down angry feelings. Try this:

• BREATHE DEEPLY, from your diaphragm; breathing from your chest won't relax you. Picture your breath coming up from your "gut."

• SLOWLY REPEAT A CALM WORD OR PHRASE such as "relax," or "take it easy." Repeat it to yourself while breathing deeply.

• USE IMAGERY; visualize a relaxing experience, from your memory or your imagination. Practice these techniques daily and remind yourself that the world is "not out to get you."

Source: American Psychological Association; http://www.apa.org

ALTERNATIVE MEDICINE

Acupuncture is based on traditional Chinese Medicine, that is, on the theory that life-force energy permeates all living things through meridian channels. Using a needle, other types of pressure or a laser beam at specific points on the skin, acupuncture promotes or unblocks energy flow.

Acupuncture may be beneficial to treat spinal cord injury (SCI). According to a National Institutes of Health conference in 1997, 340 out of 360 acupuncture cases (94.4 percent) reported in China had beneficial outcomes, including reduction in muscle spasms, some increased sensation, and improved bladder and bowel function. Authors recommend beginning acupuncture as soon as possible after SCI, even during the acute stage. The treatment was also helpful in reducing pressure ulcers. Laserponcture, as it is known in France, uses an infrared laser to stimulate energy flow and is said to restore function in some people with complete injuries. See *http://www.acupuncture.com* for more.

Magnets: Magnetic therapy is not embraced by Western doctors but it is widely used to treat many ailments related to paralysis, including pain, inflammation, circulation, infections, stress, energy enhancement, wound healing, etc.

Dolphin therapy: Many people, including those with paralysis, have reported feelings of well-being and even euphoria after swimming with these graceful marine mammals. For reasons unknown, this leads to beneficial healing effects; some with serious illnesses and depression have reported dramatic, long-term, favorable changes in their emotional state.

Massage and therapeutic touch have been linked to health and healing but mainstream doctors have been slow to utilize this hands-on approach. But recent research indicates that massage therapy is beneficial as a treatment for people with spinal cord injury. Massage reduced depression scores, improved range of motion and muscle strength and lowered the general levels of anxiety in a group of quads. Massage also has benefits in treating pain.

HEALING THERAPIES:
MAKING INFORMED DECISIONS

Many alternative therapies are available to people with chronic health issues or disability, all the more so with Internet information easy to find. Sure, many of these therapies are oversold and not supported by rigorously designed scientific studies, or by any studies at all. But it's good to remember, says alt med advocate Laurance Johnston, Ph.D., "that the Congressional Office of Technology Assessment has concluded that only 10-20 percent of medical interventions physicians practice are scientifically proven. Most conventional, as well as alternative, medicine is based on a history of use and experience."

Johnston points out that almost 2,000,000 people who enter hospitals in this country get infections that they did not have when they went there, and that of these, 80,000 die. Moreover, medical mistakes kill 44,000 to 98,000 people annually. Clearly, alternatives to that sort of grim medicine are needed.

"These statistics are especially relevant to people with spinal cord dysfunction, who are often prone to overmedication, life-threatening infections, and more hospitalization," says Johnston. "Clearly, such statistics warrant a serious consideration of alternative therapies."

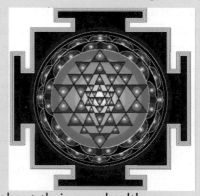

Johnston, former research director for the Paralyzed Veterans of America (which supported his writing) is the author of *Alternative Medicine and Spinal Cord Injury* (2006, Demos Publications). His goal is to help readers to make more informed decisions about their own health care.

Johnston includes sections on acupuncture; qigong; laser-based therapies; homeopathy, herbal medicine; aromatherapy, chiropractic; craniosacral therapy; dolphin-assisted therapy, Native-American healing, energy and spiritual healing; prayer, and lots more. See the Internet site *http://www.healingtherapies.info* for an overview and ordering information.

Meditation and Prayer: Clearly, meditation can have beneficial effects on health. People who meditate are said to have lower rates of cancer, heart disease, and are less likely to abuse drugs or alcohol. Meditation often involves visualization, of practicing to interrupt one's thoughts by focusing on the breath, and by using an uplifting phrase. The spirit is uplifted and well-being is restored. This has been known to be effective in treating pain.

Many large surveys have examined prayer, spirituality and health. One review of 27 studies reported a positive effect of religious involvement on health in 22 of the studies. From a scientific point of view, prayer has not been established as therapy. But many people believe that prayer may reduce anxiety and that spirituality may be beneficial for anxiety, depression, and as a tool to deal with an unpredictable disease process.

Marijuana: This drug has been used medicinally for thousands of years. It is widely used today (smoked or in pill forms, e.g. dronabinol and nabilone) for a variety of medical conditions, including paralysis. The use of this drug is complex and controversial, both medically and politically. Limited research suggests that marijuana may improve spasticity, pain, and other symptoms. Aside from its status as an illegal drug in most states, smoked marijuana may cause significant side effects, including lung cancer. Marijuana may increase the risk of seizures, memory difficulties, confusion and loss of coordination.

ALTERNATIVE MEDICINE RESOURCES

The Rocky Mountain MS Center operates MS-CAM to offer objective and accurate information on complementary and alternative medicine (CAM). Some alternatives are worth consideration, others are not. See *http://www.ms-cam.org*

The National Center for Complimentary and Alternative Medicine, part of the National Institutes of Health, explores healing practices in the context of evidence-based science, trains researchers and disseminates authoritative information to the public and professionals. NCCAM, National Institutes of Health, 9000 Rockville Pike Bethesda, Maryland 20892. See *http://www.nccam.nih.gov*

FITNESS AND EXERCISE

If not now, when? It's never too late to get a fitness program going. Exercise is good for mind and body, and almost anyone can do it, regardless of functional capabilities. Some people exercise to buff up. Others do it to get stronger, to build endurance and stamina, to help keep joints loose and flexible, to reduce stress, to get more restful sleep, or just because it makes them feel better.

No doubt about it, exercise is good for you. It prevents secondary conditions such as heart disease, diabetes, pressure sores, carpal tunnel syndrome, obstructive pulmonary disease, hypertension, urinary tract infections and respiratory disease. Research shows that people with multiple sclerosis who joined an aerobic exercise program had better cardiovascular fitness, better bladder and bowel function, less fatigue and depression, a more positive attitude and increased participation in social activities.

In 2002, Christopher Reeve demonstrated to the world that he had recovered modest movement and sensation. Reeve's recovery, coming five to seven years after his injury, defied medical expectations but had a dramatic effect on his daily life. He believed his improved function was the result of vigorous physical activity. He began exercising the year he was injured. Five years later, when he first noticed that he could voluntarily move an index finger, Reeve began an intense exercise program under the supervision of Dr. John McDonald, then at Washington University in St. Louis, who suggested that these activities may have awakened dormant nerve pathways, thus leading to recovery.

Reeve included daily electrical stimulation to build mass in his arms, quadriceps, hamstrings and other muscle groups. He rode a Functional Electrical Stimulation (FES) bicycle, did spontaneous breathing training and also participated in aquatherapy. In 1998 and 1999, Reeve underwent treadmill (also known as locomotor) training to encourage functional stepping. See page 112 for more on FES bicycle ergometry and treadmill training.

Not everyone can or should expect to get function back by exercising. But here's another great reason to get fit: Exercise helps us stay smart, and it keeps the brain healthy. The latest neuroscience research supports the idea that exercise enhances brain cells, fights degenerative disease and improves memory. A number of human studies have shown that exercise increases alertness and helps people think more clearly.

Whatever motivates you to exercise is a good reason. Weight loss is a start. According to health officials, there is an epidemic of obesity in the United States. Unfortunately, people with disabilities are even more prone to carrying excess weight due to a combination of changed metabolism and decreased muscle mass, along with a generally lower activity level.

There are compelling reasons to shed the extra pounds. Research shows that people in wheelchairs are at risk for shoulder pain, joint deterioration and even painful rotator cuff tears, due to the amount of stress they place on their arms. Quadriplegics, too, have pain in their shoulders: The more weight to push, the more stress on the shoulder. Plus, extra pounds cause risk to the skin: As people gain weight, the skin traps moisture, greatly increasing the risk of skin sores. Inactivity can also result in loss of trunk control, shortening or weakness of muscles, decreased bone density and inefficient breathing.

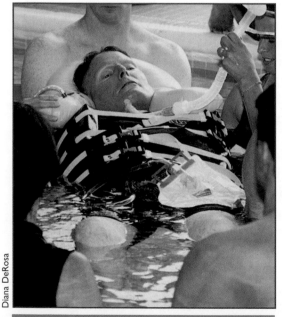

Diana DeRosa

CHRISTOPHER REEVE IN THE THERAPY POOL; HIS DOCTOR CREDITED FUNCTIONAL IMPROVEMENT TO A RIGOROUS EXERCISE PROGRAM

But people with paralysis may not be hearing the message. According to the President's Council on Physical Fitness and Sports, people with disabilities are less likely to engage in regular moderate physical activity than people without disabilities. It's the same as in the general population: It's often the "work" part of working out that keeps people from getting a fitness program going.

FITNESS VIDEOS

MS Chair Workout: Exercises designed to improve balance, coordination, flexibility, and strength. Made for MS but may be beneficial to others with extremity weakness, $15 from New York City Chapter, National Multiple Sclerosis Society, 30 West 26th Street, 9th Floor, New York, NY 10010-2094, 212-463-7787.

All Sitting Video: An energetic, balanced workout done completely seated; nonprofit program offers videos for MS, post-polio, many others, $24.95. To purchase call 509-448-9438; *www.sitandbefit.com*

Seat-A-Robics: A cardiovascular and muscle tone workout. $52.50. To purchase, *www.lifehome.com/1093.htm.*

Core and Stability Exercises for Stroke Survivors and People with Multiple Sclerosis, plus **How to Prevent Rotator Cuff Injuries** for Wheelchair Users, a compilation of exercises produced by **National Center on Physical Activity and Disability (NCPAD)**. Funding from The Christopher and Dana Reeve Foundation. $9.95. Order from NCPAD, *www.ncpad.org*; see site for numerous other exercise and activity products.

The following are available for loan from the Paralysis.org interlibrary loan program:

The ROM Dance: A Range of Motion Exercise and Relaxation Program: A mind/body exercise and rest program that features slow, gentle movements with quiet music.

Wheelchair Recovery Exercise Video: A 30-minute video for those whose primary transportation depends on arms. The advanced portion of the video is for younger, more athletic people.

Wheelercise: Exercises for seated people, including those requiring the use of a wheelchair.

Basic Strength Training for Wheelchair-Users: Why and how wheelchair users should participate in a resistance exercise program.

Physical activity, however, need not be strenuous to achieve health benefits. You don't have to be an athlete. Significant health benefits can be obtained with a moderate amount of physical activity, preferably daily. Adequate activity can be obtained in longer sessions of less intense activities (such as 30–40 minutes of wheeling oneself in a wheelchair) or in shorter sessions of more strenuous activities (such as 20 minutes of wheelchair basketball).

Additional health benefits can be gained through greater degrees of physical activity. People who can maintain a regular routine of physical activity that is of longer duration or of greater intensity are likely to derive greater benefit.

Previously sedentary people who begin physical activity programs should start with short intervals of physical activity (5–10 minutes) and gradually build up to the desired level of activity.

For paralyzed people unable to perform voluntary exercise, functional electrical stimulation (FES) has been shown to build muscle mass, improve circulation and metabolism, and favorably

❝It's the 'work' part of working out that keeps people from getting a fitness program going. But you don't have to be an athlete - moderate activity produces significant benefits.❞

alter muscle fiber composition. According to a team at The Miami Project to Cure Paralysis, FES cycling reverses cardiac muscle atrophy in quadriplegics. FES works, but it's not available widely and it's not for everyone. See your doctor about it.

Set realistic fitness goals but stick with your program. Stop exercising if you feel any pain, discomfort, nausea, dizziness, lightheadedness, chest pain, irregular heartbeat, shortness of breath or clammy hands. Always drink plenty of fluids, especially water.

People with any symptoms of paralysis should consult a physician before beginning a new program of physical activity. Over-training or inappropriate activity can be counterproductive. For example, in people with multiple sclerosis, exercise can lead to

FES FOR FUNCTION?

Functional Electrical Stimulation (FES) bikes have established themselves as a very good means of exercising paralyzed muscles. FES builds muscle mass, is good for the heart and lungs, may help with bone strength and immune function. Some people have used FES to walk with braces.

FES or any physical activity improves overall health and well being. Is there more to exercise than that? Can activity promote recovery? John McDonald, MD, who runs the International Center for Spinal Cord Injury at the Kennedy Krieger Institute in Baltimore, believes it does. "Maximizing spontaneous recovery of function is something that is possible in the majority of those paralyzed, including the most severe," he claims. Proof? Well, the evidence that FES = function is still more or less speculative. But it's coming, McDonald says.

McDonald clearly likes the concept: he helped start a company, Restorative Therapies, Inc. (*http://www.restorative-therapies.com*) to bring FES technology more into the mainstream. His bike, the RT300, competes with the original FES bike, the Ergys (*http://www.musclepower.com*). The primary difference is that the RT300 is smaller, is "ridden" without transferring from a wheelchair and is electrically powered to facilitate leg movement. Both cost about $15,000; some insurance carriers will pay this amount. The bike companies are hopeful about Medicare coverage. McDonald says it comes down to this: "Allow

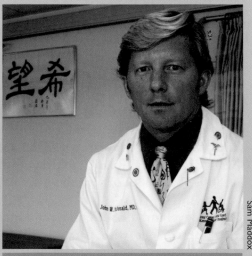

JOHN MCDONALD, MD, PHD

hope and the power of possibility to prevail. The progression of regenerative science is breathtaking and more and more scientists are joining to put their shoulder to the wheel. We will solve this problem – paralysis – and it will be done sooner rather than later."

a condition called cardiovascular dysautonomia, which lowers heart rate and decreases blood pressure. Also, because exercise tends to warm up the body, sensitivity to heat (especially in people with MS) can induce fatigue, loss of balance and visual changes; use cooling aids as needed (cool vests, ice packs: *www.steelevest.com,* or *www.coolsport.net*).

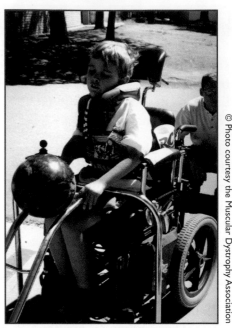

© Photo courtesy the Muscular Dystrophy Association

Sources

National Center on Physical Activity and Disability, President's Council on Physical Fitness and Sports, National MS Society, Craig Hospital, Paralyzed Veterans of America

---

FITNESS AND EXERCISE RESOURCES

National Center on Physical Activity and Disability (NCPAD) is a collaborative effort of the University of Illinois at Chicago, the Rehabilitation Institute of Chicago and the National Center on Accessibility at Indiana University. NCPAD features in depth resources on fitness, exercise and recreation for people with disabilities. A good place to start when you decide to get fit. NCPAD, 1640 W. Roosevelt Road, Chicago, IL 60608-6904; toll-free 1–800–900–8086; or visit the Internet site *http://www.ncpad.org*

The Cleveland FES Center promotes techniques to restore function for persons with paralysis. FES Information Center, 11000 Cedar Avenue, Cleveland, OH 44106; telephone 216-231-3257; or visit the Internet site *http://fescenter.case.edu*

The President's Council on Physical Fitness and Sports has information on making exercise an important part of your life. *http://www.fitness.gov/disab.htm*

RECOVERING QUADRIPLEGICS

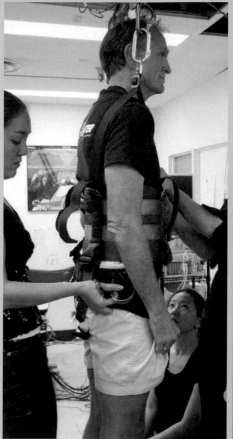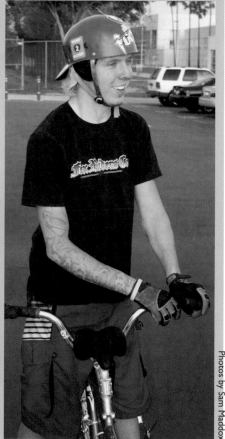

Photos by Sam Maddox

Michael Thomas (left) C7 injury, car wreck 1998. "After six years of different exercises and working out and development, I'm able to walk. I use walking sticks to keep my balance, which has also been affected. But essentially, I walk on my own." Mike was the first client at Project Walk near San Diego. See *http://www.projectwalk.org*

Aaron Baker, C4/5/6, motocross crash, 1999. "At the one year mark my insurance company deemed me pretty well rehabilitated; however, I was still in my electric wheelchair. I haven't used a wheel-chair now in...I'd say...eight months to a year. Who knows what's possible? I've been told that I'm not supposed to do anything. I'm not supposed to feed myself. Well...I'm ridin' a tandem bike across the country. I'm stoked." For his recovery Aaron teamed with trainer Taylor Isaacs in Northridge, CA. See *www.aaronbakers.com*

NUTRITION

It goes without saying, or at least it should, that good health depends on good nutrition. Food affects how we look and feel, and how our bodies work. Eating right provides energy, boosts our immune system, keeps us at the proper body weight, and keeps all body systems in harmony. Eating wrong can cause weight gain, diabetes, heart disease, cancer and other "ailments of civilization."

Eating well is even more essential for persons who are paralyzed. Because of changes that occur to the body after trauma or disease, it's more important than ever to understand the role nutrition plays in maintaining health.

After a spinal cord injury most people lose weight. The injury puts stress on the body as the body uses its energy and nutrients to repair itself. Stress ramps up the metabolic rate: the body burns calories faster. Moreover, many newly injured people are not able to eat a regular diet. As muscles atrophy, the weight loss continues — for about a month. Later, the problem isn't too few pounds, it's too many.

Compared to the general population, people with spinal cord injuries are prone to two other diet-related problems: heart disease and diabetes. For reasons that are not fully understood, blood chemistry becomes impaired: Insulin tolerance is too high (the body produces more and more of the hormone insulin to transport energy to the body tissues; this is one of the pathways to diabetes), "bad" cholesterol and triglycerides are too high, and "good" cholesterol is too low. Advice: don't smoke, don't get heavy.

For some it isn't just the food, it's the way the food is presented. People with amyotrophic lateral sclerosis and other conditions who have problems swallowing must regulate the consistency and texture of foods. Food should be softer and cut into smaller pieces that can slide down the throat with minimum chewing. If food or drinks are too runny, some of the liquid can run into the airway to the lungs and cause coughing. If food is too dry, such as toast, it tends to irritate the throat and causes coughing. This problem can often be solved by adding butter, jam, etc. Foods that may be easier to manage include custards, sherbet, puddings, plain yogurt, canned fruit, applesauce, crust-less toast with butter, dark chicken, salmon, thick soups, scrambled eggs, and mashed potatoes. Avoid extra-spicy or acidic foods, soft bread, cookies, crackers, dry cereal, graham crackers, peanut butter, lettuce, celery, rice, and fruits and vegetables with skin or seeds (peas, corn, apples, berries).

Bowel management is directly related to diet. Since the messages from the brain that control the muscular movements of the bowel are out of order, it's difficult for food to move through the intestinal system. A high fiber diet — 25-35 grams of fiber every day – and plenty of fluids is recommended. True, that's a lot of fiber. Where does it come from? Vegetables, fruits, nuts, popcorn. Some people take supplements, such as Metamucil. What to avoid: high-fat foods. They don't easily move through the system.

For some people with paralysis due to disease, diet and nutrition become almost a religious issue, though certainly not without some confusion, and controversy. There are many adherents, for example, of special diets for people with multiple sclerosis. The National Multiple Sclerosis Society recommends the standard food pyramid, with a low-fat, high-carbohydrate program with a variety of grains, fruits and vegetables. The Swank MS diet, originated by an Oregon doctor about 40 years ago, prescribes a strict no-fat, no-dairy routine. Roy Swank has claimed to reduce the frequency and severity of recurrences in his MS patients by cutting out animal fat – this being the one essential first step for anyone with MS, he says.

Roger MacDougall, a prominent Hollywood writer in the 1950s, had a severe case of MS – his legs were paralyzed, he was almost blind, he had no voice. Using a high-protein, low-carbohydrate diet that has become known as the "Paleolithic diet," he

NUTRITION RESOURCES

Nutrition.gov is a resource on diet and food, including ways these relate to disease, activity, etc. See *http://www.nutrition.gov*

National Institutes of Health: Office of Dietary Supplements offers reliable information on nutritional supplements. See *http://www.ods.od.nih.gov*

says he got completely better. "I have not been cured. I am simply experiencing a remission — but a remission which I firmly believe to be self-induced." MacDougall's premise is that until the advent of agriculture, 10,000 years ago, we were all hunter-gatherers and ate meats and nuts and berries from natural sources;we have not evolved to deal with the processed food products of modern agriculture and thus we can become allergic to certain types of foods – wheat and other glutens, refined sugar and high-fat meat. He suggests that these allergies can lead to autoimmune disease, such as MS, arthritis, etc. MacDougall's answer: Eat like a caveman.

Sources

Spinal Cord Injury Information Network; Rehabilitation Research and Training Center on Aging and Spinal Cord Injury, Rancho Los Amigos; National ALS Association

DIETARY CONCERNS RELATED TO PARALYSIS

• **pressure ulcers:** An active pressure ulcer requires a diet high in protein, vitamins, and minerals.

• **kidney or bladder stones**: Some individuals with spinal cord dysfunction may be prone to stones. Certain beverages are more likely to create calcium crystals in the urine (beer, coffee, cocoa, cola drinks). Dairy products (milk, cheese, yogurt, ice cream) can also lead to trouble. The best way to avoid kidney or bladder stones is to drink a lot of water.

• **urinary tract infection**: Carbonated beverages (soda), orange juice and grapefruit juice can cause the urine to become alkaline, a breeding ground for bacteria that can cause UTI.

• **weight control**: Obesity is on the rise in the United States and people with disabilities are part of the picture. Extra weight decreases mobility, endurance and balance. It can make transfers difficult and increases the risk of pressure sores. There are dangers to being underweight, too; it increases the risk for infections and pressure sores, resulting in less energy and more fatigue.

- **general guidelines:** Most nutritionists stick pretty close to the standard food pyramid (most calories from complex carbohydrates — breads and starches – with plenty of dairy and avoidance of refined sugars and fat). This foundation of American eating habits has been challenged in recent years by many popular high-protein diets. Going against prevailing dogma, there is research suggesting that carbohydrates are also a problem in obesity, diabetes and heart disease. Nonetheless, the usual rehab nutrition program will recommend a carbohydrate intake representing 50-60 percent of total calories, with protein being 20 percent of total calories.

- **protein:** People with mobility limitations generally need more protein in their diets to help prevent tissue or muscle breakdown. At least 2 4-ounce servings of a high-protein food should be consumed every day; make that 4 4-ounce servings if there is an active pressure sore.

- **fiber:** To promote normal bowel functioning and prevent constipation and diarrhea, nutritionists recommend whole grain breads and cereals, fresh fruits and vegetables, raw nuts and seed mixes with dried fruits and peanut butter.

- **fluids:** A lot of water is necessary to prevent dehydration and to keep your kidneys and bladder flushed.

- **minerals and vitamins:** Fruits and vegetables are good sources of vitamin A and the family of B vitamins. There is evidence that taking extra vitamin C and a zinc supplement helps keep the skin healthy.

- **antioxidant vitamins:** These round up free radicals that can damage the body's cells, and may stimulate the immune system. Many people with chronic neurological disease take supplements, including vitamins A (beta-carotene), C and E. Fruits and vegetables are good sources. Grape seed extract, co-enzyme Q 10 and pycnogenol are other sources.

Sexual Health
FOR MEN

Paralysis affects a man's sexuality both physically and psychologically. Men wonder, "Can I still do it?" Men worry that sexual pleasure is a thing of the past. They worry that they can no longer father children, that mates will find them unattractive, that partners will pack up and leave. It is true that, after disease or injury, men often face changes in their relationships and sexual activity. Emotional changes occur, of course, and these too can affect a person's sexuality.

Erections are the number-one issue after paralysis. Normally, men have two types of erections. Psychogenic erections result from sexual thoughts or seeing or hearing something stimulating. The brain sends these arousing messages through the nerves of the spinal cord that exit at the T10–L2 levels, then relays them to the penis, resulting in tumescence. The ability to have a psychogenic erection depends on the level and extent of paralysis. Generally, men with an incomplete injury at a low level are more likely to have psychogenic erections than men with high-level, incomplete injuries. Men with complete injuries are less likely to experience psychogenic erections.

A reflex erection occurs when there is direct physical contact to the penis or other erotic areas such as the ears, nipples or neck. A reflex erection is involuntary and can occur without sexual or stimulating thoughts. The nerves that control a man's ability to have a reflex erection are located in the sacral segments (S2–S4) of the spinal cord. Most paralyzed men are able to have a reflex erection with physical stimulation unless the S2–S4 pathway is damaged.

Ejaculation is the number-two issue. Researchers report that ejaculation occurs in up to 70 percent of men with incomplete lower-level injuries and in as many as 17 percent of men with complete lower-level injuries. Ejaculation occurs in about 30 percent of men with incomplete upper-level injuries and almost never in men with complete upper-level injuries.

While many men who are paralyzed can still "get it up," the erection may not be hard enough or last long enough for sexual activity. This condition is called erectile dysfunction (ED). Numerous treatments and products (pills, pellets, shots and

"While it may be that the largest sex organ is the brain, it's not always easy to make major adjustments in one's sexual persona. Professional counseling can help."

implants) are available for treating ED but paralyzed men may have special concerns or problems with their use. It is important to see your doctor or urologist for accurate information on the various treatments as they relate to specific conditions.

Newer drugs have come on to the market in recent years. Research shows that Viagra, Cialis and Levitra significantly improve the quality of erections and the satisfaction of sex life in most men with ED who have spinal cord injuries between T6 and L5. Men who have low or high blood pressure or vascular disease should not take these drugs. Some medications cannot be taken with ED drugs — review this with the prescribing physician.

Penile injection therapy is an option that involves injecting a drug (papavarine or alprostadil) or a combination of drugs into the side of the penis. This produces a hard erection that can last for an hour or two. If not used correctly, these drugs can result in a prolonged erection, called priapism, which can damage the penile tissue. Other risks from the injection are bruising, scarring or infection. An injection erection is a more difficult option for those with limited hand function.

Another option is called medicated urethral system erection (MUSE), wherein a medicated pellet is placed into the urethra for absorption into the surrounding tissue. This causes the blood vessels to relax and allows blood to fill the penis. The drug, alprostadil, is the same one used in penile injection therapy. Reported side effects include infection, burning sensation, decreased blood pressure and fainting.

Beyond drug options, vacuum pumps produce an erection. The penis is placed in a cylinder and the air is pumped out, causing blood to be drawn into the erectile tissues. Tumescence is maintained by placing an elastic constriction ring around the base of the penis. It's important to remove the ring after intercourse to avoid the risk of skin abrasion or breakdown. A battery-operated vacuum model is an available option.

A penile prosthesis, often the last treatment option for ED because it is permanent and requires surgery, involves inserting an implant directly into the erectile tissues. There are various types of implants available, including semi-rigid or malleable rods and inflatable devices. There are risks of mechanical breakdown, though, and the danger that the implant could cause infection or push out through the skin.

Paralyzed men with ED should have a thorough physical exam by a urologist familiar with their condition before using any medications or assistive devices. Men with spinal cord injuries above the T6 level must be watchful for signs of autonomic dysreflexia (AD). Signs include flushing in the face, headaches, nasal congestion and/or changes in vision. See page 61 for more on AD.

Fertility is the third biggest issue: Men with paralysis usually experience a change in their ability to biologically father a child, due to the inability to ejaculate. Some men experience retrograde ejaculation, when semen travels in reverse: back up the tube and into the bladder. The number of sperm a man produces does not usually decrease in months or years after paralysis. However, the motility (movement) of the sperm is considerably lower than for non-paralyzed men. There are options, though, for improving the ability to father children.

Penile vibratory stimulation (PVS) is an inexpensive and fairly reliable way to produce an ejaculation at home. A variety of vibrators/massagers are available for this purpose. Some are specifically designed with the output power and frequency required to induce ejaculation while minimizing skin problems.

Rectal probe electroejaculation (RPE) is an option (albeit in a clinic with several technicians around) if the vibratory method is not successful. RPE, borrowing from animal husbandry, places an electrical probe in the rectum; a controlled electrical stimulation produces an ejaculation. Electroejaculation is generally a safe and effective way to obtain a sperm sample. These sperm are healthy but usually not strong swimmers, and often not hardy enough to penetrate the egg. Because of their reduced motility, the sperm need a little high-tech help. The recent development of intracytoplasmic sperm injection (ICSI), which involves the direct injection of a single mature sperm into an oocyte (egg), can often solve the problem of conception.

If sperm cannot be retrieved using PVS or RPE, minor surgery can be performed to remove sperm from the testicle.

Once sperm are collected they can be used in various means of artificial insemination, including in vitro techniques and micro-manipulation. There are lots of success stories but high-tech, assisted fertility is not a slam-dunk. It can be emotionally draining and also quite expensive. Get the facts and treatment options from a fertility specialist experienced in issues of paralysis.

Some couples grappling with infertility have successfully utilized donor sperm (from a sperm bank) to impregnate the woman. Couples may want to explore the very rewarding options available to adopt children.

Sex after stroke: Heart disease, stroke or surgery doesn't mean that a satisfying sex life must end. After the first phase of recovery is over, people find that the same forms of lovemaking they enjoyed before are still rewarding. It is pure myth that resuming sex often causes a heart attack, stroke or sudden death.

Still, fears about performance can greatly reduce sexual interest and capacity. After recovery, stroke survivors may feel depressed. This is normal, and in 85 percent of the cases it goes away within three months.

To be sure, a man can continue or initiate a romantic and intimate relationship with a partner after a paralyzing disease or injury. Good communication with his partner is essential. It is important for both partners to understand the physical changes that have occurred, but it is equally important to talk about each other's feelings. The couple can talk about, explore and experiment with different ways to be romantic and intimate. Many couples consider oral-genital intercourse a good option. Whatever seems satisfying and pleasurable is acceptable as long as both partners mutually agree.

While it's been said that the largest sex organ is the brain, it's not always easy to make major adjustments in one's sexual persona. Professional counseling can help in working through feelings of fear or anxiety over establishing or continuing a healthy relationship after paralysis. A counselor can also work with couples on healthy ways to communicate their needs and feelings.

Safe sex: The risk of sexually transmitted disease (STD) is the same both before and after paralysis. STDs include diseases such as gonorrhea, syphilis, herpes and the HIV virus; these can cause other medical problems, such as infertility, urinary tract infections, pelvic inflammatory disease, vaginal discharge, genital warts and AIDS. The safest, most effective way to prevent sexually transmitted diseases is to use a condom with a spermicidal gel.

Sources

The American Urological Association, University of Alabama/Birmingham — RRTC on Secondary Conditions of Spinal Cord Injury, University of Miami School of Medicine

SEXUALITY AND DATING RESOURCES

University of Miami School of Medicine offers details on sexual physiology and functioning, orgasm, fertility, etc. See *http://calder.med.miami.edu/pointis/sexuality.html*

Sexual Health is an Internet site on sexuality and pleasure pertaining to men and women with paralysis or disability. Operated by Mitch Tepper, Ph.D., a sexuality counselor who is quadriplegic. See *http://www.sexualhealth.com*

Dateable is a computerized matchmaking and dating service founded in 1987 "to combat the isolation and social discrimination often experienced by people with disabilities." Dateable claims to have made over 37,000 matches with more than 260 resulting in marriage. See *http://www.dateable.org*

Lovebyrd is a disabled dating and social networking service to individuals living with a condition that makes it difficult to meet and connect with other people. There are journals, poetry, article and advice archives (including horror stories), chatrooms, instant messaging, etc. Browse by disability, including paraplegia, quadriplegia, multiple sclerosis, amputee, depression, etc. On the Internet see *http://www.lovebyrd.com*

FOR WOMEN

Paralysis itself doesn't affect a woman's libido or her need to express herself sexually, nor does it affect her ability to conceive a child. Generally speaking, sexuality in the paralyzed female is less affected than in the male; it is physically easier for the woman to adapt her sexual role, even though it may be more passive than that of a non-disabled women. The main difference in sexual functioning between women with disabilities and those without can be accounted for by the difficulties women with disabilities have in finding a romantic partner. Their level of sexual desire may be the same, but the level of activity is less because fewer women with disabilities have partners.

There are no physiological changes after paralysis that prevent women from engaging in sexual activity. Positioning can be an issue but can usually be accommodated. Autonomic dysreflexia can be anticipated and controlled. Many women experience a loss of vaginal muscle control and many are unable to produce vaginal lubrication. Both problems are likely the result of the interruption in normal nerve signals from the brain to the genital area. There is no remedy for muscle loss. Lubrication, of course, can be improved.

Typically, lubrication occurs as a psychogenic (mental) and reflex (physical) response to something sexually stimulating or arousing. It has been suggested that lubrication in women is the physiological equivalent of the erection in the male, and is probably innervated in the same way. Women can substitute water-based (never use oil-based, such as Vaseline) lubricants such as KY Jelly.

Low sex drive is common among women with paralysis; indeed, it is reported among all women. Meanwhile, Viagra has been clinically tested by a group of women with spinal cord injuries; almost all reported that the drug stimulated arousal. In some, it enhanced lubrication and sensation during intercourse. In some conditions of paralysis, such as multiple sclerosis, cognitive problems can undermine sexuality. People with short-term memory or concentration loss may drift off during sexual activities in a way that can be disheartening to the partner. It requires love and patience, with lots of communication, to bring this out in the open and to seek the needed psychological or medical treatment.

Women who are paralyzed often fear bowel and bladder accidents during times of intimacy. There are a number of ways to reduce the chance of accidents. The first is to limit fluid intake if a sexual encounter is planned. Women who use intermittent catheterization should empty the bladder before beginning sexual activity. Women who use a suprapubic or Foley catheter find that taping the catheter tube to the thigh or abdomen keeps it out of the way. The Foley can be left in during sexual intercourse because, unknown to many men and even women, the urethra (urinary opening) is separate from the vagina.

The best way to avoid a bowel accident is to establish a consistent bowel program. Women may also want to avoid eating right before engaging in sexual activity. With good communication, a little urine or occasional excrement won't destroy a rewarding sex life.

Sexual success is often measured, wrongly, by whether or not partners achieve orgasm. A woman with paralysis, like men with similar levels of function, can achieve normal orgasm if there is some residual pelvic innervation. Dr. Marca Sipski of the University of Alabama/Birmingham School of Medicine thinks paralyzed women may retain an orgasm reflex that requires no brain input. Her research indicates the potential is still there, she says, but women may give up trying to have orgasms because they lack the ability to feel touch in the genital area. Still, orgasm is relatively rare. Some paralyzed men and women, with practice and focused thought, are able to experience a "phantom orgasm," through reassignment of sexual response; this involves mentally intensifying an existing sensation from one portion of their body and reassigning the sensation to the genitals.

Women with paraplegia or quadriplegia who are of childbearing age usually regain their menstrual cycle; nearly 50 percent do not miss a single period following injury. Pregnancy is possible and generally not a health risk. While most paralyzed women can have normal vaginal deliveries, certain complications of pregnancy are possible, including increased urinary tract infections, pressure sores and spasticity. Autonomic dysreflexia (AD) is a serious risk during labor for those with the injuries above T6 (see page 61). Also, loss of sensation in the pelvic area can prevent the woman from knowing that labor has begun.

Another potential risk of pregnancy is the development of thromboembolism, in which blood vessels become blocked by clots. With high thoracic or cervical lesions, respiratory function may be impaired with the increased burden of pregnancy or the work of labor, requiring ventilator support.

Women with disabilities often do not receive adequate health care services. For example, routine pelvic exams are not done due to lack of awareness of the need, problems getting onto the exam table, or not being able to find a doctor with knowledge about their disability. Providers might wrongly assume that women with disabilities are not having sex, especially if their disability is severe, and therefore may neglect to screen these women for sexually transmitted diseases (STDs) or even perform a full pelvic exam. Unfortunately, some health care providers even suggest to women with disabilities that they abstain from sex and not bear children, even if they can conceive children.

Breast health: Women with disabilities must be aware that they are among the one in eight women who will get breast cancer. Screening is essential. Women with limited use of their arms and hands may may need to perform exams using alternate positions or with the help of an attendant or family member. In the clinic, getting a wheelchair in the door is the easy part; services or programs provided to patients with disabilities must be equal to those provided for persons without disabilities.

Birth control: since paralysis does not usually affect fertility in the female, contraception is important. There are also some special considerations. Oral contraceptives are linked to inflammation and clots in blood vessels, and the risk of these is greater with SCI. Intrauterine devices cannot always be felt in the paralyzed woman and may cause undetected complications. Use of diaphragms and spermicides can be difficult for those with impaired hand dexterity.

Sexuality does not disappear after paralysis. Explore sexuality with an open heart and an open mind.

Sources
The Center for Research on Women with Disabilities, Spain Rehabilitation Center, Paralyzed Veterans of America

WOMEN'S RESOURCES

The Center for Research on Women with Disabilities (CROWD) focuses on issues related to health (including reproduction and sexuality), aging, civil rights, abuse and independent living. CROWD's purpose: To expand the life choices of women with disabilities to fully participate in community life. Offers information in English and Spanish on weight management, depression, living well with physical limitations, smoking cessation, etc. The basic tips include believe in oneself, honor the body, defy the myths, demand answers. CROWD, One Baylor Plaza, Houston, Texas 77030; telephone 713-798-5782 or toll-free 1-800-44-CROWD; you can also visit the Internet site *http://www.bcm.tmc.edu/crowd*

National Resource Center for Parents with Disabilities from Through the Looking Glass, a resource on childbirth and parenting, adaptive equipment for childcare, networking and support groups. Through the Looking Glass, 2198 Sixth Street Suite 100, Berkeley, CA 94710–2204; toll-free 1–800–644–2666; or visit the Internet site *http://www.lookingglass.org*

Health Promotion for Women with Disabilities, addresses issues shared by women with various types of disability. Villanova University - College of Nursing, 800 Lancaster Avenue, Villanova, PA 19085; telephone 610-519-6828; on the Internet see *http://nurseweb.villanova.edu/womenwithdisabilities/*

Women with DisAbilities, from the National Women's Health Information Center, helps women deal with architectural barriers and lack of adequate transportation; financial restraints; and lack of reliable health information. Includes information on aging, parenting, plus much disability-specific detail, including information for girls with disabilities. Call toll-free 1-800-994-WOMAN; or visit the Internet site *http://www.4woman.gov/wwd*

MobileWomen is an Internet magazine for women with disabilities. The site features articles, resources and a bullet board to share experiences and solutions. Founded by Wendy Crawford; see facing page for profile. Contact c/o W. M. Keck Center for Collaborative Neuroscience, 604 Allison Road, D-251, Piscataway, NJ 08854; see *http://carecure.rutgers.edu/mobilewomen*

WENDY CRAWFORD: MOBILE WOMAN

Can a disabled woman find medical professionals who treat her with the same respect that they would a nondisabled woman? Well, lets say the answer is more affirming than it once was but such parity remains a work in progress.

Wendy Crawford and her MobileWomen project hopes to close the gap, using education and the power of shared experience. "Mobile women face the same issues as other women," says Crawford. "We experience regular menstrual cycles and many of us are sexually active. We want to know about birth control, sexually transmitted diseases, pregnancy, ovarian and cervical cancer." She notes, however, that in a recent study, disabled women are less likely to receive reproductive health care and often are denied services because of their disability. Medical facilities and equipment are inaccessible; medical staff has no experience, and in many cases, operate with antiquated social attitudes about disability.

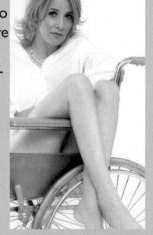

"The good news, says Crawford, "is that you can get the quality reproductive health care you deserve by educating yourself and your health care providers."

Crawford had just emerged on the international fashion circuit when a drunk driver rendered her a C5/6 quad – which means she has to work harder to be taken seriously as a woman. "My dream is for equality – physicians' offices with accessible examination tables and mammogram machines, resources and accessible abuse shelters."

MobileWomen is supported, in part, by a grant from the Christopher and Dana Reeve Foundation. See http://carecure.rutgers.edu/mobilewomen

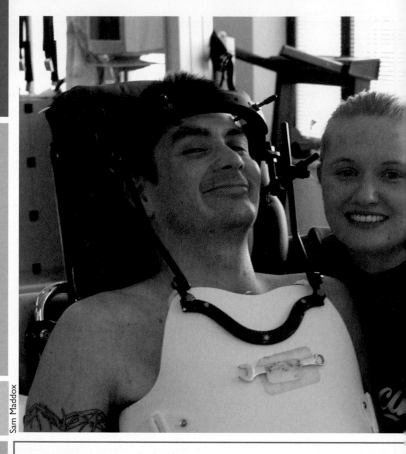

Sam Maddox

REHABILITATION

Rehabilitation centers are not all the same; they can be compared but you need to know what you're looking for.

CHOOSING A REHABILITATION SETTING

How can you predict the quality of care you or a loved one will receive when entering a rehabilitation program? How do you know what facility to choose? Is there really a choice? Does rehab really matter?

Most people have no experience with rehab or the effects of paralysis, so assessing the quality of a rehab program can be stressful and complex. The final choice may come down to which program is covered by insurance or by which one is closest to the support systems of one's family and community, but it is possible to make an informed decision. Rehabilitation centers are not all the same; they can be compared.

At the top of the list of qualifying factors is experience in rehabilitation for your specific needs. Medical rehab is increasingly specialized; the more patients a facility regularly treats with needs similar to yours, the higher the expertise of the staff. How do you know what a facility is best at? Ask the facility how many beds are dedicated to your rehab situation. For example, if 85 percent of a unit's beds are dedicated to stroke survivors, this may not be the ideal place for a young person with a spinal cord injury. Get a sense of the facility's reputation and standing. Ask around; connect to others by way of support groups (e.g., American Stroke Association, National Spinal Cord Injury Association, National Multiple Sclerosis Society, or the Internet — turn to page 302 for a list of online communities).

High-quality programs are often located in facilities devoted exclusively to providing rehabilitation services or in hospitals with designated units. Here are a few questions to consider in choosing a facility:

- Is the place accredited, that is, does it meet the professional standards of care for your specific needs? Generally speaking, a facility with accredited expertise is preferable to a general rehabilitation program. For example, recognition by the Commission on Accreditation of Rehabilitation Facilities (CARF) for spinal cord injury indicates that the facility meets a minimum standard level of care, has a wide range of specialized services and is well connected in the local community.

CARF also accredits programs in assisted living, mental health and substance abuse, brain injury, and pediatric rehab.

- For those with a spinal cord or brain injury, there are groups of specialized hospitals called Model Systems Centers. These are well-established facilities that have qualified for special federal grants to demonstrate and share medical expertise (see page 43 for connections to these centers).

- Does the place offer a wide variety of specialized personnel who offer therapies with a coordinated team approach? Rehab teams should include doctors and nurses plus social workers, occupational and physical therapists, recreational therapists, rehabilitation nurses, rehabilitation psychologists, speech pathologists, vocational counselors, nutritionists, respiratory experts, sexuality counselors, rehab engineering experts, case managers, etc.

- Does the facility offer connections to peer support and contact with others with a similar disability? Peer support is often the most reliable and encouraging source of information as people make their way in the new world of rehab.

You might also ask these types of questions: What have been the results for people like me who have used your services? How will services be individualized? How much can my family participate in the program? Are you close to public transportation? Is there bilingual staff or sign language interpreters?

The ultimate measure of good rehab is the breadth and quality of the professional staff on hand. The professions you can expect to find represented on a rehabilitation team are as follows:

Physiatrist

A physiatrist (pronounced fizz-ee-AT-trist, or more commonly, fizz-EYE-a-trist) is a doctor with a specialty in physical medicine and rehabilitation. Physiatrists treat a wide range of problems from sore shoulders to acute and chronic pain and musculoskeletal disorders. Physiatrists coordinate the long-term rehabilitation process for people with paralysis, including those with spinal cord injuries, cancer, stroke or other neurological disorders, brain injuries, amputations and multiple sclerosis. A physiatrist must complete four years of graduate medical education and four years of postdoctoral residency training. Residency includes one year spent developing fundamental clinical skills and three years of training in the full scope of the specialty.

Rehab Nurse

Rehab nurses begin to work with individuals and their families soon after the onset of injury or illness. They have special training in rehabilitation and understand the full range of medical complications related to bladder and bowel, nutrition, pain, skin integrity and more, including vocational, educational, environmental and spiritual needs. Rehab nurses provide comfort, therapy and education and promote wellness and independence. The goal of rehabilitation nursing is to assist individuals with disabilities and chronic illness in the restoration and maintenance of optimal health. Nurses are the hands-on people who carry out the directives of the medical team.

Occupational Therapist

Occupational therapists (OT) are skilled professionals who have studied the social, emotional and physiological effects of illness and injury. An OT helps individuals learn—or relearn—the day-to-day activities they need for maximum independence. OTs offer treatment programs to help with bathing, dressing, preparing a meal, house cleaning, engaging in arts and crafts or gardening. They recommend and train people in the use of adaptive equipment to replace lost function. OTs also evaluate home and job environments and recommend adaptations. The occupational therapist guides family members and caregivers in safe and effective methods of home care; he or she will also facilitate contact with the community outside of the hospital.

Physical Therapist

Physical therapists (PT) treat people with motor and/or sensory impairments, helping to increase strength and endurance, improve coordination, reduce spasticity and pain, maintain muscles, protect skin from pressure sores, and gain greater control of bladder and bowel function. PTs also treat joints and help expand their range of motion. PTs use a variety of equipment including weights, pools and bikes (including the functional electrical stimulation types). When pain is an issue, physical therapy is often the first line of defense; therapists use a variety of methods including electrical stimulation and exercise to improve muscle tone and reduce contractures, spasticity and pain.

PTs will also demonstrate techniques for using assistive devices such as wheelchairs, canes or braces. Physical therapy is not a passive activity that is "done" to you; a PT program requires active participation from both practitioner and patient—it's hard work to restore body function lost to injury or disease. Once a maintenance program has been developed by a physical therapist, it is the client's responsibility to follow it at home.

Recreation Therapist

Recreation therapists help people discover the wide range of options for active living in their community. It has been well established that exercise, fitness and relaxation reduce stress and contribute to improved cardiovascular and respiratory functioning, increased strength, endurance and coordination. Activity demonstrably reduces secondary medical complications arising from paralysis. Skin sores and urinary tract infections, for example, are significantly reduced in wheelchair athletes, as compared to non-athletes. Rec therapists push physical activity for social as well as medical reasons. Active involvement in recreation leads to improved life satisfaction, better social relationships and lower levels of depression.

Vocational Counselor

Vocational counselors perform many of the same functions that career counselors do—they assess a client's job skills and help with a smooth reentry into the workforce or school. Then they work with various government agencies to obtain equipment, training and placement. Vocational therapists also educate disabled individuals about their rights and protections under the Americans with Disabilities Act, which requires employers to

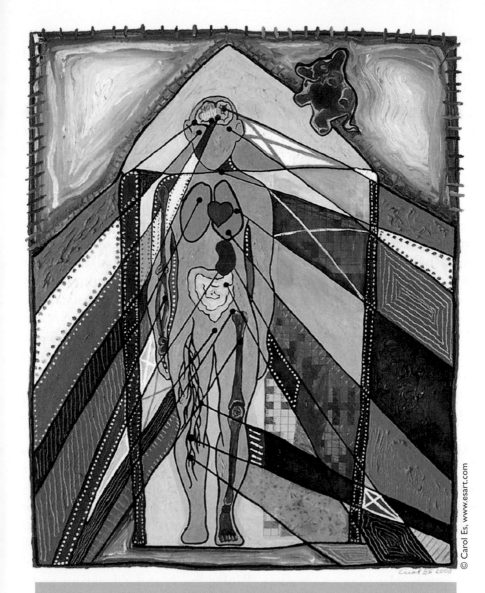

POINT BLANK RANGE

16 x 20 INCHES, OIL & COLLAGE ON CANVAS, 2000

"WHAT HAPPENED TO ME AND ALL MY YOUTHFUL COOL? A GAMUT OF TESTS, DOCTORS AND UNRELIABLE DIAGNOSES. MY PROGNOSIS UNCERTAIN, MY BODY PARTS VIEWED WITH MAGNETS AND DYES - IT'S ENOUGH TO MAKE ONE FEEL SHOT DOWN, DRUNK, CRAZY AND CONFUSED ... AND NOT IN A *GOOD* WAY."

— CAROL ES

make "reasonable accommodations" for disabled employees. Vocational therapists may mediate between employers and employees to negotiate reasonable accommodation.

Speech-Language Pathologist

Speech-language pathologists help people with aphasia or other communication problems relearn language or develop alternative means of communication. They also help people improve their ability to swallow. Sometimes, changing body position and posture while eating can bring about improvement. The texture of foods can be modified to make swallowing easier. Speech-language pathologists help people with paralysis develop strategies for language disabilities, including the use of symbol boards or sign language. They also share their knowledge of computer technology and other types of equipment to enhance communication.

Neurologist

A neurologist is a doctor who specializes in the diagnosis and treatment of disorders of the nervous system (brain, spinal cord, nerves and muscles). A neurologist makes an initial evaluation, diagnoses the injury and consults on one's immediate care.

Rehabilitation Psychologist

A psychologist helps people deal with life-changing injury or disease, offering tools to cope with the effects of disability. A psychologist offers support for families as well. Therapy might be offered individually or in a group to speed the adjustment to changes in physical, cognitive and emotional functioning. The psychology team also offers marital and family therapy and sexual or family planning counseling. Biofeedback and relaxation techniques may be included.

Case Manager

A case manager oversees many aspects of rehab, including preparing a discharge plan and working with insurance companies to communicate the rehab team's goals. A case manager may arrange for purchases of special equipment and/or home modifications.

Social Worker

A rehab social worker connects many of the aspects of the recovery process, delving into the person's personality, lifestyle, emotional behavior, past relationships, education and work history, special interests and financial background in order to help the rehab team create an optimal rehabilitation program within the hospital and back home in the community.

Sources

American Occupational Therapy Association, American Physical Therapy Association, American Academy of Physical Medicine and Rehabilitation, Commission on Accreditation of Rehabilitation Facilities, Association of Rehabilitation Nurses, American Therapeutic Recreation Association

REHABILITATION RESOURCES

The American Academy of Neurology (AAN) is a medical specialty society established to advance the art and science of neurology and to promote the best possible care for patients with neurological disorders. American Academy of Neurology, 1080 Montreal Avenue, Saint Paul, MN 55116; toll-free 1–800–879–1960; or visit the Internet site *http://www.aan.com*

The American Academy of Physical Medicine and Rehabilitation is the national medical society for more than 6,400 physicians who are specialists in the field of physical medicine and rehabilitation (physiatrists). The website includes a physician directory by state. Contact the American Academy of Physical Medicine and Rehabilitation, 330 North Wabash Avenue, Chicago, IL 60611; telephone 312–464–9700; or visit the Internet site *http://www.aapmr.org*

The American Congress of Rehabilitation Medicine serves people with disabling conditions by promoting rehabilitation research and the transfer of technology. American Congress of Rehabilitation Medicine, 6801 Lake Plaza Drive Suite B-205, Indianapolis, IN 46220; telephone 317–915–2250; or visit *http://www.acrm.org*

NEURORECOVERY NETWORK

Rehabilitation therapy is vital for maintaining the general health of spinal cord injured people. Moreover, there is evidence that shows how vigorous repetitive exercise can exploit neural plasticity both above and below the injury site, leading to an improvement in walking and standing capacity. It is possible this type of body-weight supported locomotor training program may also bring about changes at the molecular level, improving axon regeneration and neural communication.

To further the research and application of this sort of intensive activity based rehab, the Christopher and Dana Reeve Foundation launched the **NeuroRecovery Network** grant program. This includes the establishment of specialized centers that provide standardized care based on scientific and clinical evidence. The program is funded by a joint agreement between the CDRF and the Centers for Disease Control and Prevention.

Initially the NeuroRecovery Network supports programs involving locomotor training using body weight support on a treadmill. The Network's longer-term goals include: maximizing the availability and quality of rehabilitative care for patients with spinal cord injuries and other neurological disorders; developing a comprehensive database to track the success of activity-based therapies; identifying the optimal locomotor training regimens for specific patient populations; and maintaining an administrative network that can supply logistical, technical and personnel-based support for rehabilitaton programs.

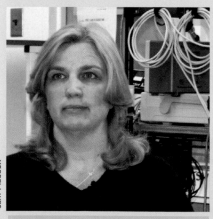

Sam Maddox

SUSAN HARKEMA, PH.D.

NRN Director Susan Harkema, PhD, of the Department of Neurological Surgery, Kentucky Spinal Cord Injury Research Center, University of Louisville and Frazier Rehab Institute, explains the methodology, and the science:

"We developed a model where you essentially move the legs of the person as they would when they were walking. It turns out, the nervous system can learn from that. So, by doing the activity that you want to learn, showing that to the nervous system by helping to move the legs, you're able to reteach, in a sense, the nervous system to do something that it did before the injury.

"We all know that the brain can learn, the brain can remember, the brain can forget and what's really accepted is that the brain tells the spinal cord what to do. Well, what was found in animal studies was that even without the brain, there were behaviors that showed the spinal cord could learn, could forget, could remember. And actually could make decisions. The spinal cord really is smarter than we think.

"And it's not only important for the recovery of standing and walking; it's important for other reasons. For example, cardiovascular changes that can occur after an injury; heart rate and blood pressures can change dramatically after spinal cord injury. We believe these can be improved with treadmill ambulation."

For more information about NRN, visit *www.christopherreeve.org*

When he was two, Chase Ford hit his head on a sofa arm. He gradually lost all function from the neck down. His parents were told that Chase would never walk again. The Fords learned about the CDRF NeuroRecovery Network locomotor training program in Louisville. After just one session, Chase began to move his legs. At four, he continues his therapy, and continues to gain function and sensation. In photo Chase zips across a New York stage to accept warm wishes at a CDRF event.

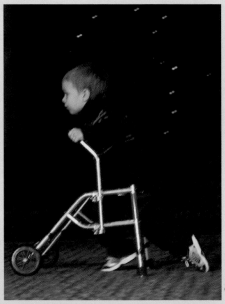

Denise Creiger

CHASE FORD

REHABILITATION RESOURCES

The American Occupational Therapy Association (AOTA) is a professional society that advances the field of occupational therapy through standard setting, advocacy, education and research. The American Occupational Therapy Association, 4720 Montgomery Lane, Bethesda, MD 20824; telephone 301–652–2682; or visit the Internet site *http://www.aota.org*

American Physical Therapy Association is the main membership organization for the PT profession, furthering the prevention, diagnosis and treatment of movement dysfunction. American Physical Therapy Association, 1111 North Fairfax Street, Alexandria, VA 22314; toll-free 1–800–999–2782; or visit *http://www.apta.org*

American Speech-Language-Hearing Association (ASHA) is the professional association for audiologists, speech-language pathologists, and speech, language and hearing scientists. American Speech-Language-Hearing Association, 10801 Rockville Pike, Rockville, MD 20852; toll-free 1–800–638–8255; or visit the Internet site *http://www.asha.org*

The American Therapeutic Recreation Association (ATRA) represents the interests of recreational therapists and promotes recreation as a means of improving health and well-being. The American Therapeutic Recreation Association, 1414 Prince Street Suite 204, Alexandria, VA 22314; telephone 703–683–9420; or visit the Internet site *http://www.atra-tr.org*

Association of Rehabilitation Nurses promotes and accredits rehab nurses and sets forth the philosophy of care of the nursing professional. Association of Rehabilitation Nurses, 4700 W. Lake Avenue, Glenview, IL 60025; toll-free 1–800–229–7530; or visit the Internet site *http://www.rehabnurse.org*

Commission on Accreditation of Rehabilitation Facilities (CARF) is an independent, nonprofit accrediting body that establishes rigorous standards to assure the quality, value and outcome of rehab services. CARF International, 4891 E. Grant Road, Tucson, AZ 85712; telephone 520–325–1044; or visit *http://www.carf.org*

The National Center for Medical Rehabilitation Research (NCMRR), a component of the National Institute of Child Health and Human Development (NICHD), supports research on enhancing the functioning of people with disabilities in daily life. NCMRR hopes to improve mobility, assess the effectiveness of various rehabilitation therapies and practices, develop improved assistive technology devices and train research scientists in the field of rehabilitation. NCMRR, 6100 Executive Boulevard, Room 2A03, MSC 7510, Bethesda, MD 20892; telephone 301–402–2242; on the Internet see *http://www.nichd.nih.gov/about/ncmrr/ncmrr.htm*

The National Institute on Disability and Rehabilitation Research (NIDRR) supports research aimed at improving the lives of individuals with disabilities from birth through adulthood. NIDRR's focus includes employment, health, technology, independent living and community integration. National Institute on Disability and Rehabilitation Research, 400 Maryland Avenue, S.W., Washington, DC 20202; telephone 202-205-8134; on the Internet see *http://www.ed.gov/about/offices/list/osers/nidrr*

Spinal Cord Injury Model Systems comprise 14 federally funded medical and/or rehabilitation centers across the United States. See page 43 for full list. The SCI Care System collects and studies acute, rehabilitation and follow-up data on approximately 25,000 people with SCI who received care in the centers since 1973. The Department of Rehabilitation Medicine in the School of Medicine at the University of Washington manages the Model Systems Knowledge Translation Center for the National Institute on Disability and Rehabilitation Research (NIDRR); visit the Internet site *http://www.mscisdisseminationcenter.org/*

Traumatic Brain Injury Model Systems consist of 16 comprehensive systems of care distributed throughout the United States. See page 13 for full list. These centers conduct research and provide "model" care to persons with traumatic brain injury. The Traumatic Brain Injury Model Systems National Data and Statistical Center is located at Craig Hospital in Englewood, Colorado. On the Internet see *http://www.tbindsc.org*.

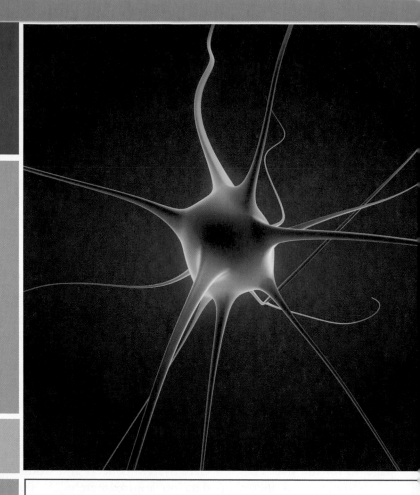

RESEARCH

Researchers are developing dozens of new therapies to treat symptoms, slow progression or even repair damage to the brain and spinal cord.

Paralysis is the result of some sort of disconnection between the central nervous system (the brain and spinal cord) and the body. Sometimes it's not hard to know why this happens, as in cases of stroke or trauma, wherein nerve cells are knocked out directly by extraordinary forces or events. In many other cases, including diseases such as multiple sclerosis or transverse myelitis, the breakdown of the nervous system comes from within, and this makes for a very complex mystery.

Hope for restoring function after paralysis continues to rise, and for good reason. Researchers in the United States and abroad are developing dozens of new therapies to treat symptoms, slow progression or even repair damage to the brain and spinal cord. These include drugs, cell transplants, growth factors, gene therapy, neural and new rehabilitation therapies. But paralysis from disease, stroke or trauma is still considered one of the toughest of medical problems. In fact, just over a generation ago, any damage to the brain and spinal cord that severely limited motor and/or sensory function was thought to be untreatable. In recent years, though, the word "cure" in this context has not only entered the vocabulary of the science community but also that of clinicians. Restorative neuroscience is bubbling with energy and expectation.

To be sure, scientific progress is a slow but steady march. One day in the not too distant future there will be some sort of procedure or treatment to mitigate the effects of paralysis. But it is not reasonable to expect a "magic bullet" for fully restoring function. Progress usually occurs in increments. Our knowledge of the nervous system extends far beyond what it was just a few years ago, but it's still quite limited. The brain and cord are incomprehensibly intricate — they are fragile tissues encased in bone, bathed in fluid and set apart from the rest of the body by the blood-brain barrier. Most importantly, these tissues on their own are unable to heal after injury.

While funding by federal grants, nonprofit groups, or even private biotech companies may be targeted toward specific diagnosis or cause of paralysis, there is a great deal of research overlap.

Understanding progressive nerve cell death relates to all neuro-logical disease or trauma categories; for example, ALS may share common biological mechanisms with Alzheimer's, Parkinson's and other neurodegenerative diseases. Understanding nervous system signaling mechanisms or the role of growth factors and cell support systems cuts across all areas of neuroscience. Stem-cell research holds much promise for all causes of nerve dysfunction. Indeed, there is tremendous expectation that stem-cell research holds "the" answer. While the stem-cell field is still in a fundamental data-gathering mode, many extraordinary claims are being made for these cells in the popular press and science literature, most of which have yet to be validated and few have moved to human clinical trials.

What follows is an overview of major research initiatives for several types of paralysis:

Amyotrophic Lateral Sclerosis Research: ALS (Lou Gehrig's disease) involves a cascade of cellular events leading to the death of neurons (called apoptosis). Research is keying in on several clues, including the role of excess glutamate (a chemical needed for nerve signal transmission), faulty mitochondria (the part of the 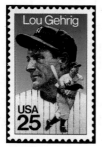 cell that provides energy), nerve cell transport problems (signals and growth factors transported by proteins) and the possible role of viruses. Here is a sample of some work being done to treat ALS:

Replacing damaged nerve cells is a tantalizing and hugely promising idea, one that has already been exploited by unscruplous psuedoclinics. It's not clear that new cells would resist the source of damage that caused ALS in the first place, but it seems that experimental stem cells can take on the identity of motor neurons and form function-restoring contacts with muscle. This could be because the stem cells act as delivery vehicles for neurotrophic factors, which are proteins found in the brain and muscle that support growth and survival of neurons. Although large-scale tests of several nerve growth factors failed to improve ALS symptoms, scientists continue working with other growth factors and new ways to deliver them. Insulin-like Growth Factor-1 (IGF-1, or myotrophin) is essential for normal development of the nervous system and appears to protect motor neurons in animal models. It is thought to block cell death pathways and pro mote muscle reinnervation and axonal growth and regeneration. Clinical trials have been inconclusive. Several biotech companies hope to establish enough clinical trial data for FDA approval to treat ALS.

A drug called arimoclomol, originally developed to treat diabetic complications, inhibits progression of ALS in a mouse model of the disease. Arimoclomol is thought to amplify "molecular chaperone" proteins, normally found in all cells of the body. These cells may in turn boost a motor nerve cell's protection against toxic proteins, repairing those that are believed to cause diseases such as ALS. Arimoclomol appears to accelerate the regeneration of previously damaged nerves in animals. Early phase clinical trials have shown the drug to be safe in humans; more tests are planned for dose and treatment.

Drug cocktails: Recent mouse model studies of ALS showed dramatic benefits using a combination of drugs, including riluzole (the only drug now approved by the FDA to treat ALS), nimodipine (a calcium channel blocker used in the treatment of acute stroke and migraine headache) and minocycline (an antibiotic that may block inflammation). The compounds given together appear to delay cell death, prevent nerve cell loss and reduce inflammation. Scientists are looking at other drugs that help nerve cells survive, including protease inhibitors that prevent cell death and antiviral drugs. Several people with HIV and ALS showed improvement (two with complete recovery) after taking an "AIDS cocktail" drug that targets viruses. This supports the theory that ALS might be caused by a virus.

Drugs approved by the FDA for other reasons are being tested in ALS. The breast cancer drug tamoxifen (Nolvadex) has also shown benefit in ALS tests with mice; clinical trials are ongoing. Previous research has shown that an immune-system compound TNF-alpha is elevated in ALS. Thalidomide, a drug which was notorious 40 years ago for causing birth defects in women who took it for morning sickness, may reduce the synthesis of TNF-alpha. Minocycline, an antibiotic, is being studied for its

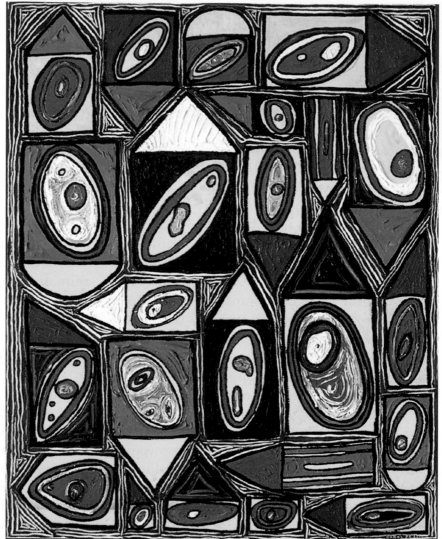

MYELIN HOUSES
16 x 20 INCHES, OIL ON CANVAS

"I AM A HOUSE OF RIDICULOUS NERVE, SILLY IDEAS, CURIOSITY,
ANGER, LOVE AND PAIN. I REFUSE TO BE NUMB.
MY AXONS ARE MADE FROM CREATIVITY. IF THE SHEATH WEARS
AWAY, WATCH OUT! I WILL MOVE INTO YOUR NEIGHBORHOOD AND SHAKE
SHIT UP WITH MY FLARE-UPS OF VISIONS AND IMAGINATION!"

- CAROL ES

antiinflamatory effect in ALS. Ceftriaxone is another antibiotic getting a look for ALS. It appears to have an effect on glutamate, a nerve messenger suspected to have a role in the disease process.

A drug called Neurodex (dextromethorphan/quinidine) is in clinical trials for the treatment of emotional lability (unwanted laughing and crying) in people with ALS. Trials are also continuing for creatine, a naturally occurring chemical involved in the energy metabolism of muscle, which may help people with ALS.

Umbilical cord blood/stem cells: Animal research suggests a clinical role for intravenous umbilical cord blood/stem cells and in some clinics these cells are already being provided to people with ALS. There have been no conclusive, long-term safety tests or beneficial results reported. Some people have told the ALS Association of their improved strength and function after the infusion. ALSA has set aside funds for further study.

Cerebral Palsy Research: Biomedical research has led to better prevention of cerebral palsy and to better diagnosis and treat people with CP. About 70 percent of cerebral palsy occurs prior to birth; 20 percent occurs in the birthing process; and 10 percent occurs during the first two years of life. Risk factors have been identified in each of these situations and include intrauterine infection, bleeding in the brain, seizures, breathing and circulation problems, and stroke, trauma or other causes of damage to the brain of the unborn baby. Certain conditions known to cause cerebral palsy include rubella (German measles) and jaundice; these can now be prevented or treated.

Low birth-weight babies are 100 times more likely to develop CP than normal weight infants. Scientists are looking for ways to reduce this risk factor, including a closer look at the role of tobacco, alcohol, prescription drugs (e.g., antidepressants), environmental toxins, etc. Researchers are also learning how to monitor the function or loss of function in the brain of the fetus while still in the mother's uterus, with the goal in mind for intervention before birth.

The role of cytokines is an active research area. Cytokines are chemical messages that regulate the metabolism of a cell and other tissues and influence their activity (i.e., activate immune system cells). Cytokines, released in response to bacterial invasion, low levels of oxygen (hypoxia), and decreased blood flow (ischemia) play a role in the cascade of events that lead to developmental brain injury; their early detection can be important in preventing brain damage in newborns.

Researchers are exploring early interventions such as hypothermic therapy (cooling), which has shown experimentally to reverse brain injury similar to that seen in CP infants. Other promising therapies include the administration of growth or trophic factors and the use of stem cells. There have been cases reported of parents taking children with CP to clinics in Mexico and abroad for stem cell treatments; there is insufficient data to support this.

There have also been many reports in the media of the effectiveness of using a baby's umbilical cord blood (by transfusion) as a treatment for CP. This is another active area of study.

Hyperbaric oxygen continues to be looked at to treat CP, stroke or brain injury. Some clinics and manufacturers promote its use for CP but there is no consensus that it is effective.

Better brain imaging and gait analysis has led to better physical, psychological and behavioral therapies. Medications, surgery and braces can often improve nerve and muscle coordination, help treat secondary medical problems and reduce contractures and deformities. Physical therapy is widely used to manage cerebral palsy; evidence is emerging to help doctors or parents choose the best approach. Elastic body suits (e.g. Therasuit) seem to help kids with CP develop muscle strength; constraint-induced movement therapy (restricting a stronger limb to improve the other) also shows benefits for some kids. Body-weight supported gait training and functional electric stimulation are also being studied.

Multiple Sclerosis Research: MS is a disease of the immune system; the body in effect turns against itself, setting forth a process that destroys the insulation on nerve fibers called myelin. Without this lining, nerve fibers cannot conduct signals. There are two main lines of research in MS—first, to alter the function to the immune system itself. This might stop or slow progressive MS and allow self-repair of damaged nerves. The second line of work aims to replace or regrow myelin on nerves. Progress is

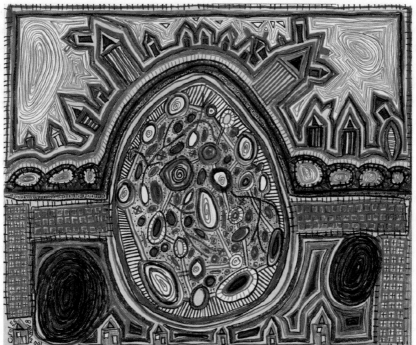

© Painting by Carol Es, www.esart.com

CELLS AND HOUSES
14 x 17 INCHES, MIXED MEDIA ON PAPER, 2001

"I BELIEVE WE OCCUPY OUR BODIES MUCH THE SAME WAY WE LIVE INSIDE A HOUSE. GOOD CELLS AND BAD CELLS ALIKE, WE LIVE TOGETHER AND ARE BOTH GROWING AND DYING AT THE SAME TIME. IT'S HUMBLING AND BEAUTIFUL."   - CAROL ES

being made in both areas.

Until recently, the primary treatments for MS were anti-inflammatory steroids, which don't alter the course of MS but can reduce the duration and severity of attacks in some people. Because of adverse side effects (acne, weight gain, seizures, psychosis), steroids are not recommended for long-term use.

There are now six approved drugs on the U.S. market for people with the more common forms of MS. Avonex, Betaseron, Copaxone, Novantrone, Rebif and most recently, Tysabri act in various ways to suppress the immune system; these drugs, which range in cost from $15,000 to $40,000 a year, are only modestly effective and can be associated with side effects (flu-like symptoms, depression and toxicity), often causing people to delay or stop taking them. (Most drug companies have programs to assist eligible patients who cannot afford these treatments.) In the search for drugs that are easier to tolerate, scientists have begun combination trials. For example, Copaxone plus albuterol, a common asthma medicine, might work better than Copaxone alone. Other combination trials include Avonex plus methylprednisolone (a steroid), Avonex plus Prozac (an antidepressant with immune system effects), Betaseron plus Copaxone, and Novantrone plus Betaseron, etc.

Numerous other trials testing for better MS treatments are occurring. Here are a few:

- Rituxan, a drug that is already used to treat cancer and rheumatoid arthritis, reduced by more than half the chance that people with MS would have symptom flare ups over a six-month period. Early studies also showed that people taking Rituxan had fewer brain lesions than those on placebo.
- The immune system modulator fingolimod reduced the number of lesions detected on MRI and also reduced disease activity in MS patients. Large scale clinical trials continue.
- Immune system defenders called T cells erode myelin by producing small chemical signals (cytokines) that activate cells known as macrophages, which destroy the myelin. A manmade antibody called Zenapax (approved for use in people with kidney transplants) attaches itself to the rogue T cells, blocking their role in the damage process. Results have been encouraging in early relapsing/remitting MS trials.
- Rolipram, developed as an antidepressant, has been shown to reduce levels of several destructive cytokines in animal models of MS with minimal side effects.
- Interleukin 4 (IL-4) appears to reduce demyelination and improve the symptoms of mice with an MS-like disease called experimental allergic encephalomyelitis (EAE), apparently by influencing T cells to become more protective than harmful.
- Oral estradiol, a form of the female sex hormone estrogen, protects mice from developing an MS-like disease. It apparently inhibits movement of immune cells into the brain and blocks cytokines related to inflammation.

- Antibiotics against infection may decrease MS disease activity. Various infectious agents have been proposed as potential causes for MS, including Epstein-Barr virus, herpes virus and coronaviruses. Minocycline (an antibiotic) showed promising results in early trails with relapsing–remitting MS.

Plasmapheresis is a procedure in which a person's blood is removed to separate plasma from other blood substances that may contain antibodies and other immune-sensitive products. The purified plasma is then transfused back into the patient. Plasmapheresis is used to treat myasthenia gravis, Guillain-Barré and other demyelinating diseases. Studies of plasmapheresis in people with primary and secondary progressive MS have had mixed results. It may only be effective for acute attacks.

Bone marrow transplantation has also been studied in MS. It is a high-risk and expensive procedure in which marrow from a healthy donor is infused into a person who has undergone drug or radiation therapy. It suppresses the immune system so the recipient will not reject the donated marrow.

Scientists are hoping to develop an MS vaccine. If myelin-attacking T cells are removed, inactivated and injected back into animals with EAE, the immune system cells attacking myelin basic protein are destroyed. In a couple of small human trials, the vaccine was well tolerated and had no side effects, although benefits did not last beyond two years.

On the cellular level, the MS process causes oxidation, which damages cells. Researchers are looking at natural anti-oxidants, including ginkgo biloba, alpha-lipoic acid/essential fatty acids and vitamin E/selenium as potential treatments.

Remyelinization: Several people with MS have undergone a procedure that transplants their own Schwann cells—the cells that produce myelin in the peripheral nervous system—into their brains with the hopes that the Schwann cells will remyelinate the nerves damaged by the disease. The transplants were tolerated; no results were released on whether they were beneficial.

Other studies are focusing on ways to reverse the damage to myelin and oligodendrocytes (the cells that make and maintain myelin in the central nervous system), both of which are destroyed during MS attacks. Oligodendrocytes proliferate and form new myelin after an attack; certain monoclonal antibodies and immunosuppressant drugs (e.g., cyclophosphamide and azathioprine) may accelerate remyelination; steroids may inhibit it.

There is excitement about stem cells in treating MS. There is experimental work being done with embryonic stem cells, olfactory ensheathing glia (a type of adult stem cell) and with umbilical cord blood stem cells. Some clinics outside the U.S. offer treatments with various cell lines; no solid data exists to evaluate these clinics.

There are many other areas of research for treatments for MS, including the use of bee venom, testosterone and thalidomide.

Polio Research: Polio is caused by a virus that attacks certain motor neurons. Until recently, research was mainly in the rehabilitation and symptom management areas, especially in light of increasing fatigue, pain and premature aging many years after the initial infection. There are also several viral theories for so-called Post Polio Syndrome (PPS), hypothesizing that the old poliovirus has been quietly hiding in the central nervous system or that it has mutated into a new reactivated form that destroys nerve tissue. There has been no conclusive evidence of a virus. Other causes of PPS, such as an immune response, hormone deficiencies and environmental toxins, have also been suggested.

Nerve growth factor and stem cell research may yield additional treatment options for polio survivors in the future. A drug called Insulin-like Growth Factor (IGF-1) is being tested to see if it can enhance the ability of motor neurons to sprout new branches, maintain existing branches and rejuvenate nerve synapses, the space between nerve cells where signals pass from one cell to another. It is postulated that stem cells could be coaxed to become motor neurons and replace, or restore, damaged cells in people with polio.

Supplements are also being investigated. Creatine and carnitine have helped some people with PPS and have shown benefits in research trials.

Spina Bifida Research: Research regarding spina bifida has in large part been focused on prevention. The push in recent years

THE MACHINE-BODY MERGER

The merging of machine and body is not science fiction, it's already happening. A neural prosthesis replaces or supplements nerve function by directly connecting with the nervous system. Over the years such devices have been wired into people with paralysis to help them stand and ambulate, grasp things with the fingers, control bowel and bladder and even control computers using only brain power.

At this time there is but one commercially available neural prosthetic device on the U.S. market, the Parastep system, a device that allows paraplegics to ambulate (*www.sigmedics.com*, see p. 240)

Two other FDA approved commercial devices, one that facilitated a hand-grasp in quads (Freehand), and one that allowed bladder control via an external switch (Vocare), were recently pulled from the American market due to high costs and low reimbursement rates. The bladder device is still available in Europe (called the FineTech-Brindley).

The Neural Prosthesis Program of the National Institute of Neurological Disorders and Stroke supports the development of aids for people with neurological disorders. On the Internet, see *http://npp.ninds.nih.gov/npp*.

The Cleveland FES Center studies the use of electrical currents to produce and control the movement of otherwise paralyzed limbs. See *http://fescenter.case.edu*

For an overview of many other high-tech solutions for enhancing mobility and function, see the Neurotech Network, formed by Jennifer French, a C7 quad who is flitted with a device that allows her to stand and pivot from her wheelchair. On the Internet, *www.neurotechnetwork.org*

Brain control: scientists have the ability to decode the brain signals for limb and hand movements so they can be controlled by thoughts alone. Working a computer by thought is being done. Human trials for BrainGate continue; see *www.cyberkineticsinc.com*

by the federal government to add the B vitamin folate to the diets of women of child-bearing age (including a mandate from the FDA that enriched bread, rice and cereal-grain products be fortified with folic acid) has decreased the incidence of neural tube birth defects, such as spina bifida, by about 23 percent. Studies have shown that if all women who could become pregnant were to take a multivitamin with folic acid, the risk of neural tube defects could be reduced by up to 75 percent.

The incidence of spina bifida has also decreased due to better diagnostic tests and early detection; many parents make the decision to interrupt the pregnancy.

Researchers are looking for the genes linked to a predisposition to spina bifida. They are also exploring the complex mechanisms of normal brain development to determine what goes wrong with the neural tube in spina bifida.

Since the 1930s, the first step in the treatment of babies with this condition has been to surgically close the opening in their back within a few days of birth. The surgery puts the tissues back in their normal position and prevents further damage to the nervous tissue; it does not restore function to the already damaged nerves.

In recent years, some doctors have begun operating on babies with spina bifida before they are born. Nerve function in babies with spina bifida seems to worsen through the course of pregnancy. Movement that can be observed in the legs and feet on a sonogram cannot be seen later in the pregnancy. This progressive pattern of damage to the spinal cord may be caused by contact with amniotic fluid. It suggests intervention as early as possible.

A five-year Management of Myelomeningocele Study (MOMS, funded by The National Institute of Child Health and Human Development) continues at three centers in the United States to compare the two approaches: surgery before birth (prenatal or fetal surgery) and surgery after birth (postnatal surgery).

Many children with spina bifida, up to 70 percent, may have symptoms related to a tethered cord (the cord and its membranes stick together, restricting spinal cord growth and spinal fluid movement). Better surgical techniques are available to treat this, thus reducing pain and weakness and improving bowel and bladder function. Untethering must sometimes be repeated over time.

Spinal Cord Injury Research: The biology of the injured spinal cord is enormously complex. Scientists are following numerous leads and are hopeful that laboratory experiments that seem to help animals will promote recovery in people with spinal cord trauma. The strategies for treating SCI can be categorized in six main areas: nerve protection, nerve rejuvenation, bridging, cell replacement, regeneration and rehabilitation. Here is a snapshot of the work being done in each area.

Nerve protection: As in the case of brain trauma or stroke, the initial damage to spinal cord cells is followed by a series of biochemical events that often wipe out other nerve cells in the area of the injury. Soon after injury, the spinal cord swells and proteins from the immune system invade the injured zone. The steroid drug methylprednisolone (MP) is the only FDA approved treatment for acute SCI; it is believed to reduce inflammation if people get the drug within eight hours of injury. The medical community is not entirely sold on the effectiveness of MP; research is underway to find a better acute drug.

Several trials are underway in what is called the subacute timeframe (generally, within three weeks of injury).

With partial funding from CDRF, Dr. Martin Schwab led a team of Swiss scientists to discover a protein in the myelin of spinal cord axons that caused the tips of axons that came near it to collapse and stop dead in their tracks. Schwab called this inhibitor Nogo and found that it acts by binding to a receptor molecule in the membrane of the growth cone. He eventually figured out how to block Nogo. An antibody to Nogo was found to enhance collateral sprouting and possibly axon regeneration in animals with SCI. The pharmaceutical company Novartis performed a Phase I open label (not controlled, not blinded) clinical trial in Europe, injecting the antibody (ATI-355) into the spinal fluid soon after injury. So far the drug has not caused major side effects so a Phase II trial is on the way.

Cordaneurin subacute trial: Soon after injury the spinal cord body forms a scar which blocks injured nerve cells from regrowing naturally. Cordaneurin, developed by German biotech company Neuraxo, prevents scar formation, enabling the injured nerves to regenerate over long distances in their natural nerve tract. Trials are expected in 2009. See *www.neuraxo.com*

A subacute treatment is underway involving placement electrical fields near the injury site; scientists hope to promote cellular health and nerve fiber (axon) growth. In earlier trials, participants implanted with a electric field device showed some improvement in sensation at six months and one year post surgery. For details see *www.cyberkineticsinc.com*

Cethrin is a recombinant protein that blocks the activity of rho, a signaling molecule that triggers cell death and damage after SCI. Tests in animals found that Cethrin promotes neural regeneration. In an early human trial (acute SCI, less than 15 days post injury), 31 percent of patients recovered some sensory and/or motor function below the level of their injury and converted from complete to incomplete injury. For more detail on this trial see Alseres Pharmaceutical, *http://www.alseres.com/*

Stem cells in the acute setting: The biotech firm Geron plans to begin human clinical trials for oligodendrocytes derived from human embryonic stem cells to potentially treat acute spinal cord injuries. Animal tests have shown these cells be effective.

Nerve rejuvenation: Many neurons survive spinal cord trauma but are weakened and can't conduct nerve signals properly. This is often because they have lost their myelin—the fatty, white insulation around axons. Several strategies have been considered for restoring demyelinated nerves. One is to replace or restore myelin so nerve conduction can occur normally. This is tough to do, since myelin in the central nervous system does not readily rebuild itself; it must be "seeded" with transplanted cells or cultivated using growth factors. In animal experiments, myelin-forming transplants have been enhanced using genetically modified Schwann cells that excrete growth factors.

Another pathway to remyelination is to find the "switch" to turn on the body's own myelin machinery. Researchers are working on ways to encourage support cells called oligodendrocytes to make new myelin. Mice with myelin damage caused by a virus were given injections of several different immune-system proteins (antibodies). Those that received certain antibodies or immunoglobulins showed more signs of myelin repair in their spinal cords than those given a placebo.

Rejuvenating central nerves is possible by adjusting the neurochemistry of the system to compensate for poor conduction. This is the basis for using 4-AP, a drug that basically boosts impulse conduction. Thousands of people with spinal cord injury and multiple sclerosis are already getting 4-AP by prescription from certain "compounding" pharmacies. A much more sophisticated, time-release version of 4-AP (known as fampridine) from the biotech company Acorda Therapeutics awaits FDA approval for people with MS. The drug works in one of three people—doctors can't predict who will benefit or what the effect will be until a person tries it. Some people report dramatic improvement in strength and sensation, reduced fatigue, better bladder function and, in some cases, reduced pain and spasticity and improved sexual function. Side effects may include dizziness, insomnia, numbness/tingling and, in higher doses, seizures. See *www.acorda.com*

Bridging: The idea of a bridge is conceptually easy—transplanted nerves or cells fill the damaged area of the cord (often a scar-lined cyst) and thus allow nerves of the spinal cord to cross through otherwise inhospitable terrain. In 1981, Canadian scientist Albert Aguayo showed that spinal cord axons could grow long distances using a bridge made of peripheral nerve, proving without doubt that axons will grow if they have the right environment. A variety of techniques has evolved through experiments to create a growth-enhancing environment, including the use of fetal tissue, stem cells, cells called olfactory ensheathing glia (OEG) that come from the upper nose, and Schwann cells.

Trials are going on now to test the safety and efficacy of OEG cells in Australia and China, and a doctor in Portugal is treating patients with OEG cells. In Beijing, hundreds of fetal OEG transplants (reportedly using fetal OEG cells) have been performed in people (many from the U.S.). These procedures are not part of any kind of controlled trial. The results have not been published in peer reviewed journals and there is no good evidence that patients have benefited. It is important to know what became of these transplanted cells; given the experimental evidence in animals, it is very unlikely that they became neurons.

Professir X

Back when I got injured almost 20 years ago, I was deejaying. Being that I loved music and hip hop, I had to find another way of doing it. So, a friend of mine coached me to write rhymes and to rap. It was hard for me to breathe, but he used to see me arguing with my sister; he told me to use that same energy I had when I was upset in my rapping. So, I learned how to use that energy – that determination – to get my points across and to write rhymes and rap

At one time, the music I wrote wasn't about cures. It wasn't about hope. It was about being angry and I was using that as my way of dealing with paralysis. But, Christopher and Dana opened my eyes to a new way of writing rhymes. I started with a tribute to Christopher and then I heard all the scientists talk about how hard their work is. So, I said I'm going to make songs that talk about unity and everybody getting together: the scientists, the community. We all have to be able to come together to get the funding for the research. So, with my music, I use it as part of my inner healing as well as a way to inspire other people to heal themselves. See *www.professirx.com*

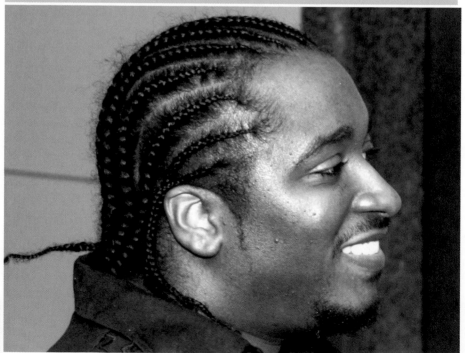

SAM MADDOX

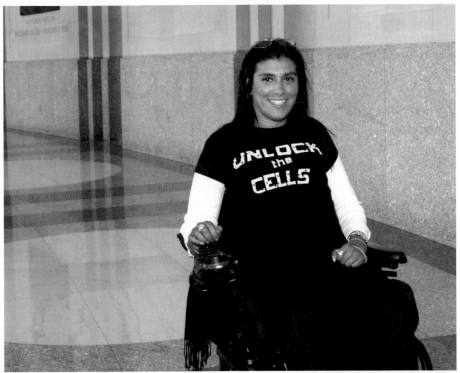

SAM MADDOX

Sabrina Cohen

We live in one of the most advanced countries in the world. Yet, when it comes to scientific research, politics is getting in the way of finding possible medical breakthroughs that could revolutionize the medical world. It's sad to hear that scientists are leaving the field because there's no money. That really sheds light on why medical research, like stem cell research, is so important and why we need to move this forward. This research is not just for paralysis but for many other diseases as well.

I've basically devoted my life to advocating and trying to advance stem cell research. I've been going around speaking to different medical facilities and colleges and educating everybody and anybody that I meet about this issue. I also have gone to the politicians and asked them to please consider helping us get the funding that we need. There are 128 million Americans in this country who are currently affected by a disease or an injury. I represent just one of them. I started a campaign "Free the Stem Cells," to educate people on the subject and fight for more funding. See *www.sabrinacohenfoundation.org*

In a spinal cord injury, stem cells might have the potential to form bridges at sites of injury over which injured connections (axons) could extend. See pages 176 - 177 for more on stem cells.

Schwann cells are support cells of peripheral nerves that contribute substantially to repair after injury. Several researchers have shown that transplants of Schwann cells to the spinal cord can support the regrowth of connections (axons) after spinal cord injury. Still, functional recovery is only modest. Combining Schwann cells with growth factors may ultimately be more useful than transplants of Schwann cells alone. For example, a team at the Miami Project found that Schwann cells alone activated nerves to grow into a bridge but they stopped short of crossing the gap in the injured spinal cord. By adding OEG cells to the Schwann cells, the axons crossed the bridge and entered the spinal cord on the other side of the lesion.

Cell replacement: Stem cells from embryonic sources have tremendous potential to repopulate spinal cord cells. It also seems possible that stem cells harvested from one's own body can be coaxed to take on new identities. OEG cells, fetal tissue, umbilical cord blood and even cells from other species have been used experimentally in animals with SCI in an attempt to restore function.

Regeneration: This is perhaps the toughest of the treatment possibilities. To restore major sensation and motor control after injury, the long axons in the white matter of the spinal cord have to grow again and connect over long distances—as much as two feet—to precise targets. It is important to note, however, that only about 10 percent of damaged axons need to be reconnected to restore significant function. Central nervous system axons cannot regenerate unless their path is cleared of poisons, enriched with vitamins and paved with an attractive roadbed. By blocking inhibitory factors (proteins that stop axon growth in its tracks), adding nutrients and supplying a matrix to grow on, researchers have indeed grown spinal nerves over long distances.

A growth factor called NT-3 appears to boost the growth activity of the long axons needed for motor function. Another growth factor that shows potential is leukemia inhibitory factor (LIF), which also appears to promote the growth of spinal cord axons needed for motor activity.

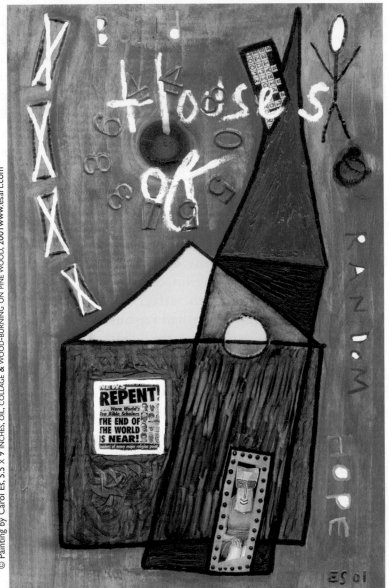

RANDOM HOPE

"IN EVERY DARK HOUR I HAVE EXPERIENCED, JUST WHEN I BEGAN TO BELIEVE THERE WERE NO IMPORTANT REASONS TO GO ON, IDEAS AND GOALS WOULD MOVE THROUGH MY MIND - LIKE THE SUN PARTING THE CLOUDS, IF JUST FOR A FAINT MOMENT. THESE ARE RANDOM HOUSES OF HOPE THAT EMBRACE ME LIKE A PARENT, JUST WHEN I NEED IT MOST. HOPE CAN MAKE YOU STRONG. THE MORE THE BETTER. IT IS THE STUFF THAT MAKE MY IDEAS HAPPEN." - CAROL ES

Gene therapy has the potential to deliver growth factors where they are needed: for example, skin cells can be genetically engineered to produce large quantities of growth factors. These modified cells can then be placed into sites of spinal cord injury. As a result, injured axons eagerly grow into the enriched territory.

Substrate and guidance molecules may improve targeting once axons have been encouraged to regenerate past the lesion site. These proteins act as roadmaps and scaffolds, steering axons to their correct targets and providing a framework for new growth. These are critical functions because even if axons do survive, they must be coaxed to reconnect with the correct targets.

Rehabilitation: Almost any treatment to restore function after paralysis will require a physical component to rebuild muscle, build bone and reactivate patterns of movement. Some form of rehab will be needed after function comes back. Moreover, it appears that activity itself can affect recovery: In 2002, Christopher Reeve showed that he had regained limited function and sensation after many years of paralysis. His doctor credits his use of functional electrical stimulation, which may have kick-started the repair process, and a program of passive electrical stimulation, aqua therapy and passive standing.

Separately, Reeve also used treadmill training, a therapy that forces the legs to move in a pattern of walking as the body is suspended in a harness above a moving treadmill. The theory is that the spinal cord itself has a "brain" called a central pattern generator (CPG) that, independent of brain input, activates the pattern of locomotion. After a prolonged period of inactivity and what scientists call "learned nonuse," the neuronal circuits needed for walking are in effect turned off. Stepping during treadmill training sends repeated sensory information to the CPG, reminding the spinal cord how to step. Scientists describe the reactivation due to stepping as plasticity—the nervous system is not "hard wired" and appears to have the ability to adapt itself to new stimulation. Treadmill training, currently being studied in clinical trials in the United States, enables some people with spinal cord injuries to recover significant function. For more, see *www.christopherreeve.org*, search for Neural Recovery Network. See also page 138.

Spinal Tumor Research: Malignant cancers of the brain or spinal cord (called tumors or gliomas) are very challenging to treat. Despite decades of advances in surgery, radiation therapy and drug development, the prognosis for people with these tumors hasn't changed much. Studies have not been translated to the clinic, partly due to the huge variety of tumor types and the relative difficulty in gathering patients, young or old, for clinical trials. Progress has been slow but that may change as the molecular mechanism of cancer becomes clearer and as new agents that target tumors while preserving normal tissue come into play.

Radiation remains the primary treatment for malignant tumors, although the overall outcome of this therapy is not always good. Researchers are looking for better ways to target radiation or enhance its effectiveness, perhaps by making tumor tissue more vulnerable to radiation. Researchers are studying brachytherapy (small radioactive pellets implanted directly into the tumor) as the optimum way to deliver radiotherapy to the tumor while sparing surrounding normal tissues.

Some cells within tumors are quite resistant to radiation. Using a gene therapy approach, scientists hope to kill these cells by inserting a "suicide" gene that could make the tumor cells sensitive to certain drugs or program the cancerous cells to self-destruct.

Blocking the formation of blood vessels (angiogenesis) is a very promising new tool for the treatment of various cancers. Since brain tumors are the most angiogenic of all cancers, blocking their blood supply might prove to be especially effective.

The gamma knife is a newer tool that provides a precisely focused beam of radiation energy that delivers a single dose of radiation on target. The gamma knife does not require a surgical incision; doctors have found it can help them reach and treat some small tumors that are not accessible through surgery.

Since tumors are more sensitive to heat than normal tissue, scientists are testing hyperthermia as a treatment by placing special heat-producing antennae into the tumor region.

While scientists are trying to understand why some nervous system tissues become cancerous, they are also looking for ways to duplicate or enhance the body's immune response to fight against brain and spinal cord cancer.

CLINICAL TRIALS

Drugs and treatments are developed—or as the research community says it, "translated" from laboratory experiments. Clinical research is usually conducted via a series of trials that begin with a few people and become progressively larger as safety and efficacy are better understood.

Because full-scale clinical trials are expensive and time consuming, only the most promising of many treatments emerging from research labs are selected in the translation process. A National Institute of Neurological Disorders and Stroke panel noted that future trials on treating paralysis should be based on minimum risk with significant benefit in a relevant animal model that has been independently replicated by other labs. Questions remain as to what the minimal clinical improvement would be to warrant various levels of risk and expectation.

Once laboratory and animal studies show promise, a Phase I clinical trial is initiated. Phase I is primarily used to test the safety of a therapy for a particular disease or condition.

A Phase II clinical trial usually involves more subjects at several different centers and is used to test safety and efficacy on a broader scale, such as to test different dosing for medications or to perfect techniques for surgery.

A Phase III clinical trial involves many centers and sometimes hundreds of subjects. The trial usually involves two patient groups comparing different treatments, or, if there is only one treatment to test, patients who do not receive the test therapy get a placebo (dummy drug) instead.

Many Phase III trials are double-blinded and randomized. Double-blind means that neither the subjects nor the doctors treating them know which treatment a subject receives. Randomization refers to the placing of subjects into one of the treatment groups in a way that can't be predicted by the patients or investigators.

Phase IV is carried out after approval in order to detect possible rare undesirable side effects which had escaped attention in the previous phases.

Informed Consent: The government has strict safeguards to protect people who participate in clinical trials. Every clinical trial in the United States must be approved and monitored by an Institutional Review Board (IRB), an independent committee of physicians, statisticians, community advocates, and others who assess risk and ensure that the trial is ethical and that the rights of study participants are protected.

Informed consent is about the learning the key facts about a clinical trial before you decide whether or not to participate. These facts include why the research is being done; who the researchers are; what the researchers want to accomplish; what will be done during the trial and for how long; what risks and what benefits can be expected; what are the possible side effects? Informed consent continues as long as you are in the study.

Before joining a clinical trial, participants must meet the study's eligibility guidelines, such as age, type of disease, medical history, and current medical condition. People may leave a trial at any time.

NACTN: To help select and move promising therapies from the lab to the clinic, the Christopher and Dana Reeve Foundation has formed the North American Clinical Trials Network, a group of eight clinical research centers and a biostatistical center.

The Network is collaborating with a similar-minded European consortium to define the natural history of spinal cord injury, create an international database of carefully selected spinal cord injured persons, and fine-tune what are now considered rather crude outcome measures for treatment. By building the infrastructure for a global cross-collaboration, it is expected that the network will speed therapeutic development based on the best evidence available. For more, contact *http://www.christopherreeve.org,*

Source: National Institutes of Health

For information about clinical trials taking place in the United States (search by condition or diagnosis), see *http://clinicaltrials.gov* or *http://www.centerwatch.com.* Be cautious before joining a trial or seeking an experimental treatment. See *www.icord.org/iccp.html*

Stroke Research: In fact a "brain attack," stroke occurs when the blood supply to part of the brain is suddenly blocked or when a blood vessel in the brain bursts, spilling blood into the spaces surrounding brain cells. Some brain cells die immediately; others remain at risk for hours and even days due to an ongoing sequence of destruction. Some damaged cells can be saved by early intervention with drugs. The search for so-called neuroprotective drugs, ongoing for more than a decade, has been difficult and frustrating, as one drug after another that showed great promise in animal studies and early human trials was found ineffective in large-scale clinical studies.

Meanwhile, the only approved clot-busting treatment, tPA (tissue plasminogen activator), is underutilized: Only 3–5 percent of those who have a stroke reach the hospital in time (less than three hours) to be considered for this treatment. It also carries a significant risk of death due to internal bleeding. New delivery methods and refinements of tPA are being developed, including intra-arterial tPA, which is infused into a main artery in the neck or even smaller arteries in the brain for faster, safer delivery.

Here are some of the research leads for treating stroke:

- An enzyme (DSPA) found in saliva from vampire bats may help dissolve blood clots in the brain for stroke survivors. This enzyme may be much more potent than existing anticoagulant drugs and may cause fewer bleeding problems because it only targets the clot itself.
- A drug called PP1, if given within six hours of stroke, protects mice from brain damage by blocking activity of a family of molecules called Src, which increase leakiness of blood vessels.
- Erythropoietin, a hormone produced by the kidney, appears to protect some neurons from executing genetically programmed "cell suicide" missions.
- A protein called fibronectin may protect against serious brain damage from stroke.
- Stroke-related bleeding in the brain unleashes dangerously high amounts of a brain chemical called glutamate, normally used for brain cell communication. Too much glutamate triggers the release of more toxic chemicals. Several drugs are known to block glutamate.

- A large multi-center clinical trial is investigating whether taking amphetamines for several weeks after stroke will help kick-start the process of self-repair in the brain.
- For many years, doctors have relied on warfarin, a drug with potentially dangerous side effects (it is also used as rat poison), to reduce the risk of stroke in people at risk for clotting in the heart. A newer drug, ximelagatran, is now being tested and appears effective and safer than warfarin.

Neural cell transplantation has shown some early-trial success in humans with small strokes. To be sure, there is great excitement for stem cells as a stroke treatment:

- A Korean team reported that human neural stem cells transplanted intravenously into adult rats during the chronic stage of cerebral ischemia migrated, became neurons and brought about functional improvement.
- Researchers at the University of Minnesota reported that transplanted adult stem cells (from bone marrow) restored function in laboratory animals with stroke.
- A British biotech company called ReNeuron has injected nerve stem-cells to the site of damage in the brain. In animal models, the new cells appear to replace the injured cells with healthy ones of the same type. The company has plans for human trials in stroke, Parkinson's disease, Huntington's disease and Type 1 diabetes. See *www.reneuron.com*
- Human umbilical cord blood cells injected into the tails of rats migrated to the animals' brains within hours after a stroke and apparently began repairing damage. Rats treated within 24 hours after a stroke had much greater recovery, and even animals treated one week after stroke showed improvement.

Research advances have led to new therapies and new hope for people who are at risk or who have had a stroke. For example, the Heart Outcomes Prevention Evaluation (HOPE) study found a 33 percent reduction in stroke in diabetics who were given the hypertension drug ramipril. Treatment with statins (cholesterol lowering drugs) decreases the risk of stroke as well as heart attacks in people with known coronary heart disease.

A clinical trial is now underway to test the safety and effectiveness of a protein called E-selectin, administered by way of a nasal spray, to prevent the formation of blood clots that could cause stroke. Animals that received E-selectin had almost no strokes compared with those that did not receive it.

The National Institute of Neurological Disorders and Stroke (NINDS) has initiated a program called Specialized Programs of Translational Research in Acute Stroke (SPOTRIAS). The goal is to reduce the disability of and mortality in stroke survivors by promoting rapid diagnosis and effective interventions. In the area of stroke rehabilitation, an approach called constraint-induced movement-based therapy has improved the recovery of people who have lost some function in a single limb. The therapy entails immobilizing a patient's good limb to force use of the weakened limb.

Traumatic Brain Injury (TBI) Research: The brain is quite fragile, though it is protected by hair, skin and skull, as well as a cushion of fluid. In the past, this protection was mostly adequate, until we developed more lethal weapons and new ways of hurtling along at high speeds.

Brain injury comprises many conditions depending on which part of the brain is injured. A blow to the hippocampus causes memory loss. A brainstem injury is similar to a high spinal cord injury. Injury to the basal ganglia affects movement, and damage to the frontal lobes can lead to emotional problems. Injury to certain parts of the cortex affects speech and understanding. Each symptom may require specialized care and treatment.

A brain injury also involves many physiological processes, including nerve cell (axon) injury, contusions (bruises), hematomas (clots) and swelling. As in stroke, SCI and other types of nerve trauma, brain injury is not an isolated process, it is a continuous event; waves of destruction can last days and even weeks after the initial damage. To repair the original injury, which may include massive loss of nerve cells, is yet beyond the realm of medicine. The spread of secondary damage to the brain can be limited however. Scientists have targeted some of these secondary factors, including cerebral ischemia (loss of blood), low cerebral blood flow, low oxygen levels, and the release of excitatory amino acid (e.g., glutamate). Edema, once thought to be the result of blood vessel leakage, is now believed to be due to continuing cell death in the injured tissue.

There have been numerous drug trials to control a wide range of secondary effects of brain trauma, including glutamate toxicity (selfotel, cerestat, dexanabinol), calcium damage (nimodipine), and cell membrane breakdown (tirilazad, PEG-SOD). Smaller clinical studies have investigated application of growth hormones, anticonvulsants, bradykinin (increases blood vessel permeability), and cerebral perfusion pressure (increases blood flow to the brain). A large trial began in 2007 to see if cooling the brains of kids (hypothermia) soon after TBI improves function. For the most part, clinical trials of potential neuroprotective agents have not been successful, even though the various therapies seemed to work well in animals. Why? For one, the gap between animal models and human clinical practice is huge, in part because human injury is poorly demonstrated in a small lab animal. Also, it is often difficult to get treatment started in humans within the proper therapeutic time frame. Animals don't always experience the same intolerable side effects to drugs as humans do, and animal models can't address the complicated, sometimes lifelong, effects of brain trauma on human mind, memory and behavior.

To be sure, the injured brain does have some capacity to recover. As scientists put it, the brain is "plastic," that is, using nerve growth factors, tissue transplantation or other techniques the brain can be encouraged to remodel itself and thus restore function. Because different mechanisms are active at different times during recovery, interventions may work better at certain times. There may be the need for a series of timed medications, each addressing specific biochemical processes in the wake of brain damage. Cell replacement (e.g. stem cells) is theoretically possible, but much research remains.

Sources

National Institute of Neurological Disorders and Stroke, ALS Association, Department of Veterans Affairs, United Cerebral Palsy, National MS Society, Spina Bifida Association of America, American Stroke Association, American Cancer Society, Myelin Project, Miami Project to Cure Paralysis, Reeve-Irvine Research Center, PVA Spinal Cord Research Foundation

RESEARCH RESOURCES

Christopher and Dana Reeve Foundation (CDRF) raises funds to develop treatments to restore function after injury or disease of the spinal cord. The foundation also works to improve the quality of life for people living with disabilities through its grants program, Paralysis Resource Center (*www.paralysis.org*) and advocacy efforts. Since 1982, CDRF has awarded nearly $50 million in research grants to the world's leading neuroscientists. The research grants are catalytic, supporting new initiatives, taking smart risks, and making sure research dollars do the most good. Through the Quality of Life Grants program, CDRF provides more than $1 million annually to nonprofit organizations that help improve the daily lives of people living with paralysis. For details, and for information on how to support the work of CDRF, write c/o 636 Morris Turnpike, Suite 3A, Short Hills, NJ 07078; toll-free 1-800-225-0292; see *http://www.ChristopherReeve.org*

Alan T. Brown Foundation to Cure Paralysis was formed to support research in spinal cord injury. The Alan T. Brown Foundation, 19 West 44th Street, Suite 1519, New York, NY 10036; telephone 212-944-8727; on the Internet see *http://www.atbf.org*

ALS Therapy Development Foundation is a nonprofit biotechnology company focused on rigorous, open-minded research and proven drug development techniques to treat ALS. ALS Therapy Development Foundation, 215 First Street, Cambridge, MA 02142, telephone 617-441-7200; on the Internet see *http://www.als.net*

ALS Association (ALSA) funds numerous projects to develop treatments for ALS (Lou Gehrig's disease). Contact ALSA, 27001 Agoura Road, Suite 150, Calabasas Hills, CA 91301-5104; on the Internet see *http://www.alsa.org/*

CenterWatch provides an extensive list of approved clinical trials being conducted internationally. CW, 22 Thomson Place, 47F1, Boston, MA 02210; telephone 617-856-5900; see *http://www.centerwatch.com*

ClinicalTrials is a user-friendly listing of all federally supported clinical trials for all conditions in the U.S., sorted by disease or condition, location, treatment or sponsor. Developed by the National Library of Medicine. On the Internet see *http://www.clinicaltrials.gov*

Coalition for the Advancement of Medical Research (CAMR), comprised of patient organizations, universities, scientific societies, foundations, and individuals with life-threatening disorders, advocates for the advancement of research and technologies in regenerative medicine - including stem cell research and somatic cell nuclear transfer. CAMR, 2120 K Street NW, Suite 305, Washington, DC 20006; telephone 202-725-0339; see *http://www.camradvocacy.org*

Dana Foundation provides reliable, accessible information on the brain and spinal cord, including research. The Foundation offers numerous books and publications and sponsors Brain Awareness Week. Contact Dana Alliance at 745 Fifth Avenue, Suite 900, New York, NY 10151; on the Internet see *http://www.dana.org*

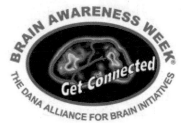

International Campaign for Cures of Spinal Cord Injury Paralysis is a group of organizations around the world that together fund about $25 million a year in SCI research. ICCP produced a key document on clinical trials and experimental treatments, available online. Members include: Miami Project to Cure Paralysis, Christopher and Dana Reeve Foundation, Paralyzed Veterans of America, Japan Spinal Cord Foundation, Rick Hansen Institute, Spinal Cure Australia (formerly Australasian Spinal Research Trust), Neil Sachse Foundation (formerly Spinal Treatment Australia), Spinal Research (International Spinal Research Trust) and French Institute for Spinal Cord Research. On the Internet see *http://www.campaignforcure.org*

Japan Spinal Cord Foundation takes aim "at the liberation from paralysis, and to promote the improvement of medical care concerning spinal cord injuries...and at the realization of a society where spinal cord injured persons can establish a life with independence and self esteem regardless of the severity of their disabilities." Telephone 81-42-366-5153; On the Internet see *www.jscf.org*

Life Rolls On Foundation was established by paralyzed surfer Jesse Billauer to support research toward treatments for paralysis. The foundation also spreads the word on motivation: life with SCI does indeed

RESEARCH RESOURCES

"Roll On." Life Rolls On Foundation, 7770 Regents Road, Suite 113-199, San Diego, CA 92122; toll-free telephone 866-939-4559; on the Internet visit *http://www.liferollson.com*.

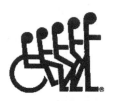 **Miami Project to Cure Paralysis** is a research center at the University of Miami dedicated to finding more effective treatments and, ultimately, a cure for paralysis. The Project has assembled a broad spectrum of researchers, clinicians and therapists whose full-time focus is spinal cord injury research. Miami Project, Post Office Box 016960 (R-48), Miami, FL 33101; toll-free 1-800-STAND-UP; on the Internet see *http://www.miamiproject.miami.edu*

Mike Utley Foundation provides financial support of research, rehabilitation and education programs on spinal cord injuries. Mike Utley Foundation, Post Office Box 458, Orondo, WA 98843; toll-free 1-800-294-4683; on the Internet see *http://www.mikeutley.org*

Muscular Dystrophy Association sponsors 400 research projects a year in the hopes of discovering therapies for muscular dystrophy and related myopathies and diseases, including ALS. For information on research, gene therapy efforts, clinical trials, etc., contact MDA, 3300 E. Sunrise Drive, Tucson, AZ 85718; toll-free 1-800-FIGHT-MD (344-4863; on the Internet see *http://www.mdausa.org/research*

Myelin Project funds research for diseases related to loss of myelin (a fatty insulation on nerve fibers) including multiple sclerosis and types of leukodystrophy. "Lorenzo's Oil" (and the 1992 movie of the same name) originated here. The Myelin Project, 1400 Wallace Blvd, Suite 258, Amarillo, Texas 79106; toll free 1-800-869-3546; on the Internet see *http://www.myelin.org*

National Institute of Neurological Disorders and Stroke is the primary funding source for all research related to the brain and spinal cord and provides authoritative research overviews for all diseases and conditions related to paralysis. On the Internet see *http://www.ninds.nih.gov*, for detail and references, click on condition or diagnosis.

National Multiple Sclerosis Society (NMSS) funds millions of dollars in research each year seeking therapies for MS. Site includes an overview of MS neuroscience, deep detail and progress reports. NMSS, 733 Third Avenue, New York, NY 10017; toll-free 1-800-344-4867; On the Internet see *http://www.nationalmssociety.org/research.asp*

Paralysis Project of America funds selected scientific and clinical studies that focus on spinal cord repair and regeneration. The Paralysis Project of America, P. O. Box 627 Glendale, CA 91209; telephone 323-663-6554; on the Internet see *http://www.paralysisproject.org*

PubMed, a service of the National Library of Medicine, provides access to over 12 million citations in the medical literature back to the mid-1960s. Includes links to many sites providing full text articles and other related resources. See *http://www.ncbi.nlm.nih.gov/entrez*, search using key word, researcher name or journal title.

PVA-EPVA Center for Neuroscience and Regeneration Research at Yale University works to develop new treatments, and ultimately a cure, for spinal cord injury and related disorders. It brings together the Paralyzed Veterans of America, Eastern Paralyzed Veterans Association, the Department of Veterans Affairs, and Yale University. PVA-EPVA Center for Neuroscience and Regeneration Research, Yale University School of Medicine, 950 Campbell Avenue, Building 34, West Haven, CT 06516; telephone 203-937-3802; on the Internet visit *http://info.med.yale.edu/neurol/pva-epvacenter*

Rick Hansen Man in Motion Foundation was created in Canada in 1988 to support spinal cord injury research, as well as wheelchair sport, injury prevention and rehabilitation programs. Man In Motion Foundation, 5th Floor, 520 West 6th Avenue, Vancouver, BC, Canada V5Z 1A1; toll-free 1-800-213-2131; see *http://www.rickhansen.com*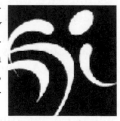

Reeve-Irvine Research Center was formed by Christopher Reeve and philanthropist Joan Irvine Smith to study injuries and diseases of the spinal cord that result in paralysis. Contact c/o University of California at Irvine, 2109 Gillespie Neuroscience Research Facility, Irvine, CA 92697-4292; telephone 949-824-3993; see *http://www.reeve.uci.edu*

RESEARCH RESOURCES

Sam Schmidt Foundation helps individuals with spinal cord injuries and other debilitating illnesses by funding research, medical treatment, rehabilitation and technology advances. Named for Schmidt, a quadriplegic former race car driver. The Sam Schmidt Paralysis Foundation, PO Box 3661, Princeton, NJ 08543-3661; telephone 317-236-9999; see *http://www.samschmidt.org*

SCORE is dedicated to finding a cure for paralysis and also allocates funds to assist young people who have been injured while participating in sporting or athletic events. SCORE helps with out-of-pocket costs for home modifications, vehicle adaptations, medical co-payments, etc. SCORE, P.O. Box 251255, Los Angeles, CA 90025; telephone 323-655-8298; on the Internet see *http://www.scorefund.org*

Society for Neuroscience is an organization of 40,000 basic scientists and physicians who study the brain and nervous system, including trauma and disease, as well as brain development, sensation and perception, learning and memory, sleep, stress, aging and psychiatric disorders. SFN, 1121 14th Street NW, Suite 1010, Washington DC 20036; telephone 202-962-4000; on the Internet see *http://apu.sfn.org*

The Spinal Cord Injury Project at Rutgers University seeks the rapid movement of therapies from laboratory to clinical trial. This includes research to test and confirm the efficacy and safety of promising therapies, training of laboratories to do spinal cord injury research and animal care, and community outreach/education. Home of Wise Young and the CareCure community. W.M. Keck Center for Collaborative Neuroscience, 604 Allison Road, Piscataway, NJ 08854; telephone 732-445-2061; see *http://keck.rutgers.edu*

Spinal Cord Research Foundation of the Paralyzed Veterans of America (PVA) funds research to treat spinal cord dysfunction and to enhance the health and quality of life of people who are paralyzed. PVA SCRF, 801 Eighteenth Street, NW, Washington, DC 20006; toll-free 1-800-424-8200; on the Internet see *http://www.pva.org*, click on "Research and Education."

Spinal Cord Society (SCS) is a research advocacy organization that raises money to cure spinal cord injuries. SCS, 19051 County Highway 1, Fergus Falls, MN 56537; 218-739-5252

Spinal Cure Australia (formerly Australasian Spinal Research Trust) was established in 1994 to fund scientific research to find a cure for paralysis; telephone 61-2-9660-1040; on the Internet see *www.spinalcure.org.au*

Spinal Research (formerly International Spinal Research Trust) is a United Kingdom charity funding research to end the permanence of paralysis. Founded in 1980 by Stewart Yesner, a young lawyer paralyzed in a car accident in Zambia in 1974. Diana, Princess of Wales became the charity's Royal Patron in 1989. On the Internet see *http://www.spinal-research.org*

StemCellAction is a grassroots group of people with chronic medical conditions and their families and friends who believe that stem cell research has the potential to treat Parkinson's, Alzheimer's, juvenile diabetes, MS, ALS and spinal cord injury. A Portraits of Hope project tells the stories of people affected by such diagnoses. See *http://www.stemcellaction.org*

Stem Cell Research Foundation raises funds to support basic and clinical research of stem cell therapy. Stem Cell Research Foundation, 22512 Gateway Center Drive, Clarksburg, Maryland 20871; toll free 1-877-842-3442; see *http://www.stemcellresearchfoundation.org*

Travis Roy Foundation, named for the injured Boston University hockey player, helps people with spinal cord injuries and funds research for a cure. The foundation has awarded grants for wheelchairs, assistance with van purchases, vehicle and home modifications, exercise equipment and other adaptive gear. Travis Roy Foundation, c/o Palmer & Dodge, LLP, 111 Huntington Avenue at Prudential Center, Boston, MA 02199; telephone 617-239-0556; see *http://www.travisroyfoundation.org*

Veterans Affairs Rehabilitation Research and Development Service advances knowledge to optimize health care for veterans. The VA has an active research agenda that includes the study of pain, bowel and bladder function, FES, nerve plasticity, prosthetics, numerous clinical issues and more. Publishes the *Journal of Rehabilitation R&D*, hosts the biannual International Symposium on Neural Regeneration at the Asilomar Center in Pacific Grove, CA. Contact VA RRDS, 810 Vermont Avenue, NW, Washington, DC 20420; telephone 202-254-0255; on the Internet see *http://www.vard.org*

THE BIOLOGY OF STEM CELLS: A PRIMER

In 1998, scientists isolated pluripotent stem cells from early human embryos and grew them in culture. In the few years since this discovery, evidence has emerged that these stem cells can become almost any of the 200 known specialized cells of the body and, thus, may generate replacement cells to repair or replace cells or tissues that are damaged or destroyed by diseases and disabilities.

Meanwhile, as the political process limits research in many areas of stem cells and therapeutic cloning, a flurry of information suggests great potential for adult stem cells.

There is tremendous expectation for stem cell therapy; at this time it's too soon to say just how or when stem cells from any source will be useful for the treatment of disease or trauma. More research for all types of stem cells is needed. What follows is a brief primer on stem cell terminology.

Stem cell: a cell from the embryo, fetus, or adult that has, under certain conditions, the ability to reproduce itself for long periods or, in the case of adult stem cells, throughout the life of the organism. It also can give rise to specialized cells that make up the tissues and organs of the body.

Pluripotent stem cell: can give rise to the cells that develop from the embryonic germ layers, from which all the cells of the body arise.

Induced pluripotent stem cell: A type of pluripotent stem cell derived from an adult cell such as a skin cell, by inducing an expression of certain genes that reprogram the cell. iPS cells are believed to be identical in many respects to embryonic pluripotent stem cells, including the ability to form all cells in the body and to reproduce themselves indefinitely.

Embryonic stem cell: derived from an early (4- to 5-day) embryo called the blastocyst. Cells of the inner cell mass can be cultured into embryonic stem cells. Current challenges: to direct differentiation of embryonic stem cells into specialized cell populations; to devise ways to control their proliferation once placed in people.

Embryonic germ cell: derived from fetal tissue, specifically from the primordial germ cells that develop into the testes or ovaries. Embryonic stem cells and embryonic germ cells are pluripotent, but they are not identical in their properties.

Differentiation: the process by which an unspecialized cell (such as a stem cell) specializes into one of the many cells in the body.

Adult stem cell: an undifferentiated (unspecialized) cell that occurs in a differentiated (specialized) tissue, renews itself, and becomes specialized for the cell types of the originating tissue. Adult stem cells are rare and difficult to identify, isolate, and purify but are capable of making identical copies of themselves for the lifetime of the organism. Currently used to treat leukemia.

Plasticity: an adult stem cell from one tissue generates the specialized cell type(s) of another tissue, e.g., adult stem cells from bone marrow generate cells that resemble neurons.

Progenitor or precursor cell: occurs in fetal or adult tissues and is partially specialized. When a progenitor/precursor cell divides, it can form similar cells or it can form two specialized cells, neither of which is capable of replicating itself.

Somatic cell nuclear transfer (therapeutic cloning): removing the nucleus of an unfertilized egg cell, replacing it with the material from the nucleus of a "somatic cell" (e.g. a skin, heart, or nerve cell), and stimulating this cell to begin dividing. Stem cells can be extracted five to six days later.

Most evidence that stem cells can be directed into specific types of cells for transplantation comes from mice experiments. Mouse and human cells differ in significant ways. Another issue to work out is any immune response that would reject a cellular transplant.

Source: NIH, Genetics Policy Institute

On the Internet see *http://stemcells.nih.gov/info/basics/*; see also *http://www.stemcellfunding.org* or *http://www.genpol.org*

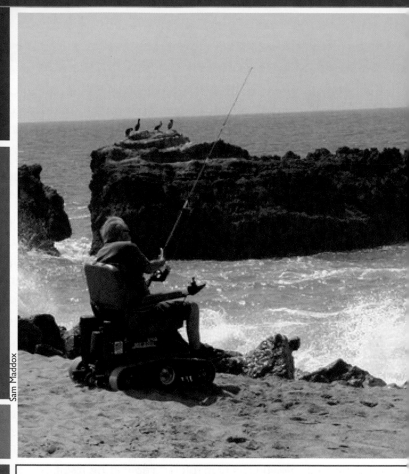

Sam Maddox

SPORTS AND RECREATION

Challenge the world, explore your own limitations. Escape the ordinary, take risks. Most of all, have fun with friends and family.

Recreation. The word says it all. We all need to get away from our day-to-day routines, to recreate mind and body with fun activities, sports and games with friends and family. Paralysis is a ready excuse to stay indoors and inactive. But the benefits of escaping the ordinary, of being challenged, of exploring the boundaries of limitation, are fulfilling and meaningful.

The physical benefits of active living promote health and wellness, reduce stress and help us think more creatively. The social and psychological reasons add balance to life with disability. We need to do things that focus on activity and not limits. Recreation and adventure enable people to explore themselves, to take risks, to get the blood going, to gain a fresh perspective.

We're here to discuss fun, though, not therapy. Many recreational activities, sports and competitions are inclusive and accessible. Here's the real story: No matter your level of function or your physical limitations, if you want to try something — anything — there's almost always a way to do it.

Jump out an airplane … hooked up to a ventilator? Been done. Climb the rock face of El Capitan in Yosemite, with just arm power? Done. Bag an elk with a large caliber rifle, by a high quad sitting in a wheelchair? Sure, if that fits your notion of recreation. Surf the waves off Malibu, with no hand or leg power? Yep. Bungee jumping, swimming the English Channel, riding the rapids in the Grand Canyon, skiing the black diamonds in Vail, sailing or flying solo around the world – all done by people with paralysis.

The point isn't to raise the recreation bar to the level of the extreme achiever. Recreation doesn't have to be measured or scored, or even noticed by anyone but the participants. There is something for everyone. Find your own rec groove.

Below is a list of some popular individual activities that for the most part can be shared with families and friends (see team sports listed on page 193). Some require adaptive gear, such as cycles, skis and clubs. Some require a bit of fitness going in. All require a spirit of fun and a readiness to recreate.

RECREATION SPORTS

Billiards

This is a great game for wheelchair users. The rules and regulations are basically the same as in the stand-up game; individuals with upper body limitations must stay seated (one bun on the chair at all times) during play and are allowed to use adaptive devices for shooting control. Modified pool cues or a roller attachment at the end of a cue stick allow players with limited hand use to enjoy the sport and be competitive with the best players. Some wheelchair players compete quite well against nondisabled players. For further detail, contact the National Wheelchair Pool Players Association, 820 Coastal Beach Road, Henderson, NV 89002, telephone 703-817-1215; or on the Internet visit *http://www.nwpainc.org*

Bowling

Wheelchair bowling, like basketball, emerged as part of social and physical rehab programs for disabled World War II vets. The sport is

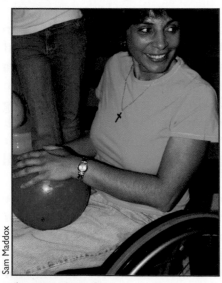

Sam Maddox

easy to learn and does not require enormous strength. It is played just as the stand-up version, with the exception of special push tools and ball-drop ramps for bowlers with limited arm mobility. Special snap handle balls are available for those who can't get a good grip on the ball. Can you do well against nondisabled bowlers? Ask Walt Roy, a para from Redding, California. He came within one pin of a perfect game once, and he sports a respectable average of 200. To find out about leagues and adaptive bowling gear, contact The American Wheelchair Bowling Association (AWBA), Post Office Box 69, Clover, VA 24534, telephone 434-454-2269; or visit the Internet site *http://www.awba.org*

Camping

Some people's idea of roughing it is being far enough from home that Domino's will no longer deliver. While "rough" is a relative term, there is more to camping than getting out of the city service area. It's a way to be close to nature, to simplify, to cut the electronic umbilical cords and conveniences we take for granted. Getting away might mean car or motorhome camping within a designated site. It might mean getting off the beaten path and deep into the woods. Wheeling into the wilderness isn't easy for people who are paralyzed, but it's not impossible with a bit of preparation and determination.

Where to go? State and national parks are a good place to start.

> **"Roughing it is a relative term but there's more to camping than getting outside the Domino's delivery area. Go lightly as you escape the mundane."**

As mandated by the Americans with Disabilities Act, these parks have accessible accommodations, bathrooms and level ground — usually. Progress toward accessibility continues but you can find many camp areas that are inclusive. Be prepared and be creative. To get started, check with your state's outdoor recreation or state parks agency. You may need reservations.

What to bring? There may be no way to avoid the necessities of mobility, medications and hygiene. But go lightly – you don't need the handheld satellite TV or the Swiss Army microwave. Remember, the idea is to escape the mundane and the routine.

Resources: National Parks Visitor Facilities & Services is available from the National Park Hospitality Association, 129 Park Street, Vienna, VA; telephone 703-242-1999. See the Internet site for the U.S. National Parks, *http://www.nps.gov*. Note: residents of the United States who are blind or permanently disabled can obtain a Golden Access Passport, a lifetime entrance pass to national parks, monuments, historic sites, recreation areas and wildlife refuges. The Passport also provides a 50 percent discount on fees for camping, swimming, parking, boat launching and tours. Note: You can only get a Passport in person at a national park, historic site, etc. where an entrance fee is charged.

Flying

By its very nature flight is restrictive – by gravity, of course, and by licensing agencies and cost, but not necessarily by paralysis. If a person has normal health and has either quick reflexes or a suitable alternative control, most likely he or she can fly. Flying does not require great strength although good headwork is a must. Hundreds of paraplegics, quadriplegics and amputees have successfully flown over the years, having proven their abilities to the FAA and other controlling authorities throughout the world.

The best resource is the International Wheelchair Aviators, which began in 1972 as a monthly "fly to lunch" group of four paraplegic aviators from the Southern California area. IWA has information and resources on adaptive flying. IWA, P.O. Box 2799, Big Bear City, CA 92314; telephone 909-585-9663; or visit the Internet site *www.wheelchairaviators.org*

Freedom's Wings International, a New Jersey based organization, has a fleet of specially adapted sailplanes. These motorless gliders are towed into the sky by a regular airplane and then released for a quiet ride back to the airport. When conditions permit, sailplane pilots ride the natural thermal currents to stay aloft for hours. People with disabilities can come along either as passengers or by joining the flight training program. For more information contact FWI, Post Office Box 7076, East Brunswick, NJ 07076; toll-free telephone 800-382-1197; or visit the Internet site *http://www.freedomswings.org*

Gardening

Digging in the dirt, planting seeds and growing flowers or food is pleasurable and rewarding. Gardening provides exercise and mental stimulation. Many people claim it's also therapeutic – there's an organization called the American Horticultural Therapy Association that promotes physical and mental health through gardens and plants. Gardening can relieve tension. With its clear cause-and-effect nature, it can foster a sense of expectation, of accomplishment, self-reliance and responsibility. Moreover, with some adaptations (raised beds and special tools, for example), gardening can be barrier-free and fully inclusive. The Paralysis Resource Center library carries several books on accessible gardening. Go to *www.paralysis.org*, click on library, search for gardening; books available by way of interlibrary loan.

Golf

Such a simple game. Maddeningly simple. Simply maddening. Hit the ball down the grassy fairway, get it on the green, and sink it in the hole. Easier to say than do, but that's part of the fun of it. The game is quite adaptable to the seated player. Custom clubs and special carts, some with single-passenger swivel seats and tires that won't damage the greens, open the game to players who have limited leg function.

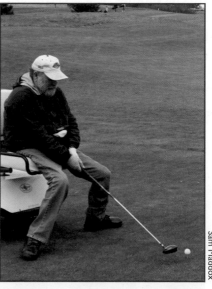

Sam Maddox

Golf is growing in popularity among disabled players, not only because of equipment innovation but also because of the changes in law. The Americans with Disabilities Act requires all public accommodations, including golf courses, to provide goods and services to people with disabilities on an equal basis with the rest of the general public. Public entities, such as states and local governments, must make golf courses and other facilities accessible to people with disabilities and all new golf course facilities must be accessible. The ADA also requires removal of architectural barriers in existing facilities when "readily achievable," or when it can be done without much difficulty or expense for that facility. Before you show up at a golf club expecting an equal basis experience, check ahead. You may need to work with the management and perhaps enlist the help of national organizations such as the United States Golf Association. USGA/Resource Center for Individuals With Disabilities, 1631 Mesa Avenue, Colorado Springs, CO 80906; telephone 719-471-4810, ext. 15; or log on to *http://www.resourcecenter.usga.org.*

Hand Cycling

Hand cycling really took off in the early 1990s, once the technology came of age with sophisticated three-wheel, multi-geared cycles. Hand cranking has become quite popular across the country and abroad, and for good reason. It's fun, fast and family oriented. It's great for fitness, too. A rider can move the three-wheelers along at a steady 20 mph pace, enough to keep up with nondisabled bike riders. Many riders have hand-powered over the thin air of Colorado's highest mountain passes, or even around the world. Hand cycling has emerged as an elite competitive sport,

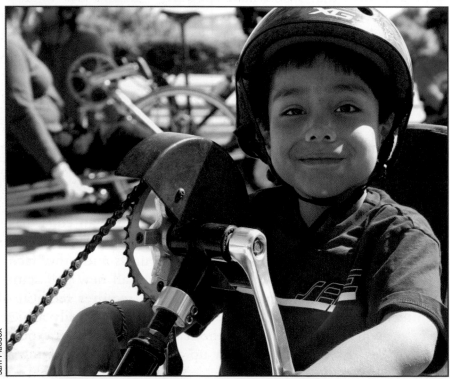

Sam Maddox

too; it's included in the Paralympics.

There are several variations on the hand-power theme: Some cycles clamp on to a standard manual wheelchair, with a chair-driven front wheel to more or less pull the chair along. Clamp-ons are best for cruising around the neighborhood. Serious road travel or competition requires a trike: they are lighter and deliver more power to the drive wheel, have greater stability at speed, and offer much less wind resistance. For more information about products on the market visit these Internet sites: *www.freedomryder.com, www.varnahandcycles.com* or *www.bike-on.com*

The United States Hand Cycling Federation (USHF) is the official governing body for recreational and competitive hand cycling in America. USHF, Box 3538, Evergreen, CO 80437; *www.ushf.org*.

Pinball

The game of pinball has been out of reach to many players. The machines are usually too high for wheelchair users and for those with less than normal hand function there just isn't any way to activate the flippers. But a New Jersey company has made pinball accessible. Ron Kochel and Gene Gulich created a game that a disabled player and 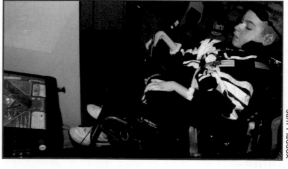 nondisabled player can share on equal terms. Using the U Can Do controls, players can become wizards whether they use one hand or two, or one foot or two. Players can use fists, elbows, head switches or even a sip and puff method, moving the steel ball around the game by blowing or sucking air out of a straw. Every independent living center and accessible recreation program should have one. See *www.ucando-central.com* or call toll-free 866-822-6362.

Riding

Horseback riding is an exhilarating recreation that's doable for many people who are paralyzed, using padding or specially made saddles and a mounting ramp. While riding can be done simply because it's pleasurable, for some people the goal is therapeutic.

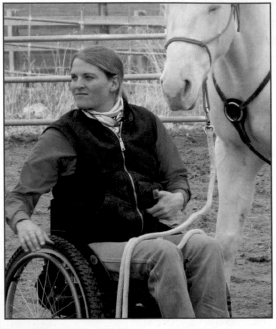

The rhythmic motion and warmth of a horse can be helpful. Riding can facilitate cognitive as well as sensory and motor development. Moreover, it can help foster a sense of responsibility and self-confidence while reducing spasticity and improving strength, stimulating good posture, balance and flexibility for more functional independence off the horse. There are many riding programs across the United States that cater to disabled riders. The best source of information is the North American Riding for the Handicapped Association, P.O. Box 33150 Denver, CO 80233; toll free 1-800-369-RIDE; or visit the Internet site *http://www.narha.org*

Sailing

Sailing can be a peaceful and relaxing way to explore and enjoy the world of water. The sport also offers great adventure and challenges to instincts we forgot (or never knew) we had. It's a lot of fun if you're along for the ride, but it is especially so if you're the skipper, reading the wind, setting the course and piloting the boat. Sailboats can accommodate people with varying degrees of paralysis. There are boats that are quite accessible for the wheelchair sailor (a transfer box helps with the hardest part – getting aboard). In fact, there are boats that can be single-handed by people with no hand function whatsoever. A sip 'n puff control has been adapted to a fleet of Canadian boats called the Martin 16. These were originally designed to be quad friendly, with inspiration from Sam Sullivan, a high-quad sailor from British Columbia (who is now mayor of Vancouver). These boats are affordable, comfortable, safe and accessible to anyone. For more contact Inventure Management Limited, 5917–1A Street, SW,

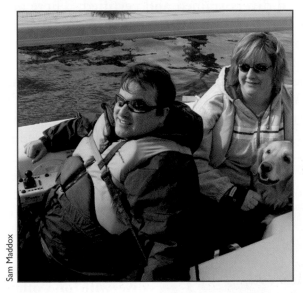

Sam Maddox

Calgary, AB T2H 0G4; telephone 403-870-7210; or visit *www.martin16.com*.

A newer, unsink-able and quite accessible boat called an Access Dinghy, which can be con-trolled using a joystick, is available for rent at many sail-ing centers. Sailors are seated low in the boat for added stabil-ity. A servo-assist joystick can operate the electric winches and can be controlled by hand, foot, chin or any moving body part. The Access Dinghy brings full inclusion to the marina, *http://www.accessdinghy.org*.

For some, the most fulfilling way to enjoy sailing is to see who's got the fastest boat. Sailing is something of an aquatic equalizer – nondisabled sailors have no particular advantage when it comes to boat handling and navigation skill. There are also many disabled-only races, including the Paralympic Games. For information on racing, contact The United States Sailing Association, Box 1260, Portsmouth, RI 02871; telephone 401-683-0800; or see the Internet site, *www.ussailing.org/swsn*

There are numerous sailing programs across the country that offer boats and instruction for people with disabilities. These are included on the USSA Website.

Scuba

Scuba diving opens a fantastic new world to the gravity-bound. And for those with limitations of mobility, underwater sports offer an exhilarating "aquatic equality" unsurpassed on land. With training and some assistance getting in and out of equipment, even high-quads can enjoy the clear, 85-degree water of the beautiful reefs of the Caribbean.

There are dive programs all over the United States that specialize in getting disabled divers trained and certified. There are special tour companies that target the wheelchair diver, and there are even resorts in such exotic places as Bonaire in the Caribbean that offer fully "walk 'n roll" accessible dive vacation packages.

Many divers have been trained by instructors certified by the Handicapped Scuba Association, a California nonprofit that's been running scuba and underwater education programs for 20 years. HSA bases diving proficiency on one's ability to assist another diver in the water. Level A divers are certified to dive with one other person; a Level B diver must dive with two other nondisabled divers. Level C

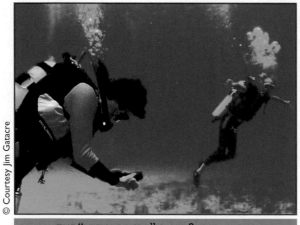

© Courtesy Jim Gatacre

THE "LIVELY DIVERS," DON & GAIL LIVELY, BOTH QUADRIPLEGICS

divers require two dive buddies and one must be trained in diver rescue. Says HSA fournder Jim Gatacre, "Virtually everyone I've ever trained will tell you that their lives have been changed by the diving. Just about anybody can do it; if a person has fair respiratory function, even if they can't move at all, there are ways to teach them to dive so they can have a wonderful diving experience."

Contact HSA International, 1104 El Prado, San Clemente, CA 92672-4637; telephone 949-498-4540; or visit the Internet site *http://www.hsascuba.com*. Site includes a list of dive instructors across the United States.

Skiing

This is a sport that's been well adapted for people with disabilities, thanks to technology. Depending on one's level of function, there are three ways a person can get from the top of the mountain down the snowy trails to the bottom. At the highest end of the tech scale is the mono-ski, best for those with good upper body strength and trunk balance. The skier sits in a molded shell mounted to a frame above a single ski with a shock absorber linking the frame to the ski. Two ski poles with outriggers are used for balance and turning. Mono-skiing closely resembles stand-up skiing – the skier can become highly skilled, carving turns in tight formation and taking on the deep and the steep. Ski all day without anyone's help: the mono-ski is self-loaded onto the chairlift.

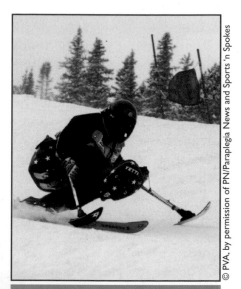

The bi-ski is similar to a mono-ski except the skier sits above two skis for better balance. The bi-ski can be skied independently with the use of two outriggers for balance and turning. For those needing more assistance, a ski instructor may tether the bi-ski to keep it under control.

MONOSKIER RUNNING SLALOM GATES. TECHNOLOGY HAS OPENED THE ENTIRE MOUNTAIN TO SIT-DOWN SKIERS.

© PVA, by permission of PN/Paraplegia News and Sports 'n Spokes

The sit-ski, akin to a toboggan, works for people with even more significant limitations. Those with some hand function can steer the sit-ski with short ski poles and by leaning. For quads and others with no hand function, the sit-ski is tethered to an instructor. There are many disabled ski programs across the United States. Among the largest is the National Sports Center for the Disabled, which runs recreation programs year-round. NSCD, P.O. Box 1290, Winter Park, CO 80482; telephone 970-726-1540; or visit the Internet site *http://www.nscd.org/*. See also the National Ability Center, P. O. Box 682799, Park City,

UT 84068; telephone 435-649-3991; on the Web at *http://www.discovernac.org*. A full scale California program can be found at Alpine Meadows, in the Tahoe region. Contact *http://www.dsusafw.org/winter.html*

Skiing has a very active competitive and Paralympic side. Contact the U.S. Ski and Snowboard Association for information. USSA, 1500 Kearns Boulevard, Park City, UT 84060; telephone 435-649-9090; or visit the Internet site *http://www.usskiteam.com*

Surfing

Well, dude, it's gnarly, that's why. Jesse Billauer, a quad after a surfing accident, started Life Rolls On (LRO) to raise awareness about quality of life and research related to spinal cord injury. Jesse, of course, got back on his board, riding huge waves on his stomach, with help from some standup surfers to get in and out. To share the joy, he started They Will Surf Again, a LRO program that gets people in wheelchairs out riding the waves, on surfboards. For more, contact LRO, 7770 Regents Road, Suite 113-199, San Diego, CA 92122, toll-free 866-We Will Walk (866-939-4559) or visit *www.liferollson.org*

Tennis

Wheelchair tennis is played by the same rules as stand-up tennis, except the wheelchair player is allowed two bounces of the ball. Decent wheelchair players can actively compete against stand-up players, making this one of the best activities to share with friends and family.

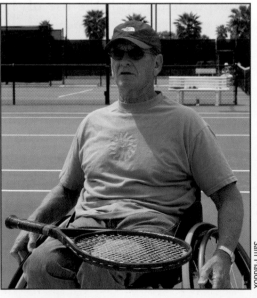

In wheelchair tennis, the player must master the game as well as the wheelchair. Learning mobility on the court is exciting and challenging, and it helps build strength and cardiovascular fitness. The competitive side of tennis is robust and international in scope. Contact the United States Tennis Association for details. USTA, 4 West Red Oak Lane, White Plains, NY 10604; telephone 914-696-7000; or online visit *http://www.usta.com*, search under "wheelchair."

Table tennis is a fast and fun indoor/outdoor option, too. For information on competitive action, contact USA Table Tennis, USOC Paralympics, One Olympic Plaza, Colorado Springs, CO, 80909; telephone 719-866-2048; or visit the Internet site *http://www.usatt.org*

Video games

The modern video game has better graphics, better games, better interactivity than ever before. No problem for anyone with decent hand function to join the action. But can a high quad play? If you can sip and puff, the answer is yes. A company called KY Enterprises has been in the accessible gaming business for 20 years and makes a joystick controller for Playstation 1 and

Video games: Better graphics, better action, better interactivity. Now, better access for players of all abilities.

Playstation 2 games. It takes a bit of practice to become skillful with six switch modes on the sip and puff unit, which doubles as a joystick, and two buttons operated by the lip. But if a gamer is motivated, this popular activity is wide open. There are some PS2 games that are not compatible (those that require analog-only control – that's the mushroom thumb control on a regular control unit. See the box of the video game; it will indicate if analog is required). Most driving games, sports games and other popular titles don't require analog. The system is compatible with X-Box. For more, contact KYE, 4040 Graf Street, Bozeman, MT 59715; telephone 406-586-2376; or visit the Internet site, *http://www.quadcontrol.com*

GimpGear offers a sip n puff video game controller for

PlayStation 2, Xbox, GameCube, PC Computer, or Xbox 360, and limited game support on PS3. The company also has many other accessible joystick options, including a voice activated system well-suited for flight sim games and solo shooter gigs. *See www.gimpgear.com*

Water Skiing

Water skiing is a terrific heat-beating summer sport that's been adapted so that skiers of almost all abilities can participate with family and friends. If skiers get good at it and have the urge to compete, there are various water ski meets around the United States. Using a sort of sit-ski that's wider than the mono-ski used by stand-up skiers, paraplegics, and even quads who have a little bit of arm strength, can hook up to a boat and thrill to the speed and wake-crashing fun of water skiing. Skis are available commercially; many have been added to recreation programs in many communities across the country.

Water ski tournaments for skiers with mobility limitations include slalom, tricks and jumping events. Competition is organized by the Water Skiers with Disabilities Association, a division of USA Water Ski, the National Governing Body for the sport in the United States. WSDA promotes the recreational aspects of the sport by way of clinics, teaching materials, equipment development and maintenance of a national network of water ski resources. For more information, contact WSDA, 1251 Holy Cow Road, Polk City, Florida 33868; telephone toll-free 1-800-533-2972; or visit the Internet site *http://usawaterski.org*

Weightlifting

Granted, many don't hear the calling for this strenuous, get-pumped recreation, but it is not hard to adapt lifting weights to people with lost function due to paralysis. The activity has clear benefits for fitness but lifting has also emerged as a very competitive activity at the international level. Buff enough: Kim Brownfield, a paraplegic, bench presses 602 pounds, just 75 pounds shy of the Olympic world record for nondisabled lifters in his class. Contact Wheelchair Sports USA, P.O. Box 5266, Kendall Park, NJ 08824, 732-422-4546; *http://www.wsusa.org*

Basketball

Basketball is probably the most well-developed sport for wheelchair users in the United States, for good reason. The game has been played for 60 years, originated by World War II vets in rehab on the East and West coasts. There are teams and divisions all over the country for men, women and juniors. Some colleges suit up wheelchair hoops teams. The game is fast and fun, and quite entertaining to watch. For the full story contact the National Wheelchair Basketball Association, 6165 Lehman Drive, Suite 101, Colorado Springs, CO 80918; telephone 719-266-4082; or visit the Internet site *http://www.nwba.org*

Quad Rugby

Quad Rugby, or murderball, is a combination of soccer, keepaway and demolition derby that emerged from the cold northern winters of Winnipeg, Manitoba, to become an international sport whose fans say it's the fastest growing wheelchair sport in the world. There are dozens of very competitive teams in the United States. Each team utilizes four players, mostly quads. A player has 15 seconds to advance the ball into the opponent's half-court. The player with the ball must pass or dribble every 10 seconds or a turnover is awarded. The idea is to cross the end line on the court

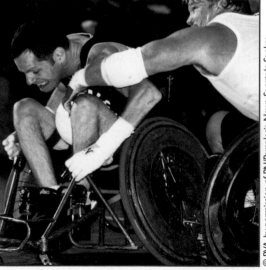

© PVA, by permission of PN/Paraplegia News, Sports 'n Spokes

and score a point. The other guys do what they can to stop you. It's not a game for polite recreation. United States Quad Rugby Association, 5861 White Cypress Drive, Lakeworth, FL 33467; telephone 561-964-1712; or visit *http://www.quadrugby.com*

Sled hockey

Sled hockey is played by people who use their arms to propel themselves by digging picks on the ends of two short hockey sticks into the ice. Players are seated on sleds, which are affixed to two hockey skate blades under the seat. The sleds are about 3 inches off the ice and are anywhere from 2 to 4 feet long, depending on the size of the player. There are few differences between this and the stand-up game. The puck is the same, as are the pads. Protection is needed, as there

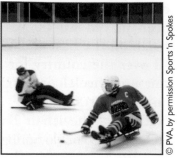

is a lot of checking. International competition is fierce, including the Paralympic Games. See USA Hockey, 1775 Bob Johnson Drive, Colorado Springs, CO 80906; 719-576-USAH (8724); see *http://www.usahockey.com/*

Softball

It's not easy to field full teams of wheelchairs for a Saturday afternoon pick-up game. The best chance for action occurs at an annual tournament sponsored by the National Wheelchair Softball Association, where 30 or so teams show up to compete. The game is much the same as slow pitch softball, using a 16-inch slow pitch ball, with base paths shortened to 50 feet. There is no adaptive equipment. For more, contact NWSA, 6000 West Floyd Avenue #110, Denver, CO 80227; 303-842-12292; or see the Internet site *http://www.wheelchairsoftball.org*

Volleyball

Volleyball has been adapted as a team sport that includes seated persons of many types of disability. The net is about three feet high and the court is smaller than a standard volleyball setup. The only major differences between the standing game and the sitting game are that players can block the serve and that one bun must be in contact with the floor when a person makes contact with the ball. For more, contact USA Volleyball, 715 S. Circle Drive, Colorado Springs, CO 80910; telephone 719-228-6800; or see the Internet site *http://www.usavolleyball.org*

ART AND CREATIVITY

The arts enrich our lives in countless ways, whether we create art or appreciate its beauty, truth or abstraction. The worlds of creative endeavor and artistic expression are inclusive; there are no limitations on imagination. There are only a few restrictions on accessing the tools of art; musical instruments, paintbrushes, pencils or video cameras are fairly adaptable. Because art is infinite and unconditional, people with disabilities are free to express themselves without physical, social, or attitudinal barriers.

The arts are not recreation, per se, but they can be uplifting, refreshing and socially involving. The arts provide unlimited possibilities for personal, academic, and professional success.

By engaging in the arts, people with disabilities are able to greatly contribute to their communities, help extinguish old stereotypes regarding disability, and create a culture truly representative of all people. The arts help forge a collective identity. People with disabilities share common experiences through the expression of their struggles and histories.

Below are resources for art, dance, music and other performing arts, including motion pictures and television.

Resources:

VSA (formerly Very Special Arts) creates learning opportunities through creative writing, dance, drama, music and the visual arts for people with disabilities. There are affiliates in 39 states and 67 countries. VSA, 818 Connecticut Avenue, NW, Suite 600, Washington, DC, 20006; toll-free 800-933-8721; or visit the Internet site *http://www.vsarts.org*

The National Arts and Disability Center (NADC) is an information, technical assistance and referral center specializing in arts and disability. NADC is dedicated to full inclusion of children and adults with disabilities into the visual, performing, media, and literary arts communities. NADC, Tarjan Center for Developmental Disabilities; 300 UCLA Medical Plaza Suite #3310, Los Angeles, CA 90095-6967; telephone 310-794-1141; or see the Web site at *http://nadc.ucla.edu*

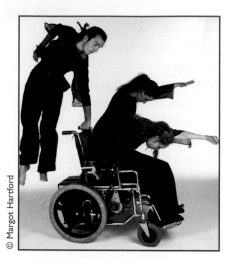

© Margot Hartford

AXIS Dance Company has performed its innovative body of work throughout the U.S. as well as overseas. AXIS has become an internationally known resource for physically integrated dance and is one of a handful of companies setting a standard for professionalism in this emerging field. AXIS Dance Company, 1428 Alice Street, Suite 200, Oakland, CA 94612; telephone 510-625-0110; or visit *http://www.axisdance.org*

Full Radius Dance explores the sweep of the human experience in a world that contains a diversity of attitudes, actions and outcomes. Full Radius Dance, Post Office Box 54453, Atlanta, GA 30308; telephone 404-724-9663; or visit the Internet site *http://www.fullradiusdance.org*

Ballroom Dancing: This graceful and dramatic style is catching on with wheelchair dancers. On the Internet visit *www.americandancewheels.com*

Coalition for Disabled Musicians, Inc. introduces disabled musicians to each other, offers an accessible rehearsal and recording studio and helps with adaptive techniques for pain, endurance, and other limitations. Coalition for Disabled Musicians, Inc., Post Office Box 1002M, Bay Shore, NY 11706; telephone 631-586- 0366; or visit the Internet site *http://www.disabled-musicians.org*

Creative Growth Art Center provides art programs, educational and independent living training, counseling and vocational opportunities for adults who are physically, mentally and emotionally disabled. Creative Growth Art Center, 355 24th Street, Oakland, CA 94612; 510-836-2340; *www.creativegrowth.org*

Arts and Healing Network is an Internet resource considering the connection between art and healing. Post Office Box 276, Stinson Beach, CA 94970. See *http://www.artheals.org*

The National Institute of Art and Disabilities (NIAD) is a visual arts center serving adults with developmental and physical disabilities. NIAD, 551 23rd Street, Richmond, CA 94804; telephone 510/620-0290; on the Internet see *http://www.niadart.org*

Association of Foot and Mouth Painting Artists is a 50-year-old international organization that offers significant financial support to develop the talents of painters who are accepted in the group. The American affiliate is Mouth and Foot Painting Artists Inc., 2070 Peachtree Industrial Court, Suite 101, Atlanta, GA 30341; telephone 770-986-7764; or visit the Internet site *http://www.amfpa.com*

That Uppity Theatre Company produces the Disability Project, an ensemble of conversation, writing, sound, movement and theatrical exercises to empower individuals, honor their stories, spark imaginations and enhance public awareness about disability. TUTC, 4466 West Pine Boulevard, Suite 13C, St. Louis, MO 63108; telephone 314-995-4600; or visit the Internet site *http://www.disabilityproject.com*

Stunts-Ability trains disabled persons for stunts, acting and effects for the entertainment industry. Stunts-Ability, P.O. Box 600711, San Diego, CA 92160; telephone 619-542-7730; see *http://www.stuntsability.com*

Media Access Office promotes the employment and accurate portrayal of persons with disabilities in all areas of the media and entertainment industry, ensuring that people with disabilities are part of the cultural diversity. The Media Access Office is currently administered with assistance from the State Employment Development Department. Media Access Office/EDD, Verdugo Jobs Center, 1255 S. Central Avenue, Glendale, CA 91204; 818-409-0448 or see *http://www.disabilityemployment.org*

RECREATION RESOURCES

Sports 'N Spokes is the guide to sports and recreation for people with paralysis. The bi-monthly magazine, published by the Paralyzed Veterans of America, offers details on wheelchair athletics and competition, recreation, exercise, training, nutrition, event schedules and other topics of interest to the active person in a wheelchair. Contact SNS, 2111 East Highland Avenue, Suite 180, Phoenix, AZ 86016; toll-free 888-888-2201; 602-224-0500; or visit the Internet site *http://www.sportsnspokes.com*

The National Center on Physical Activity and Disability (NCPAD) offers multimedia information on recreation and sports programs, equipment vendors, etc., across the nation. Contact NCPAD, 1640 W. Roosevelt Road, Chicago, IL 60608; telephone toll-free 1-800-900-8086; or visit the Internet site *http://www.ncpad.com*

Paralympics: United States Olympic Committee manages the U.S. Paralympic team. With minor exceptions, services provided disabled

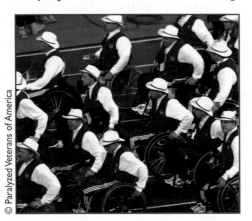

© Paralyzed Veterans of America

athletes are comparable to those provided nondisabled Olympic athletes. The USOC is dedicated to the integration and advancement of elite disabled athletes into open competition whenever possible. The Paralympics are open to elite athletes who meet the rigid qualifying standards of their sport. Athletes are categorized by a combination of functional and medical determinations. The Paralympic Games have been contested since 1960 and now feature competition in 19 sports. The Paralympic Winter Games showcase four sports, and were first held in 1976. The 2008 summer Games will take place in Beijing, just after the Olympic Games. The 2010 Winter Games will be held in Vancouver. Contact U.S. Paralympics, 719-471-8772; or see *http://www.usparalympics.org*. Also see the Internet site for the International Paralympic Committee, *http://www.paralympic.org*

U.S. Disabled Athletes Fund (USDAF) is an outgrowth of the 1996 Paralympic Games held in Atlanta, Georgia. USDAF hopes to develop a national program of adaptive sports in every community, including programs for military veterans. The program is named BlazeSports after the Atlanta Paralympics mascot Blaze. U.S. Disabled Athletes Fund, Inc., 280 N. Interstate Circle, SE, Atlanta, GA 30339, telephone 770-850-8199; on the Internet see *http://www.blazesports.com*

Disabled Sports USA was formed in 1967 by a group of disabled veterans. DS/USA now offers nationwide sports rehabilitation programs to anyone with a physical disability. Activities include winter skiing, water sports, summer and winter competitions, fitness and special sports events. Participants include those with visual impairments, amputations, spinal cord injury, dwarfism, multiple sclerosis, head injury, cerebral palsy and other neuromuscular and orthopedic conditions. DSUSA National Headquarters, 451 Hungerford Drive, Suite 100, Rockville, MD 20850; telephone 301-217-0960; or visit *http://www.dsusa.org*

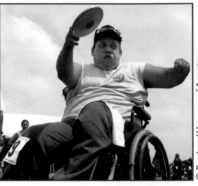
© Paralyzed Veterans of America

World T.E.A.M. Sports brings individuals with and without disabilities together in unique athletic events (ride around the world, rides through Vietnam, etc.). The program promotes diversity and increased awareness, acceptance and integration of those with disabilities. Contact World T.E.A.M. Sports, 150 Mount Vernon Street, Dorchester, MA 02125; 617-282-6104, or visit the Internet site *http://www.worldteamsports.org*

The Achilles Track Club (ATC) is an international nonprofit group that encourages disabled people to participate in long-distance running. ATC provides support, training and technical expertise to runners with all kinds of disabilities. Achilles Track Club, 42 West 38th Street, NY, NY, 10018; telephone 212-354-0300; or visit the Internet site *http://www.achillestrackclub.org*

RECREATION RESOURCES

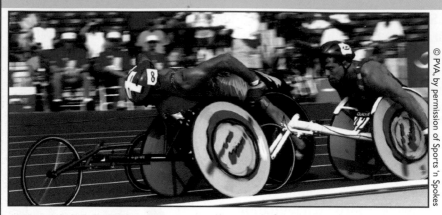

© PVA, by permission of Sports 'n Spokes

Wheelchair Sports USA was founded in 1956 as the National Wheelchair Athletic Association to provide mobility-limited athletes the chance for recreational and competitive sports. WSUSA offers national sports programs and linkage to the Paralympics through a widespread regional structure. WSUSA, P.O. Box 5266, Kendall Park, NJ 08824; 732-422-4546; or visit the Internet site, *http://www.wsusa.org*

The National Disability Sports Alliance (NDSA) is the gateway to big time athletics and competitive sports for individuals with cerebral palsy, traumatic brain injuries or survivors of stroke. NDSA was originally formed as the United Cerebral Palsy Athletic Association (USCPAA) in 1987. NDSA conducts national championships in twelve sports, disseminates safety and sports medicine information and selects the athletes to represent the United States in international competition. Contact NDSA National Center, 25 West Independence Way, Kingston, RI 02881; telephone 401-792-7130; or visit the Internet site *http://www.ndsaonline.org*

Turning P.O.I.N.T. sponsors opportunities for paralyzed people of all shapes, sizes and ages to camp, fish, sail, scuba dive, hunt, water ski or take pictures from a pontoon boat in the scenic swamps of East Texas. Based on the notion that it's okay to get together with other people with disabilities without feeling embarrassed. Contact Turning P.O.I N.T., 10 Haynes Court, Terrell, TX 75160; telephone 972-524-4231; or visit the Internet site *http://www.turningpointnational.org*

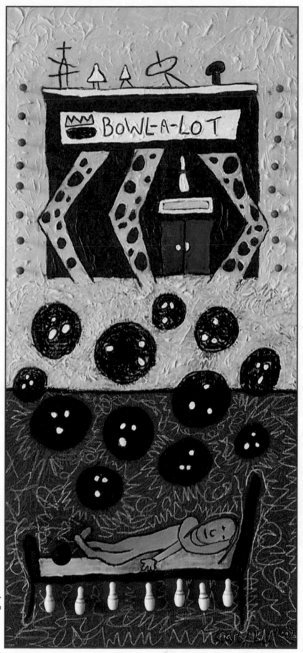

BOWL-A-LOT

7.25 × 15 INCHES, OIL, WOOD & PINS ON PINE WOOD, 2002

I MISS BEING ABLE TO BOWL. I GREW UP AROUND THE BOWLING ALLEYS OF THE SAN FERNANDO VALLEY IN LOS ANGELES AND WATCHED MY PARENTS WIN THOSE UGLY TROPHIES. I THINK A GOOD GAME SCORE IS IN MY BLOOD.

- CAROL ES

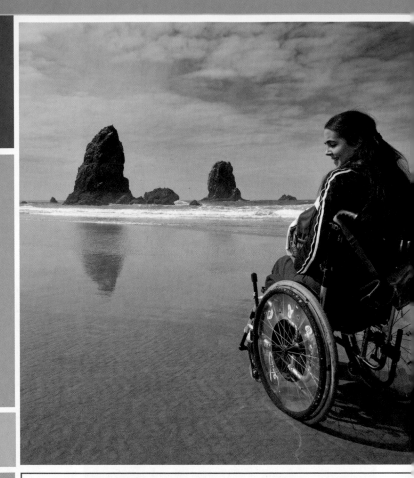

TRAVEL

It's a big planet. You should
see it. Here's how to get
ready to explore, to relax,
to savor exotic cultures.

Whether you're a tourist or a traveler, or even if you don't know the difference, there is great appeal in getting away from home to experience the global community in far-flung places across the land and sea. For the purposes of this Resource Guide, it's the trip that counts, not the purpose, or the destination, or the scenery.

Travel is a process; sometimes it's familiar and comfortable, sometimes random or perhaps unsettling. Unless you have an unusually high threshold for the unpredictable, the best travel plan is to have a plan. This is especially true for people with reduced mobility. No plan is bulletproof, of course, especially when it comes to transportation, scheduling, weather and all the unforeseen tribulations that remind you travel is an art, not a science. We'll break the planning into three steps: getting ready, getting there, and being there.

Getting ready

For those who haven't done a lot of pleasure travel with wheelchairs, walkers and all the paraphernalia of paralysis, it's a good idea to enlist the help of a travel agent who specializes in the disability travel market. These travel professionals know how to get you where you want to go and pretty much what to expect once you get there, matching your level of adventure with your need for creature comfort. In many cases, it's best to make your maiden voyage to a destination that is familiar with people with disabilities. This would include, among many other places, San Diego, Las Vegas, Disney World in Orlando, New York and Washington.

Your agent may also recommend a cruise—this is a very relaxing way to see exotic ports of call in an accessible, well-fed and friendly environment including, in many cases, cabins with roll-in showers. As a whole, the cruise business does a good job anticipating the needs of travelers with disabilities.

Your agent should know a few tricks, such as booking a direct flight whenever possible. Changing planes can be unnerving, especially if your connection is tight—you have to make absolutely sure your wheelchair and other gear make the connecting flight.

Airlines may try to seat you in one of their one-size-fits-all wheelchairs at the gate. In the name of comfort and safety, insist that your personal equipment be

> **"Generally, you don't have to give the airline notice if you're in a wheelchair. But it helps."**

brought forth. On the subject of missing baggage, here is another pro tip: Keep your meds and catheter supplies, etc. in your carry-on bag. Never pack them in your checked luggage.

Agents should know to get their mobility-restricted clients assigned to a bulkhead seat on the airplane; it is much easier to transfer in and out. Your travel pro should also know about general accessibility of your destination, public transportation, rental cars with hand controls and other details once you arrive. Book your van well ahead of time. Where the agent is going to be most helpful is in arranging lodging on the other end. Just because a hotel's brochure has the little wheelchair symbol that says it has accessible rooms doesn't mean you can get in the bathroom. In many cases, the agent has been there ahead of you with a tape measure and knows what to expect, including accessibility of shops, restaurants, and the hotel pool. There are several experienced agencies listed at the end of this chapter.

Getting there

The airline industry in the United States must by law accommodate passengers with disabilities. The compliance record for all airlines is spotty, although much improved in recent years. But here's a rule of thumb experience has taught the veteran traveler with a disability: Despite federal regulations and many years of ADA sensitivity, don't assume that anyone who wears the airline's uniform knows what to do with you or your gear. It may not be necessary to pack a copy of the Air Carrier Access Act (you can get a summary online at *http://www.faa.gov*) but you may have to tap into the deep reserves of your patience.

Generally, you don't have to give any notice to the airline if you have a disability and intend to fly, but there are some exceptions. Air carriers may require up to 48 hours advance notice if you plan to use oxygen or the plane's power supply to operate a respirator. If the plane has fewer than 60 seats, power chair users may also be required to give a two-day notice. A note on oxygen: Most U.S. airlines can accommodate passengers requiring oxygen, although the FAA requires a physician's statement. Also, regulations pro-

THE BEACH BECKONS

Thinking vacation? Think warm, think sand. Head for the sunny beach. It's easier now to get to the surf: Many beach towns have made ramps or paths to the waterfront. Also, there are special plastic-framed beach chairs that glide over the sand on big, puffy tires. These accessible devices are available at many public beaches from coast to coast.

According to Adam Lloyd, a quad travel maven, beach wheelchairs are fine - for sitting out on the sand. "Because of their huge tires, these chairs float – a floating wheelchair can be extremely destabilizing, and has resulted in the chair's tipping over."

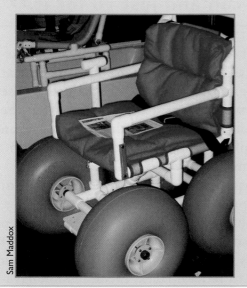

Sam Maddox

Lloyd gets carried to the water via stretcher and then placed on a float. "It is truly a spectacular feeling of freedom, especially for those of us who spend most of our time either sitting in a chair or lying in bed," he says.

To buy a beach chair, check out the Access to Recreation Catalog. Some models are aluminum, others made of plastic tubing. Telephone toll-free 1-800-634-4351; or visit http://accesstr.com

hibit the use of passenger-provided oxygen equipment during flight. Airlines will charge extra for their oxygen, and it's not cheap, so check with the carrier.

Do you need to bring an attendant? No, unless you are on a stretcher or the air carrier cites a safety issue, which you should get in writing. As the rule reads, an attendant may be required if "A person with a mobility impairment so severe that the person is unable to assist in his or her own evacuation of the aircraft."

How about bringing your service dog? No problem. Any public or private accommodation, including restaurants, hotels, stores, taxis and airlines, must allow people with disabilities to bring their service animals with them, wherever customers are normally allowed. You and your dog can't be denied any seat, either, unless the animal obstructs an aisle or other areas that would impede an emergency evacuation. When booking your ticket, tell your travel or ticket agent that a service dog is coming along. Bring the dog's health certificates with proof of vaccinations.

❝You might say the most important piece of luggage is a joyful heart. Or that the heaviest baggage is the empty purse. Prepare as best you can and just go for it.❞

It's best to get to the airport early to check in. As you are transferred to one of those skinny aisle chairs to get you to your seat (first to board, last to deplane), your chair will be tagged so the destination ground crew knows to bring it to the gate when the plane arrives. A lot of wheelchair users keep their seat cushion with them and use it on the plane. Bigger planes (more than 30 seats) must have movable armrests so you can slide in easily.

Once onboard, the travel experience is pretty much like that of everyone else on board, except for using the lavatories. Newer, two-aisle planes have accessible lavatories, as long as you can maneuver yourself in the little onboard chair or have an attendant standing by. The cabin crew is not required to help you once you reach the lavatory. According to federal rules, the accessible lavatory "shall afford privacy to persons using the on-board wheel-chair equivalent to that afforded ambulatory users." Still, it's a rather conspicuous and indiscrete hassle to use the toilet on a plane. It's common for people with dysfunctional bladders to restrict fluid intake before boarding the plane and to use airport facilities right before going aboard.

Airport personnel can be very helpful but they are not required to hand-carry passengers except in emergency evacuations. They don't have to help you eat or to help with any medical services.

Once you land, will your chair or scooter be there, and will it have survived the ride in the cargo hold? Usually there's no problem, especially for manual chairs. If you use a power wheelchair there are more reasons for concern of the well-being of your equipment. Airlines prefer that you use gel or dry-cell batteries as

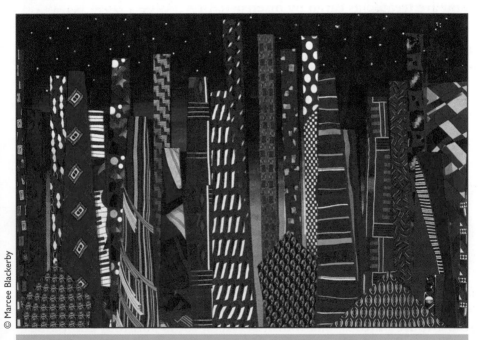

© Marcee Blackerby

TIE LAND

"FOUND OBJECTS CONTAIN THE RESIDUE OF HUMAN EMOTION....MY ARTWORK GIVES ME AN OPPORTUNITY TO BE AN ARMCHAIR TRAVELER WHERE I FEEL UNLIMITED AND WITHOUT BARRIERS."

- MARCEE BLACKERBY, WHEELCHAIR USER SINCE AGE SIX.

opposed to the more common liquid (spillable, corrosive lead acid) ones. If the chair cannot be stored upright, the lead acid battery must be packaged and stored separately. Also, the spillable battery's regular vent caps will be replaced with spill-proof vent caps. Be sure the handlers replace the regular vent caps before reconnecting the battery so dangerous pressure does not build up in the battery during later use.

Some power chair or scooter users remove their joystick controls and carry them on board. These devices are sensitive to abuse and difficult to repair away from home. Not leaving anything to chance, a Maryland company makes protective molded containers for folding manual wheelchairs and for power wheelchairs and scooters. See *http://www.haseltine.com*.

Air travel is an overwhelmingly positive experience for most passengers with disabilities. But if you are treated as cargo by insensitive personnel, or if your own cargo is mangled, always be prepared to assert your rights. Anyone who feels an airline has violated any provision of the access rules may report the incident to the Department of Transportation, Aviation Consumer Protection Division, C-75, 400 Seventh Street, SW, Washington, D.C. 20590. You can be sure that complaints are taken seriously.

> **U.S. DOT HOTLINE:**
> Travelers who experience disability-related air travel service problems may call this toll-free hotline: 1-800-778-4838.

Being there

Public transportation may work out fine. For a useful listing of local travel connections see the Project Action Accessible Traveler's Database, funded by Easter Seals. There is information on accessible airport shuttles, paratransit services, tours and tour companies, and taxi services in cities large and small across the United States. To use the database, visit *http://www.projectaction.org*.

A rental car affords more flexibility and independence. Most of the major car rental companies can supply hand controls, but it's best to give them a few days notice. Several accessible van rental companies are found in major cities. These offer daily and weekly rates on a variety of accessible, full-size cars and mini-vans. Check ahead of time with the companies, listed below, to make sure their rigs are configured to meet your specific needs.

Once you check in and make sure the accommodations are what you expected at the hotel or aboard the cruise ship, go do what travelers do: eat, shop, relax, go to a museum or just watch humanity pass by. You're on a holiday clock now.

So, what are you waiting for? There is nothing so invigorating as travel. It renews the spirit, recharges the imagination. Travel can be a challenge no matter your level of function. But the hassles and even the horror stories supply the contrast to make the good parts all the more special.

When you're ready to hit the road or the high seas, be well informed. Know what you're getting into and to some degree, what you can expect once you get there.

You might have heard that the most important piece of luggage is a joyful heart. Or that the heaviest baggage is the empty purse. The best advice is to take all advice with a grain of salt, to be prepared as best you can, and be open to the adventure. Bon voyage!

ADAM LLOYD: ON THE GO

Adam Lloyd took a passion for wanderlust and transformed it into his life platform. Lloyd, from Bethesda, Maryland, was injured during high school swim practice in 1983 and is a C4 quad. He hasn't been one for sitting on the sidelines.

The power chair, of course, adds another challenge. "The amount of research, planning, and coordination that goes into every trip makes it a chore. That's really why I started Gimp on the Go. Each of us was reinventing the wheel." (*www.gimponthego.com*)

Favorite destination? Las Vegas. "It's incredibly accessible and loads of fun." Any transformative experiences? "Germany was my first trip outside the Americas and traveling through Bavaria...the topography, architecture, history, food, people - I felt like I was living in a Grimm's fairytale. In Costa Rica, after almost 20 years in a chair, I was almost moved to tears at being able to trek through a genuine rainforest! It was such a unique experience, and one I never would have dared to dream could be a reality for me after my accident."

TRAVEL RESOURCES

Travel agents that have lots of experience with travelers with disabilities include the following:

Access Tours, based in Wyoming, specializes in tours of the Grand Canyon, Yellowstone Park, the canyons of Utah and the sights of Northern California. Call toll-free 1–800–929–4811.

Accessible Journeys, based in Pennsylvania, has nearly two decades' experience making vacations across the world accessible and comfortable. Toll-free 1–800–846–4537; *http://www.disabilitytravel.com*

Flying Wheels Travel, founded in Owatonna, MN in 1970, has arranged group tours and independent travel for well over 10,000 clients with disabilities. Visit *http://www.flyingwheelstravel.com*

Nautilus Tours & Cruises, based in California, is a full-service agency for people with disabilities that offers escorted tours and cruises, including many to Europe. Contact the agency toll-free (outside California) 1–800–797–6004 or in California at 818–591–3159. On the Internet see *http://www.nautilustours.com*

Access-Able Travel is an online resource for travelers with disabilities, operated by scooter-user Carol Randall. "All too often these travelers experience unwanted surprises or difficulties with access," says Carol. "This discourages many people from traveling. Fear and doubt keeps many people from even thinking about going somewhere." Her site offers the practical resources to make travel enjoyable for everyone. *http://www.access-able.com*

Emerging Horizons is a consumer magazine about accessible travel. It contains lots of access information, resources, news and travel tips. Editor Candy Harrington has also written several books, including *Barrier-Free Travel, A Nuts and Bolts Guide for Wheelers and Slow Walkers;* and *Inns and B&Bs for Wheelers and Slow Walkers.* Visit the Internet site *http://emerginghorizons.com*

The Society for Accessible Travel & Hospitality (SATH) is a clearinghouse for accessible tourism information, dedicated to a barrier-free environment throughout the travel and tourism industry. SATH, 347 Fifth Avenue, Suite 610, New York, NY 10016; telephone 212–447–7284; or visit the Internet site *http://www.sath.org*

Mobility International USA (MIUSA) is an exchange program clearinghouse to increase the participation of people with disabilities in international exchange programs. Since 1995, MIUSA has served as the National Clearinghouse on Disability and Exchange (NCDE), a project sponsored by the Bureau of Educational and Cultural Affairs of the United States Department of State to educate people with disabilities and related organizations about international exchange opportunities and to facilitate partnerships between people with disabilities, disability-related organizations and international exchange organizations. MIUSA, 132 East Broadway, Eugene, OR 97401; telephone 541–343–1284; or visit the Internet site *http://www.miusa.org*

ScootAround offers scooter and wheelchair rentals in dozens of North American destinations. Call toll-free 1–888–441–7575; or visit the Internet site *http://www.scootaround.com*

Amtrak has many trains that accommodate travelers with disabilities. Call toll-free 1–800–USA-RAIL for information on reservations, accessible coaches and sleeping accommodations, boarding, use of oxygen, etc., or visit *http://www.amtrak.com*, search under "accessibility."

Greyhound buses offer an alternative to trains and planes. Accessibility is much improved. Call toll-free 1–800–231–2222 for details.

Accessible Van Rentals
- **Accessible Vans of America:** toll-free 1–888–282–8267
- **Wheelchair Getaways:** toll-free 1–800–536–5518
- **Wheelers:** toll-free 1–800–456–1371

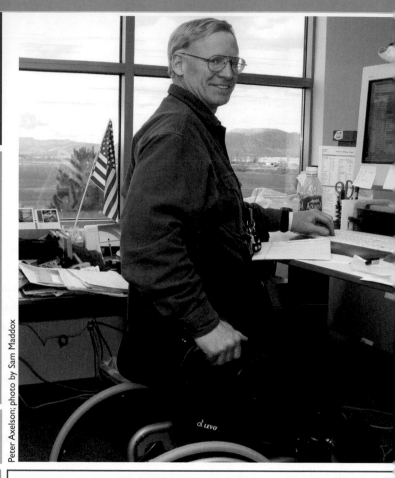

Peter Axelson; photo by Sam Maddox

TOOLS & TECHNOLOGY

With the right gear, gadgets and equipment, people with paralysis can open the doors of opportunity to self-sufficiency, work or play.

Welcome to the wonderful world of assistive technology – all the tools, the gear and gadgets that can profoundly affect the lives of people who have lost function due to paralysis. Innovation and product design offer much more than convenience, of course. There are many people thriving in their communities who would have been locked away in institutions a generation or two in the past.

Indeed, technology opens the doors of opportunity. The computer, for example, is a truly essential and empowering tool; it offers human contact and access to the community. It is a pipeline for information and a gateway to the marketplace. It can offer recreation and fun, and it can lead to gainful employment. With a variety of switches and software options, almost anyone can access the power of the PC – even people who cannot move a muscle.

There are dozens of accessories and gadgets not even listed here, such as reachers, grabbers and all the special devices to make things easier in the kitchen, bath and bedroom. A truly amazing array of products is available. See one of the big home healthcare catalogs, such as Sammons Preston (*www.sammonspreston.com*); or Mail Order Medical (*www.momsup.com*).

Still, we've taken a pretty broad view of what might be considered a tool, from microchips to velcro. We have included computers and a variety of hands-free options for using the PC. We have also featured personal mobility (wheelchairs, scooters and seating systems); environmental control systems (central switch boxes to run home appliances and electrical functions); home modification (the tools and the architectural design elements that make the home or workplace accommodating for a person with restricted mobility); automobiles and the hand controls to operate them; orthoses and bracing devices to improve function, and in some cases, ambulation; and clothing tailored for people with limited function or for those who spend all day sitting. While most of us don't normally think of a dog or a monkey as a tool, we have included service animals in this section for the high utility they offer as assistive pets.

WHEELCHAIRS

The common saying has it all wrong: People are not "confined" to their wheelchairs—they are in fact *liberated* by their wheels. A person with paralysis can get around as quickly in a wheelchair as anyone else can walking. A wheelchair offers people access to work and shopping or any other travel outside the home. For those who are interested, a wheelchair accommodates participation in races, basketball, tennis and other sports.

In some ways a wheelchair is like a bicycle: There are many designs and styles to choose from including imports, lightweights, racing models, etc. The chair is also like a pair of shoes—there are distinct styles for special purposes, such as tennis or rugged trail use. If the fit isn't just right the user can't get comfortable and therefore can't achieve maximum function.

Selecting the right chair, especially for a first-time wheelchair user, can be confusing. It's always a good idea to work with an occupational therapist (OT) who has experience with various kinds of wheelchairs. Many people choose their first chair because it was the one the insurance company was willing to pay for. The second one, though, is often selected because of styling, performance or other features. Here are some basics on wheelchairs:

Manual Chairs

People with upper body strength typically use a manual chair—it is propelled, of course, by pushing the arms forward as the hands grab the wheel rims. A generation ago the standard chair was a chrome-plated behemoth that weighed about 50 pounds. Today's standard chair comes in every color you can think of and is much less than half that weight. The modern chair is designed for far superior performance—they ride truer and are much easier to push than the clunkers of yesteryear. The lightweights, whether with a rigid frame or a folding frame, are also easier to transfer in and out of cars. Generally speaking, a rigid frame (one that does not fold up) transfers more of the rider's energy into the forward motion than does a folding unit. The primary advantage of a folding chair, however, is portability; a folding unit can even fit in the overhead bin of an airplane.

In recent years, chair makers have added suspension systems,

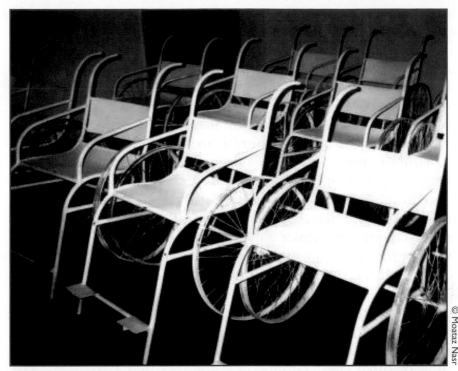

"THE WATER," HAND-MADE WHEELCHAIRS BY MOATAZ NASR, FROM THE TOWNHOUSE GALLERY, CAIRO, EGYPT, 2001

© Moataz Nasr

which smooth the ride considerably. Aftermarket products (e.g. Frog Legs, *http://froglegsinc.com*) are also available to add suspension to the front forks; these have been approved for reimbursement by Medicare. Another key innovation is the use of super-light titanium in wheelchair frames. There are also lots of options for wheels and tires, including innovations for performance, off-road traction and high style.

Power

A person who can't push may require a wheelchair or scooter powered by batteries. Power chairs come in several basic styles. The traditional style looks like a beefed-up standard issue wheelchair, along with all the extra bulk of the batteries, motor and control systems. There are also platform-model power chairs with a more ordinary-looking seat or captain's chair fixed atop a power base. Scooters come in three- and four-wheel configurations and are most often used by people who don't require them full-time.

Until just a few years ago, the power chair market was limited to just a few brands and models. Innovation has expanded the choices toward lighter, more powerful and much faster chairs. Most power chairs have rear-wheel drive, but mid-wheel and front-wheel drives have grabbed a share of the market. These are easier to turn and are quite nimble in tight spaces.

Reimbursement is a key issue for all durable medical equipment, especially for high-ticket items such as power chairs (which can cost more than a fully loaded Ford). In an attempt to curtail fraud, Medicare has changed some of its reimbursement rules, effectively limiting choice for many power users. You'll need to work with your funding sources, your OT and seating specialists, and your rehab supplier to get the best chair for your needs.

Batteries

Battery life is a crucial issue for power chair users. Failure to manage this power source can lead to sticky or annoying situations, especially if you're far from home. Power chair batteries come in three sizes: Group-22, Group-24 and Group-27. The larger the group number, the larger the battery and the more power it stores.

There are three types of battery. Lead-acid or "wet" batteries create electrical energy when lead and sulfuric acid interact. Wet means just that: These battery cells need to be periodically filled with distilled water, maybe once a month. The main advantage of a wet-cell battery is the lower cost. The main disadvantage is that they require special handling when you fly, including special packaging so they don't spill corrosive acid in the cargo hold. Gel batteries don't have liquid to spill or top off. They are more expensive than wet battery versions, but they have a longer life cycle and are much preferred for airline travel. Absorbent glass mat (AGM) batteries are newer to the market. Like gel units, AGM batteries don't require maintenance and are okay for flying. They are very rugged, hold a charge better and last twice as long as standard lead-acid batteries. They are also the most expensive.

Wheelchair batteries are the same as those used in the boating industry. If you pay for your own batteries out-of-pocket, save

IBOT: MOBILITY, WITH EMOTION
By John Hockenberry

My first impression of the machine was not positive.

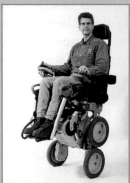

The IBOT is a cumbersome, complicated thing that makes you dread being stuck somewhere without a tool kit. But watch the IBOT balancing, making little rocking motions to keep it upright, and you feel as though you're in the presence of some humanoid intelligence.

When [inventor] Dean Kamen began testing his chair with disabled users, he discovered an eerie and unanticipated brain-machine interface. "Each person we took up the stairs said, 'Great.' They said great when we took them through the sand and the gravel and up the curb and down the curb. But when we stood them up and made them eye level with another person, and they could feel what it was like to balance, every single one of them started crying."

Kamen believes that people who use the IBOT in its two-wheel balancing mode are literally feeling the experience of walking, even though the machine is doing the work. "If you could get an MRI picture of the balance center of the brain of some person in a wheelchair who goes up on the IBOT's two wheels, I bet you'd see some lights go on," he says. "I'm convinced the brain remembers balancing, and that's why people feel so much emotion."

I felt exactly that when I used the IBOT for the first time and stood upright. The chip was making the wheels move, but my brain's own sense of balance seemed to instantly merge with the machine. Its decisions seemed to be mine. No implants. No wires. It was truly extraordinary.

— Excerpted by permission, Wired Magazine

money by purchasing marine batteries at Wal-Mart or any other non-medical retailer of deep-cycle batteries. To say something is for medical use seems to drive up its price.

Is there an IBOT in your future? This is the ultimate high-tech chair; riders claim it moves them both physically and emotionally. It rides on four wheels but can rise up on two wheels — at eye level to walking people; it goes up and down stairs and even moves through sand. Riders are mechanically balanced by gyroscopes and microprocessors. Independence Technology has FDA approval to market the IBOT. The chair will be sold directly by the company, at price point in the $30,000 range. Some insurance companies have paid for the IBOT. It is approved by the VA for some veterans. But it won't be paid for by Medicare, which considers it to be a standard power wheelchair and provides reimbursement only at that modest level. The company is vigorously challenging Medicare's determination.

Power assist: A sort of hybridization has recently occurred. The standard lightweight manual can be tricked-up with special rims that contain small, powerful motors. When the assist is turned on, a forward push on the handrim gives the chair a strong boost. The e.motion fits many types of chairs. The Xtender is available on some Quickie models in two versions, one that increases the force applied to the handrims by a factor of 1.5 and one that boosts you by a factor of 3. These assist hubs add quite a bit of weight to the chair (from 38 to almost 50 pounds) and quite a bit of expense ($6,000 to $8,000), but the advantages are terrific, especially for lower-level quads and anyone with achy shoulders who won't have to struggle up steep hills. A rider's range will increase dramatically using the assist, saving personal energy and wear and tear on the rotator cuffs. What's more, the chair doesn't look like a beefed-up power unit: It looks more or less "normal." See *www.frankmobility.com* for more on e.motion and *www.sunrisemedical.com* for more on the Xtender.

Kids Chairs

Children's bodies are growing and changing, which means their chairs must be adjusted or replaced more often than adult chairs. Since chairs are not cheap and insurance providers often place limitations on replacement, most manufacturers offer adjustable chairs to accommodate a growing child. Wheelchair companies also offer chairs for kids that don't look as "medical" as the older styles. The updated looks offer more streamlined designs, cooler upholstery and different frame colors. Colours by Permobil offers the Little Dipper, a little chair with a little attitude. Likewise, the Sunrise Quickie Kidz and the Invacare Orbit are

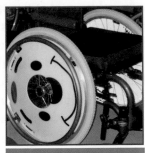

KID CHAIR

made for younger wheelers who want to ride with a bit of style.

Seating and Positioning

People with paralysis are at high risk for pressure sores and therefore usually require special cushions and seating systems to give the skin some relief. There are three basic kinds of cushion material, each with benefits for certain types of users: air, foam or liquid (e.g., gel). Work with your seating specialist to determine which is the right one to fit your body, lifestyle and budget.

The right cushion can provide comfort, correct positioning and prevent pressure sores, but it need not meet all those criteria for every user. An ambulatory person who only uses a wheelchair to go shopping doesn't have the same needs as a high-level quad who spends eighteen hours per day in a power chair, so it's important to fully understand your requirements and select the appropriate cushion, weighing the pros and cons of the different styles.

Foam is the least expensive material for a cushion. It's also lightweight and doesn't leak or lose air. It does wear out, though, losing its compression over time. Air flotation cushions, such as the popular ROHO model (see *www.rohoinc.com*), provide support using a bladder of evenly distributed air. These work well but can leak; they also require air adjustments when you change altitude. Gel cushions, such as the Jay (see www.*sunrisemedical.com*), are filled with slow-flowing gel. They are effective for skin protection, but are also somewhat heavy.

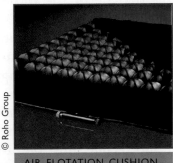

AIR FLOTATION CUSHION

Another cushion option features an oscillating pump that facilitates alternating pressure; the theory is that seating can continue for longer periods of time if pressure is alternated with no pressure. This adds weight to the chair and, because the pump runs on batteries, is not as carefree as a static cushion (for an example, see the Aquila line at *www.aquilacorp.com*). For a complete list of available cushions and seating systems see ABLEDATA (*www.abledata.com*) or see Care Catalog, *www.caremedical.com*.

Tilt or Recline

Some people use special wheelchairs to distribute pressure and thus reduce the risk of skin sores. These chairs also increase comfort and sitting tolerance. One type of chair, called "tilt in space,"

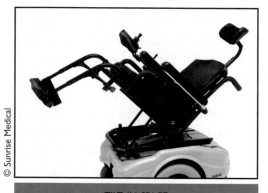

© Sunrise Medical

TILT IN SPACE

changes a person's orientation while maintaining fixed hip, knee and ankle angles. In effect, the whole seat tilts. The other chair option is a recline system, which basically changes the seat-to-back angle, flattening out the back of the chair and, in some cases, raising the legs to form a flat surface.

A tilt system redistributes pressure from the buttocks and posterior thighs to the posterior trunk and head. The system maintains posture and prevents sheering (the friction on tissues from dragging across a surface). A drawback: If a user sits at a workstation, for example, the tilt requires that he or she move back from the table to avoid hitting it with the knees or footrests.

Recline systems open the seat-to-back angle and, in combination with elevating legrests, open the knee angle. There are some advantages to a recline system for eating, making transfers or assisting with bowel or bladder programs, as all are easier when lying down. Generally speaking, the recline system offers more pressure relief than tilt, but with a higher risk of sheer. Elevating the legs may be beneficial to people with edema. Both tilt and recline must be fitted and prescribed by seating and positioning experts.

Standing

Standing chairs act as normal manual chairs but also help the rider rise to a standing position. There are many advantages to being tall at home, in school and in the workplace. Some manual chairs come with a power assist to activate the rising mechanism. Some power chairs also enable the rider to rise to a standing position, with the advantage of eye-to-eye contact with others. The drawback: They are not cheap and are heavy for an everyday chair. See *www.lifestandusa.com* or *www.levousa.com*.

Standing has physical benefits, too. It helps to prevent pressure sores, improves circulation and range of motion and, for some, reduces spasms and contractions. A few years ago the Hines VA reported that people who stand for 30 minutes or more per day "had significantly improved quality of life, fewer bed sores, fewer bladder infections, improved bowel regularity, and improved ability to straighten their legs." There are several models of standing frames available. Some, such as the Stand-Aid (see *www.stand-aid.com*) or Vertran (*www.vertran.com*), are motorized. Others are more rudimentary—basically a static frame that supports a paralyzed person in the standing position (see *www.stand-rite.com,* or *www.easystand.com*).

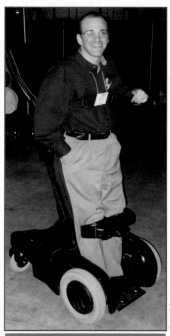

MOTORIZED STANDER/VERTRAN

Sam Maddox

There are other specialty chairs available, including ultra lightweight three-wheelers for road racing; chairs with extra camber for tennis and basketball (they don't tip over); heavy duty four-wheelers for off-road use; and even chairs with tractor treads for those who cannot resist negotiating the roughest of terrain.

Sources
American Occupational Therapy Association, ABLEDATA

WHEELCHAIR RESOURCES

WheelchairJunkie.com is a resourceful and opinionated Website owned and operated by self-described "power chair gonzo" Mark E. Smith. Says Smith, "WheelchairJunkie.com is about mobility, not manufacturers, so the voices expressed here represent only users." On the Internet see *http://www.wheelchairjunkie.com*

The TechGuide is an Internet guide to wheelchairs and assistive technology, including numerous reviews of mobility gear. Sponsored by United Spinal Association. See *www.usatechguide.org*

WheelchairNet is a federally funded virtual community for people with an interest in wheelchair technology. Home of Wheelchair University. Its primary audience is the person who uses wheeled mobility. Lots of information here on every aspect of wheelchairs, including selection guidelines, research, reimbursement, quality control, etc. See *http://www.wheelchairnet.org*

Wheelchair and scooter companies include:
Invacare (toll-free 1-800-333-6900 or *www.invacare.com*)
Sunrise Medical/Quickie (toll-free 1-888-333-2572 or see *http://sunrisemedical.com*)
Permobil (toll-free 1-800-736-0925 or see *www.permobil.com*)
Colours (1-800-892-8998 or *www.colourswheelchair.com*)
TiSport (1-800-545-2266 or *www.titaniumsports.com*)
Pride Mobility (the Jazzy brand, toll-free 1-800-800-8586, or see *www.pridemobility.com*)
Bruno makes scooters and a full line of lifts and car carriers (toll-free 1-800-882-8183 or *see www.bruno.com*)

Spinlife is one of several online dealers of durable medical equipment. See *www.spinlife.com;* other online dealers include *www.phc-online.com* and *www.medicalsupply4u.com/*

Sportaid is a discount online wheelchair and rehab goods retailer. See *www.sportaid.com*

Wheelchair accessories: Backpacks, trays, cup holders, canopies, umbrellas and other gear. Cool stuff for your chair. Contact Diestco, toll-free 1-800-795-2392 or see *www.diestco.com*

ASSISTIVE TECHNOLOGY

Technology plays a vital role in the lives of millions of people who are paralyzed. There are numerous assistive technology (AT) products on the market today that enable people with disabilities to achieve greater independence and enhance their quality of life. These products, tools and gadgets help ease people through their daily routines and assist them in communication, education, work or recreation.

Assistive technology, including the powerful personal computer, can help improve one's physical and mental functioning, strengthen a weakness, improve a person's capacity to learn, or even replace a missing muscle system. AT can help with running the household, bathing, dressing, grooming, cooking, cleaning, writing, reading and so on.

Below are links to resources on technology and tools.

ABLEDATA is a national resource database on all adaptive technology products. For specific solutions contact ABLEDATA, 8630 Fenton Street, Suite 930, Silver Spring, MD 20910; toll-free 1-800-227-0216 or visit *www.abledata.com*

RESNA (Rehabilitation Engineering and Assistive Technology Society of North America) is an interdisciplinary association with an interest in technology and disability. RESNA, 1700 N. Moore Street, Suite #1540, Arlington, VA 22209-1903, telephone 703-524-6686; *http://www.resna.org*

The Center for Assistive Technology (Project Link) offers "Link to Assistive Products" where you can learn about products and where to get them. CAT, University at Buffalo, 322 Stockton Kimball Tower, Buffalo, NY 14214-3079; toll-free 1-800-628-2281; *http://cat.buffalo.edu/*

Trace Center at the University of Wisconsin is working to make standard information technologies and telecommunications systems usable by people with disabilities. Trace

Research & Development Center, University of Wisconsin-Madison, 1550 Engineering Drive, Madison, WI 53706; telephone 608-262-6966; or *www.trace.wisc.edu*

The Computer Access Center (CAC) hopes to empower people with disabilities through technology. CAC, 6234 West 87th Street, Los Angeles, CA 90045; telephone 310-338-1597; or *http://www.cac.org*

The Alliance for Technology Access is a network of community-based resource centers that provide information and support to children and adults with disabilities. Alliance for Technology Access, 1304 Southpoint Blvd., Suite 240, Petaluma, CA 94954; telephone 707-778-3011 or visit the Internet site *http://www.ataccess.org*

Assistive Technology Training Online Project provides information on technology applications to help students with disabilities learn in elementary classrooms. *http://atto.buffalo.edu*

AbilityHub is a place to find information on adaptive equipment and alternative methods for accessing computers. Created by Dan J. Gilman, a rehab engineer and quad. See *http://www.abilityhub.com*

Technology and Persons with Disabilities is an annual conference in Los Angeles hosted by California State University, Northridge. For details contact CSUN Students with Disabilities Resources, telephone 818-677-2684 or visit the Internet site *http://www.csun.edu/cod*

AT508.com is an internet site with "the latest and greatest information on assistive technology and how it pertains to Section 508" (federal law). From AT maven John Williams. Includes Internet television archives on assistive technology. See *http://www.at508.com*

ENVIRONMENTAL CONTROL

Paralysis often restricts control over one's living space. An environmental control unit (ECU) can help people regain power over their environment and maximize functional ability and independence at home, school, work and leisure.

Generally, an ECU is a single remote control unit designed to operate a variety of switches and appliances — such as opening a door, turning on the television, dialing a telephone, adjusting the lights, etc. The ECU can operate with an array of switches, by voice command, by computer or by sip and puff. The unit can also be operated by motion detection switches; for example, one can control the environment with as little movement as an eye blink.

Below are resources on ECUs and other tools.

X-10 technology is a nifty and inexpensive remote switching system that uses existing wiring in the home or workplace. For information, contact X10 Wireless Technology, Inc., 19823 58th Place, South Kent, WA 98032; toll-free 1-800-675-3044 or visit the Internet site *http://www.x10wti.com*

Quartet Technology Incorporated (QTI) offers high-end ECU units that operate by voice, switches or computer mouse. QTI, 1934 Lakeview Avenue, Dracut, Massachusetts 01826; 978-957-4328 or visit *www.qtiusa.com/*

Mastervoice offers two set-ups, either a single- or two-user voice-activated control system for hands-free control of appliances, lights and telephones. Both "Butler-in-a-Box" systems use existing household wiring. Contact Automated Voice Systems, Inc., 17059 El Cajon Avenue, Yorba Linda, CA 92686; telephone 714-524-4488; or visit the Internet site *http://www.mastervoice.com*

Home Automated Living (HAL) makes software that turns the home computer into an ECU controllable from anywhere. HAL, Inc., 14401 Sweitzer Lane, Suite 600, Laurel, MD 20707; toll-free 1-800-935-5313; or visit the Internet site *http://www.automatedliving.com*

Able-Phone makes adaptive telephones designed for persons with little or no arm and hand function. Able-Phone, 354 Chatfield Avenue, Biggs, CA, 95917; telephone 530-846-PHONE; or visit the Internet site *http://www.ablephone.com*

Tech Act: It's a good idea to try out various ECU or computer operating systems before purchase. One way to shop for adaptive technology is to check in with your state's federal Tech Act office. The Association of Assistive Technology Act Programs supports implementation of the AT Act and promotes full access to AT devices and services. See *http://www.ataporg.org* for a list of regional resources.

Rehabtool.com features a comprehensive collection of links to the largest AT catalogs, databases and vendor directories in North America. Rehabtool.com, P.O. Box 572190, Houston, TX 77257; telephone 281-531-6106; or visit the Internet site *http://www.rehabtool.com*

United Spinal Association features an AT site with product listings and reviews. See *www.usatechguide.org/*

Closing the Gap is a national publication on assistive equipment and adaptive gear for children and adults. Great resources in print and online. Closing the Gap, 526 Main Street, Henderson, MN 56044; telephone 507-248-3294; or visit the Internet site *http://closingthegap.com*

Assistivetech.net is an online information resource providing up-to-date information on assistive technologies, adaptive environments and community resources. On the Internet see *http://www.assistivetech.net*

HANDS-FREE COMPUTING

Hands-free technology is available for quadriplegics and people with upper-body restrictions to fully and independently operate a computer and almost all software. It's also possible to navigate the World Wide Web by using only voice, eyes, head or breath. Soon the world of computing will be accessed using brain waves.

Here is a rundown on "headmice" and other hands-free cursor control alternatives.

The Cordless Gyro-HeadMouse offers an onscreen keyboard cursor control unit built into a baseball hat. The user must be able to move his or her head two inches up, down, to the right and left. Mouse function requires sip and puff action. Advanced Peripheral Technologies, Ltd. 14416 Erin Court, Lockport, IL 60441; telephone 708-301-4508.

The HeadMouse translates the movements of a user's head into movements of a computer mouse pointer using a wireless optical sensor that tracks a tiny target placed on the user's forehead or glasses. Full computer control (including portables) is facilitated by an onscreen keyboard. Prentke Romich Company, 1022 Heyl Road, Wooster, OH 44691; toll-free 1-800-262-1984; or visit *www.prentrom.com*

A **HeadMouse** model is also available from Origin Instruments Corporation, 854 Greenview Drive, Grand Prairie, TX 75050-2438; telephone 972-606-8740; or visit the Internet site *http://www.orin.com*

The Cyberlink allows hands-free control of a mouse cursor, video games and other external devices. Users wear a headband with sensors that detect electrical signals from subtle facial muscle, eye movement and brain wave activity. Brain Actuated Technologies, Inc., 1350 President Street, Yellow Springs, OH 45387; telephone 937-767-2674; or visit the Internet site *http://www.brainfingers.com*

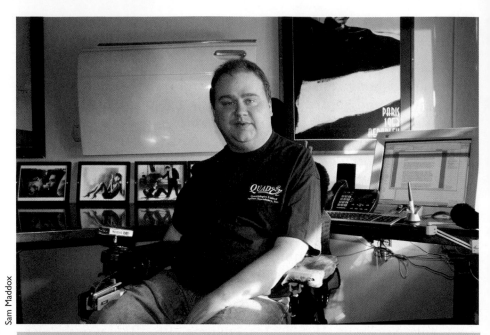

Sam Maddox

No question about it, my computer is my most valuable possession. It's an incredible tool for communication, for learning, for fun, for shopping, for running one's home environment, and best of all, for making a living. There are lots of ways to operate the computer without using hands. I use a mouth stick, which I make myself. I can type fairly quickly with it. A common approach these days is voice activation. It's inexpensive and generally very reliable. I was one of the first to try this way back when but for me there were too many glitches – I spent more time correcting my work than creating it. - *Pete Denman, C4*

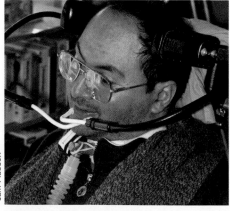

Sam Maddox

If you have access to a computer, you're able to communicate with the outside world. They won't even know you even have a disability unless you tell them. I use Morse code and a sip-n-puff. I tried a lot of ways to do this and this seems to work the best. Once you memorize the codes, it's just automatic. - *Jim Lubin, C2*

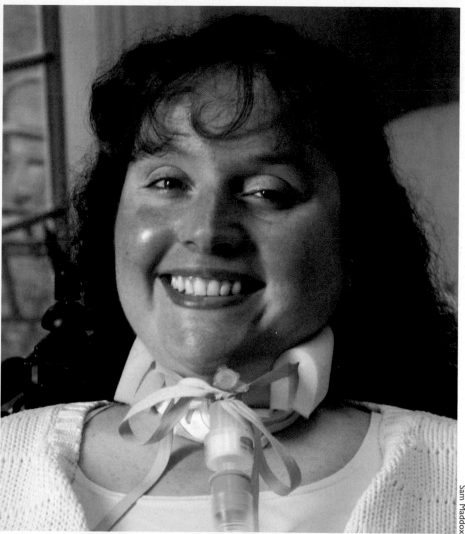

Sam Maddox

I do a lot of paper-writing, a lot of work, on the computer. I spend hours and hours every day on the computer, doing either reading or writing, or both. I use a voice-activated system, a voice-activated software program called Dragon: Naturally Speaking, which works very well for me. For me to move the mouse, which I use pretty extensively, it works through the wheelchair system. The mouse is infrared, and it sends a signal from my wheelchair to the computer. I have a little remote control that sits on the roof of my mouth, and I hit little buttons with my tongue. - *Brooke Ellison, C2*

Tracker 2000 allows smooth cursor control; the unit sits on top of the computer and tracks a tiny reflective dot worn on the forehead or glasses. Head movement is converted into computer mouse movement. Madentec, 4664 - 99 Street, Edmonton, Alberta, Canada T6E 5H5; toll-free 1-877-623-3682; or visit *http://www.madentec.com*

The NaturalPoint SmartNAV is a hands free ergonomic mouse. Increase productivity by moving your head to control the computer. Also available for Mac users. Contact NaturalPoint, P.O. BOX 2317, Corvallis, OR 97339; telephone 541-753-6645; *www.naturalpoint.com/smartnav/*

Quad-Joy is a hands-free system that uses a joystick-operated mouse controlled by sip and puff. Inventor Tom Street, a C-4 quad, targets people on a limited budget or who have no outside funding source. Street Electric Manufacturing Company, 3211 N. Koning Drive, Sheboygan, WI 53083; toll-free 1-877-736-2663; or visit the Internet site *http://www.quadjoy.com*

Dragon Systems voice activation: Prices have dropped in recent years as voice input technology keeps improving. This software is widely used at home and in the office to translate voice to text; it's easy and reliable. For information see *www.nuance.com/naturallyspeaking/*

The Talking Desktop is speech recognition software that talks back, reads text and allows hands-free computer operation. Abasoft Corporation, 37 Norton Road, Hampton, NH 03842; toll-free telephone 1-866 697-0326; or visit the Internet site *http://www.talkingdesktop.com*

RJ Cooper & Associates offers dozens of assistive technology solutions, including unique, custom adaptations. Call 1-800-RJCooper; see *http://rjcooper.com*

HOME MODIFICATION

The world isn't flat or paved, of course, and for the most part no one was thinking about people using wheelchairs or walkers when they designed all our streets and buildings. But things are changing as people with disabilities — joined by the largest ever U.S. generation heading toward its senior years – have pushed to open up access to all people, including those with paralysis or mobility problems.

The concept of universal design goes beyond ramps, retrofits and curb cuts. It isn't just about accessibility. It is a way of looking at the designed world knowing that thoughtful plans from the get-go will accommodate any user across his or her lifespan – whether it's getting in the office, the ballpark, or on the Internet.

Ron Mace, who founded the Center for Universal Design at North Carolina State University, put it this way: "Universal design is the design of products and environments to be usable by all people, to the greatest extent possible, without the need for adaptation or specialized design." What he means is that design should work for all of us, across our lifespans, transparently.

There are laws on the books making schools, transportation, housing, public accommodations and the sidewalks fully accessible in every city. For most people, day-in and day-out access has more to do with getting in and out of the house, working in the kitchen, using the bathroom.

Home modification can be as simple as a doorknob that's easy to work, a grab bar in the right place or a ramp to get in through the back door. It may involve widening a door or installing a special sink or elevator. It gets as fancy or as complicated as any architect can make it. There are solutions that don't cost much and there are money pits.

Home access and ease-of-use modifications are for the most part still viewed as an exception: Builders will not include them unless consumers ask for them, and consumers won't ask for them unless they have a significant need. So be informed, know what's out there. *What follows are resources to help you assess your needs, weigh your many product options and locate contractors to make your home or work environment accessible.*

HOME MODIFICATION RESOURCES

The Center for Universal Design is a national research, information and technical assistance center at North Carolina State University that evaluates, develops and promotes universal design in housing, public and commercial facilities, and related products. Center for Universal Design, College of Design, North Carolina State University, Campus Box 8613, Raleigh, NC 27695-8613; toll-free 1-800-647-6777; on the Internet see *www.design.ncsu.edu/cud*

The National Resource Center on Supportive Housing and Home Modification, based at the University of Southern California, promotes aging at home for frail elderly and persons aging with a disability, and they hope to equip families and individuals with the knowledge to plan for their housing, health and supportive service needs. The Center features a national directory of home-mod resources, a newsletter, library and more. Contact the Center c/o USC Andrus Gerontology Center, 3715 McClintock Avenue, Los Angeles, CA 90089; telephone 213-740-1364; or visit the Internet site *http://www.homemods.org*

ABLEDATA is a national resource database on adaptive technology products, including every sort of device and tool for home or workplace modification. For specific solutions, contact ABLEDATA, 8630 Fenton Street, Suite 930, Silver Spring, MD 20910; toll-free 1-800-227-0216 or visit the Internet site *http://www.abledata.com*

The Access Board is an independent federal agency devoted to improving accessibility for people with disabilities. The board develops and enforces accessibility requirements for the built environment, transit vehicles, telecommunications equipment and electronic and information technology. The Access Board, 1331 F Street, NW, Suite 1000, Washington, DC 20004-1111; toll-free 1-800-872-2253; or visit the Internet site *http://www.access-board.gov*

Accessibility Equipment Manufacturers Association is a trade group of companies that make elevators and lifts, stairway chairlifts and similar products. Toll-free 1-800-514-1100; or visit the Internet site *http://www.aema.com*

Adaptive Environments promotes accessibility and universal design through education programs, technical assistance, and design advocacy so that every individual, regardless of disability or age, can participate fully in all aspects of society. Adaptive Environments, 180-200 Portland Street Suite 1, Boston, MA 02114; telephone 617-695-1225; or visit the Internet site *http://www.adaptenv.org*

Center for Inclusive Design and Environmental Access (IDEA) is dedicated to improving the design of environments and products by making them more usable, safer and appealing to people with a wide range of abilities, throughout their life spans. IDEA provides resources and technical expertise in architecture, product design, etc. Center for Inclusive Design & Environmental Access, 378 Hayes Hall, School of Architecture and Planning, 3435 Main Street, University at Buffalo, Buffalo, NY 14214-3087; telephone 716-829-3485 or see *www.ap.buffalo.edu/idea*

AARP spotlights universal design for the home of the future, a home that is safer and more comfortable for people of all ages. AARP, 601 E Street, NW, Washington, DC 20049; toll-free 1-800-OUR-AARP. Or visit the Internet site *www.aarp.org/families/home_design/*

The Ramp Project, an effort of Minnesota's Rehabilitation Services Department and the Metropolitan Center for Independent Living (MCIL), offers an inexpensive, modular, reusable, easy to build wheelchair ramp design. The manual, "How to Build Ramps for Home Accessibility," contains detailed step-by-step installation instructions, and engineering drawings for ramps and stairs. It can be purchased for $15 or viewed at *http://www.wheelchairramp.org*. Contact MCIL, 1600 University Avenue, St. Paul, MN 55104-3825; telephone 651-603-2029.

Concrete Change is an Atlanta-based agency that works to make all homes visitable, that is, accessible to all. Minimum standards include at least one entrance with zero steps, 32-inch passages through interior doors and at least a half-bath on the main floor. For details, contact Concrete Change, 600 Dancing Fox Road, Decatur, GA 30032; or visit the Internet site *http://concretechange.org*

CARS AND DRIVING

There's more to having a set of wheels than getting from here to there. Jumping in a car is a ticket to freedom, independence and adventure. For people new to paralysis, driving is a sure way to get back into the swing of things. But can you do it? Can a paralyzed person get behind the wheel and handle the machine and the traffic? Driving is quite possible for many people who are paralyzed, even those with very limited hand and arm function. A wide range of adaptive driving equipment and vehicle modifications are on the market today.

Driving with a disability often means relearning to drive. The rules of the road don't change, but the controls do. Depending on one's specific needs, an adapted vehicle may include hand controls for braking/accelerating, power assist devices for easy steering, touch ignition pads and gear shifts, adjustable driver's seats, automatic door openers and even joysticks for people with extremely limited hand function (see sidebar on joystick driving, page 238). For a person who has had a stroke, a spinner knob might be attached to the steering wheel for one-hand steering. A left gas pedal may be adapted if the right foot can't operate the gas.

The first step in the process is to get an evaluation from a qualified driver trainer. This will determine your basic driving set up, specific modifications and driving equipment to match your needs. An evaluation also includes vision screening and assessment of muscle strength; flexibility and range of motion; hand-eye coordination and reaction time; judgment and decision making; and the ability to handle adaptive equipment. An evaluator may also take into account medications a potential driver is taking.

To find a qualified evaluator, visit your local rehabilitation center or contact the Association for Driver Rehabilitation Specialists (ADED – see page 237), which maintains a list of certified specialists throughout the country.

As for getting a new driver's license, most states require a valid learner's permit or driver's license to receive an on-the-road evaluation. You cannot be denied the opportunity to apply for a permit or license because you have a disability, but you may receive a restricted license, based on adaptive devices you require.

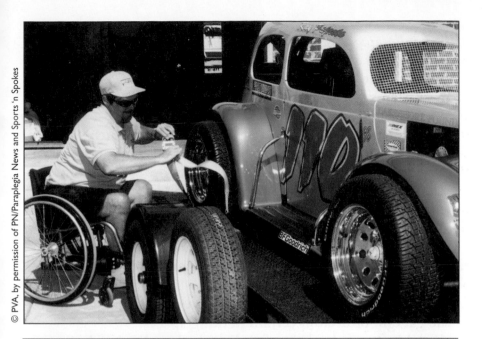

RAY PAPROTA PREPARES HIS RACE CAR FOR THE TRACK. RAY, WHO HAS A NASCAR CREDENTIAL, USES CUSTOM-DESIGNED HAND CONTROLS FOR HIS RACE CARS TO OPERATE FOUR- AND FIVE-SPEED MANUAL TRANSMISSIONS.

Once you get the green light from the evaluation and your state's motor vehicle department, it's time to think about the kinds of vehicles that suit your abilities and needs. Choosing the right car may lead you to more practical wheels than you might have chosen before paralysis (two-seater sports cars may fit the image you have of yourself but are pretty low on the practical scale; minivans, those dreaded mom-wagons you swore to avoid are of much higher utility). See what other people with similar disabilities drive. Then be sure and collaborate with the evaluator and a qualified vehicle modification dealer.

People who sit in their wheelchair while driving or riding in minivans or full-size vans need either a manual tie-down or power lockdowns for safety. The manual systems usually require help getting in and out. Power units allow for more independence – you just roll into place and the chair automatically locks down. Because there is no way a person can operate a van from a scooter, users must be able to transfer to the vehicle seat to drive; electronic seats are available to help with the transfer.

The following can help with vehicle selection and perhaps adaptation of a car you already own:

- Does the necessary adaptive equipment require a van, or will a smaller passenger car do? In other words, will you be driving from a wheelchair or can you transfer to the car seat? If you can transfer in to drive a car, your choices are much wider.
- Will you fit in a minivan? A person may sit taller in the chair and may not clear the ceiling.
- Can the vehicle accommodate the hand controls or other needed driving equipment?
- Will there be enough space to accommodate other passengers once the vehicle is modified?
- Is there adequate parking space at home and at work for the vehicle and for loading/unloading a wheelchair or walker? Be aware that full-size vans might not fit in your garage or public garages or even in certain parking spaces.
- If a third party is paying for the vehicle, adaptive devices, or modifications, are there limitations or restrictions on what is covered? Get a written statement on what a funding agency will pay before making your purchase.

If you are adapting a used van or family vehicle, make sure the technician has lots of experience. All lifts are not created equally; some just won't fit. Also, some lifts are built for wheelchair users; scooter users may not be able to use them.

The cost of modifying a vehicle varies greatly. A new vehicle modified with adaptive equipment can cost anywhere from $20,000 to $80,000. Be a savvy shopper; investigate public and private financial assistance.

There are programs that help pay part or all of the cost of vehicle modification. Contact your state's department of vocational rehabilitation or another agency that provides vocational services and, if appropriate, the Department of Veterans Affairs. Also, consider the following:

- Some nonprofit groups that advocate for individuals with disabilities have grant programs that help with adaptive devices.
- If you have private health insurance or workers' compensation, you may be covered for adaptive devices and vehicle modification. Check with your insurance carrier.

- Several auto manufacturers, including Toyota, Chrysler, Ford, Saturn and General Motors, have rebate or reimbursement plans for vehicles that will be modified.
- Some states waive the sales tax for adaptive devices if you have a doctor's prescription for their use. You may also be eligible for medical expense-related savings on your federal income tax return; consult a tax specialist.

Find a qualified dealer to modify your vehicle. Ask questions, check credentials and references. Do they work with evaluators? Will they examine your vehicle before you purchase it? Do they require a prescription from a physician or other driver evaluation specialist? Do they provide training on how to use the equipment? Do they provide service? What is the cost? How long will it take to do the work? What is the warranty? Have fun. Be safe.

Sources

U.S. Department of Transportation, Association for Driver Rehabilitation Specialists

DRIVING RESOURCES

The Association for Driver Rehabilitation Specialists (ADED) certifies driver trainers who are experts in adaptive driving and vehicles. The organization offers several fact sheets for drivers with various types of disabilities. Call toll-free 1-800-290-2344 or visit the Internet site *http://www.driver-ed.org*

National Mobility Equipment Dealers Association (NMEDA) is a trade group of companies that sell adaptive driving equipment. Call toll-free 1-800-833-0427 or visit *http://www.nmeda.org*

National Highway and Transportation Safety Administration offers advice on driver training, vehicle selection and modification. See *http://www.nhtsa.gov/cars/rules/adaptive*

Disabled Dealer is a publication featuring used vehicles (and all sorts of other rehab and medical gear). Regional editions feature numerous pre-owned adapted vans and cars. On the Internet visit *http://www.disableddealer.com* for more.

ONE-HANDED DRIVING

The joystick has enabled a fleet of quads who'd otherwise be riding shotgun to hit the freedom freeway.

Joystick car systems have been around long enough to establish their safety, reliability and performance. You may face a choice between a mechanical/hydraulic system (like an airplane) or electronic system (like a PlayStation). It may come down to your comfort level with electronics and any worries about a total power shutdown at 70 mph.

A California company called dSi custom fits its Scott mechanical system to each driver. The firm says mechanical is more reliable and more refined than electronic. They like to use big Ford vans and have drivers who've logged more than 300,000 miles on the system.

EMC offers an electronic solution called Aevit. A main advantage is that Aevit does not require modification of original equipment brakes, steering and airbag assemblies. This means you can resell the vehicle without the mods. Also, an Aevit system can be operated by a non-disabled driver. The Scott system, by contrast, is joystick only.

If you're thinking about going joystick, you can't get one without a referral from a driving instructor (see ADED, page 237). Also, the importance of training cannot be overstated. Oh, you may need to line up a trunkload of money, too. A joystick system will run you $40,000 to $65,000, plus the cost of the van. Third parties, including private insurance, voc rehab and the VA, have paid for lots of these, so investigate your options.

For details, ask each manufacturer for user references and if at all possible, check out each system yourself. Contact EMC, telephone 225-927-5558 or visit *http://www.emc-digi.com;* contact dSi-Scott, telephone 818-782-6793, or visit the Internet site *http://www.drivingsystems.com*

ORTHOSES AND BRACES

Orthoses and braces are tools common in rehabilitation, though somewhat less so than in years past. This is due in part to cost cutting, limited clinical expertise and reduced patient time in rehab. There is also a general feeling among many users that orthoses are cumbersome and appear too bionic or "disabled" looking.

An orthosis might be used for positioning a hand, arm or leg, or to magnify or enhance function. The orthosis could be as simple as a splint or as complex as a functional electrical stimulation (FES) brace that facilitates a walking maneuver in paraplegics.

Here are several options for orthoses:

The **Wrist-Hand Orthosis** (WHO) transfers force from an active wrist to paralyzed fingers; this offers prehension (grasping) function for those with cervical injuries (usually between C4 and C7). The WHO, also called a tenodesis splint, has been modified over the years with the addition of CO_2 or batteries for power; current designs are more simple and easier to maintain.

There are several types of orthoses for lower limb function:

The **Ankle-Foot Orthosis** (AFO) is commonly used in people who've had strokes, multiple sclerosis and incomplete spinal cord injury to assist the ankle and allow the foot to clear the ground during the swing phase of walking. There are many varieties of AFO; most have a molded heel cup that extends behind the calf.

The **Knee-Ankle-Foot Orthosis** (KAFO) allows a paralyzed person (usually L3 and above) to stabilize the knee and ankle. While it's very hard work, people using KAFOs, even those with no hip flexion, can ambulate by swinging their legs through steps while supported by forearm crutches. There are many varieties of KAFO, including both plastic and metal braces.

The **Reciprocating Gait Orthosis** (RGO) originated in Canada to help children with spina bifida. After various evolutions, the RGO now consists of a pair of KAFOs with solid ankles, locking knee joints, and leg and thigh straps. Each leg of the brace is attached to a pelvic unit with a hip joint; this permits hip flexion and extension. A steel cable assembly joins the two hip joints to limit step length. By rotating the torso, the user shifts the weight to the forward leg; this permits the opposite leg to move forward.

This kind of walking is stable and balanced, but very slow and requires great energy. Some clinicians have added FES to the RGO to assist walking. For more: The Center for Orthotics Design, 1-800-346-4746; *http://www.centerfororthoticsdesign.com*

ORLAU Swivel Walker is suitable for kids with spina bifida or paraplegia. It produces a back-and-forth walking action similar to that of a walking doll and is operated by leaning forward slightly and by shifting the weight from side to side by arm or shoulder movement. From the U.K. See *http://www.masseruk.com/*

Parastep is a "neuroprosthesis," a device that affects both the structure of the body (as a brace) and the nervous system (a substitute for damaged nerves). It is a portable FES system that facilitates reciprocal walking by stimulating leg muscles on cue. Users hold on to a front-wheeled walker fitted with a keypad that is wired to a microprocessor worn on the belt.

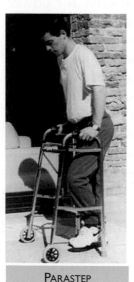

PARASTEP

Surface electrodes are placed on the quadriceps, the gluteal muscles and the peroneal nerve. The user initiates stepping by firing muscles in the proper sequence. Stimulation of the quadriceps causes a contraction that results in knee extension, enabling the user to stand. Stimulation of leg nerves initiates a contraction to flex the hip, knee and ankle; this lifts the foot off the floor as the quadriceps are stimulated. The cycle continues to extend the knee for taking a step. The movement is a bit robotic, but independent and functional for short periods. Some people prefer to use them for exercise.

Most people with spinal cord injuries between T4 and T12 are suitable for Parastep; those with lower motor neuron injuries are generally not good candidates. The Parastep runs about $12,000, not including a required physical therapy regimen of 32 training sessions. Private insurance will sometimes pay for the device. Parastep is covered by Medicare for qualified users.

For information contact Sigmedics, telephone 937-439-9131, or on the Internet visit *http://www.sigmedics.com*

CLOTHING

For a person with limited mobility or who may be sitting a great deal of the time, dressing can be a challenge. Off-the-rack clothing presents problems: seams may be placed in areas that could cause skin breakdowns; trousers may not be long enough or may bunch up in the lap; jackets bunch up; buttons and fasteners might not be handy. There are, however, options.

Here are several companies that cater to the apparel market for people with paralysis:

Ableapparel offers a line of clothing, outerwear and accessories for children and adults; 516-873-6552; *www.ableapparel.com*

Adaptive Clothing offers tops, pants, sleepwear, shoes and custom service. Toll-free 1-800-572-2224; on the internet see *www.adaptiveclothing.com/index2.ivnu*

Adrians Closet designs capes, pants, sweatshirts, jackets; toll-free 1-877-623-7426; *www.adaptationsbyadrian.com*

Easy Access Clothing has pants, jeans, outerwear. Call toll-free 1-800-775-5536; *www.easyaccessclothing.com*

Professional Fit Clothing features alterations, as well as capes and clothing protectors. Call toll-free 1-800-422-2348; *www.professionalfit.com*

Specially For You markets gowns, dresses, pants, etc. Call 605-765-9396; on the Internet see *www.speciallyforyou.net*

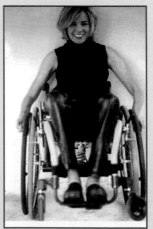

© Wendy Crawford

USA Jeans offers a line of jeans friendly to the seated body. Call toll-free 1-800-935-5170; on the Internet *www.wheelchairjeans.com*

Wheelyglam features high fashion for the wheeler, including special occasion and bridal gowns. Also consultancy service for wheelchair brides-to-be. Based in U.K. See *www.wheelyglam.com*

SERVICE ANIMALS

You may not think of an animal as an assistive device or tool, but it's easy to see that dogs, and even less conventional animals such as monkeys, can make a real difference in peoples' lives. Service animals increase their owner's independence and enhance their quality of life. A dog can help to turn on a light switch, pull a wheelchair, pick up dropped keys or open a cupboard door. Dogs are great companions in general, and from what people who own service animals report, they are great ice-breakers when meeting the public. Most service dogs are mild-mannered golden retrievers or Labrador retrievers, although some dogs without pedigree are rescued from shelters and trained to be service dogs.

There are numerous organizations across the United States and abroad that train service dogs or provide training for people to use their own dogs.

Here are several sources of information:

Assistance Dogs International maintains a list of assistance dog centers across the U.S. and abroad. On the Internet visit *www.adionline.org*

Canine Companions for Independence is a nationwide program that provides assistance dogs at no cost to the person with a disability. All the expenses of breeding, raising and training are funded through private donations. Canine Companions for Independence, P.O. Box 446, Santa Rosa, CA 95402; toll-free 1-800-572-BARK; *www.caninecompanions.org*

PAWS with a Cause, 4646 South Division, Wayland, MI 49348; toll-free 1-800-253-PAWS; or visit the Internet site *www.pawswithacause.org*

National Education for Assistance Dogs Services provides service dogs for people who are deaf or who use wheelchairs. P.O. Box 213, West Boylston, MA 01583; telephone 978-422-9064; or visit *www.neads.org*

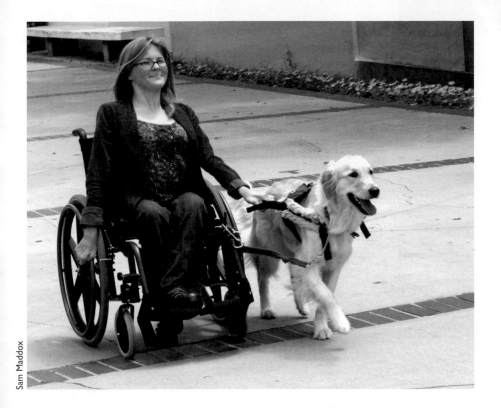

Sam Maddox

Service Monkeys: Helping Hands provides capuchin monkeys at no cost to people with disabilities. These animals (small organ-grinder-type monkeys) can fetch things, turn on switches, and help with grooming. They are very cute, and very friendly. Candidates must be at least one year post-injury, must spend most of their time at home and must be able to control a power chair. Kid-free homes only. Program offers foster placement to train the animals. Monkey Helpers for the Disabled, 541 Cambridge Street, Boston, MA 02134; 617-787-4419. See *www.helpinghandsmonkeys.org*

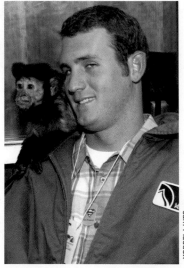

Sam Maddox

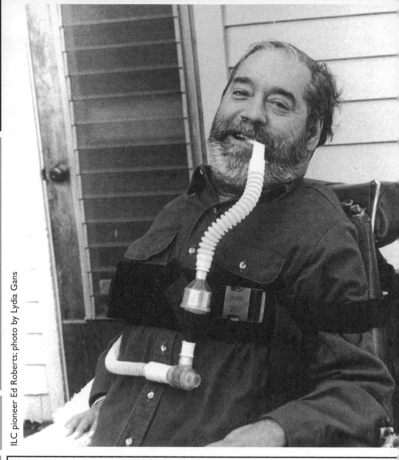

ILC pioneer Ed Roberts; photo by Lydia Gans

WORKING THE SYSTEM

To get what you need and what you are entitled to, you have to know how the system works. Know your rights.

Coming to grips with "the system" is a fact of life in the world of paralysis. This system is a complex and formidable weave of regulation, red tape and mostly good intentions; it directly affects people who want to exercise their rights as citizens, get an education, find jobs or get medical care.

What it really comes down to is getting what you are entitled to, getting what you paid for, getting what you deserve. Forewarned is forearmed: Federal and state policies regarding disability must be understood and sometimes challenged in order for people to succeed. Know your rights.

This chapter focuses on the policies, legalities and practicalities of surviving paralysis; it also looks at the agencies that write and enforce the rules. Underpinning much of the discussion are the basic civil rights of people with disabilities set forth by the Americans with Disabilities Act.

The Medicare section looks at healthcare benefit programs in both the private and public sectors. We will look at how Part A (hospital insurance) works, and when Part B (medical insurance) comes into play. We'll go over the basics of Medicaid and Medigap. Also, the steps for filing an appeal of a denial will be outlined.

The section on Social Security makes sense of the rather complex rules for getting and keeping benefits under the entitlement of federal law, for both Supplemental Security Income (SSI) and Social Security Disability Insurance (SSDI). Again, we'll go over the appeals process.

If getting a job is your goal, there are programs to help. Vocational Rehabilitation exists in all states to help people with disabilities train for or find work. Also, there are government programs that allow people to work and keep healthcare benefits. Programs such as PASS (Plan for Achieving Self-Support) and Ticket to Work help people join the workforce without fear of losing health insurance.

Education benefits are the cornerstone of public policy regarding children with disabilities. Herein is a primer. Also, resources are listed for college-age people with disabilities.

Lastly, we list the best contacts to help explain disability policies and assure that the laws are enforced fairly.

BASICS OF THE ADA

The Americans with Disabilities Act (ADA), which became law in July 1990, is the cornerstone of civil rights for people with disabilities. The law guarantees full participation in American society for all people with disabilities, just as the Civil Rights Act of 1964 guaranteed the rights of all people regardless of race, sex, national origin or religion.

The ADA covers every person with a disability, defined as a person who has a physical or mental impairment that substantially limits one or more major life activities, has a record of such an impairment, or is regarded as having such an impairment.

The law is written in several sections, or titles. Title I of the ADA prohibits private employers, state and local governments, employment agencies and labor unions from discriminating against qualified people with disabilities regarding job applications, hiring, firing, advancement, pay scale, job training, and other conditions and privileges of employment. A qualified employee or applicant with a disability is someone who, with or without reasonable accommodation, can perform the essential functions of the job in question.

Reasonable accommodation may mean making existing facilities accessible and usable by persons with disabilities. It may also include job restructuring, modifying work schedules, acquiring or modifying equipment or devices, modifying training materials or policies, and providing readers or interpreters.

An employer is required to make an accommodation to the known disability of a qualified applicant or employee unless it imposes an "undue hardship" on the operation of the business. Undue hardship would indicate significant difficulty or expense considering an employer's size, financial resources and the nature of its operation. An employer is not required to lower quality or production standards to make an accommodation.

Employers are not allowed to ask a job applicant about the existence, nature or severity of his or her disability. Applicants may be asked about their ability to perform specific job functions. A job offer may be conditioned on the results of a medical examination, but only if the examination is job related and required for all employees entering similar jobs.

Title II of the ADA prohibits discrimination against qualified individuals with disabilities in all programs, activities and services of public entities. This applies to all state and local governments, their departments and agencies, and any other special districts of state or local governments, including public transportation.

Title III of the ADA prohibits discrimination on the basis of disability by "private entities" operating places of "public accommodation." Businesses governed by Title III include banks, restaurants, supermarkets, hotels, shopping centers, privately owned sports arenas, movie theaters, private daycare centers, schools and colleges, accountant or insurance offices, lawyer and doctor offices, museums and health clubs.

If you feel your rights under the ADA have been abused, contact the U.S. Department of Justice. For job-related discrimination, contact the U.S. Equal Employment Opportunity Commission. To protect your rights you must know what they are.

Sources

U.S. Equal Employment Opportunity Commission, U.S. Department of Justice, National Institute on Disability and Rehabilitation Research

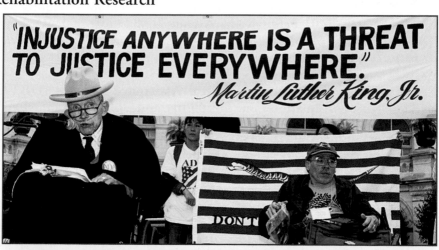

© Steve Higgins/MetroWest Center for Independent Living

"INJUSTICE ANYWHERE IS A THREAT TO JUSTICE EVERYWHERE." *Martin Luther King, Jr.*

JUSTIN DART (1930 - 2002), 'THE GODFATHER OF THE DISABILITY RIGHTS MOVEMENT,' ADDRESSING A RALLY ON THE STEPS OF THE U.S. CAPITOL, JULY 26, 2000, CELEBRATING THE ANNIVERSARY OF THE ADA.

WORKING THE SYSTEM ADA RESOURCES

The U.S. Department of Justice (DOJ) enforces the laws, including the ADA. Businesses, state and local governments, or others can ask questions about general or specific ADA requirements, including questions about the ADA Standards for Accessible Design. ADA specialists are available daily. Spanish language service is available. Call toll-free 1–800–514–0301. Contact the U.S. Department of Justice, 950 Pennsylvania Avenue, NW, Disability Rights Section, Washington, D.C. 20530. The DOJ ADA homepage features volumes of information on the law, including the full text of the ADA. Also offers many materials regarding business compliance. Includes full instructions for filing complaints. Visit the Internet site *http://www.ada.gov*

U.S. Equal Employment Opportunity Commission (EEOC) enforces the laws against employment discrimination. If you believe you have been discriminated against by an employer, labor union or employment agency when applying for a job or while on the job because of your race, color, sex, religion, national origin, age, or disability, you may file a charge of discrimination with the EEOC. U.S. Equal Employment Opportunity Commission, 1801 L Street, N.W., Washington, D.C. 20507; toll-free 1–800–669–4000; or visit the Internet site *http://www.eeoc.gov*

ADA Watch is an information network that activates grassroots responses to threats to the ADA. National Coalition for Disability Rights, ADA Watch, 1201 Pennsylvania Avenue N.W., Suite 300, Washington, D.C. 20004; telephone 202–661–4722; or visit the Internet site *http://www.adawatch.com*

Disability and Business Technical Assistance Centers (DBTACs): The National Institute on Disability and Rehabilitation Research (NIDRR) funds 10 regional centers to provide technical assistance on the ADA. In addition to the ADA, the DBTACs deal with disability legislation, the Family Medical Leave Act, the Workforce Investment Act, the Telecommunications Act and others. To reach your local branch, call toll-free 1–800–949–4232; or visit the Internet site *http://www.adata.org*

Federal Communications Commission (FCC) offers technical assistance on ADA telephone relay service requirements. Federal Communications Commission,445 12th Street S.W., Washington, D.C. 20554; toll-free 1–888–CALL–FCC; or visit the site *http://www.fcc.gov*

The U.S. Access Board (or Architectural and Transportation Barriers Compliance Board) is an independent federal agency devoted to accessibility for people with disabilities. It offers technical assistance on the ADA Accessibility Guidelines. The U.S. Access Board, 1331 F Street, N.W. Suite 1000, Washington, D.C. 20004–1111; toll-free 1–800–872–2253; or visit the Internet site *http://www.access-board.gov*

The U.S. Department of Housing and Urban Development offers assistance with issues related to housing, including public housing, vouchers for renters, etc. U.S. Department of Housing and Urban Development, 451 7th Street S.W., Washington, D.C. 20410; telephone 202–708–1112; or visit the Internet site *http://www.hud.gov* (click on "Information for People with Disabilities").

The Law, Health Policy, and Disability Center, based at the University of Iowa College of Law in partnership with the colleges of education and public health, concentrates on public policy and its impact on persons with disabilities. The Law, Health Policy, and Disability Center, University of Iowa College of Law, Iowa City, IA 52242-1113; telephone 319-335-8469; or visit the Internet site *http://disability.law.uiowa.edu*

The World Institute on Disability promotes independence and inclusion of people with disabilities in society, and works to strengthen the disability movement through research, training, advocacy, and public education. World Institute on Disability, 510 16th Street, Suite 100, Oakland, CA 94612; telephone 510-763-4100; or visit *http://www.wid.org*

The Disability Rights Education and Defense Fund (DREDF) is a national law and policy center for disability rights. DREDF offers advocacy, education, training and technical assistance to persons with disabilities, lawyers, service providers and policy makers about disability civil rights laws and policies. DREDF, 2212 Sixth Street, Berkeley, CA 94710; telephone 510-644-2555; or visit *http://www.dredf.org*

Disability Rights Advocates is an international non-profit dedicated to protecting and advancing the civil rights of people with disabilities. Disability Rights Advocates, 2001 Center Street Berkeley, CA 94704; telephone 510-665-8644 or visit *http://www.dralegal.org*

SOCIAL SECURITY AND DISABILITY

There are two main Social Security programs that support people with disabilities: Social Security Disability Insurance (SSDI) and Supplemental Security Income (SSI).

SSDI

Social Security Disability Insurance benefits are available to workers who have "medically determinable" impairments that prevent them from staying on the job or from performing any "substantial gainful activity." SSDI is the safety net for workers who cannot be helped by adjustments and adaptations called "reasonable accommodations" set forth by the Americans with Disabilities Act (ADA).

Disability under Social Security is based on one's inability to work. Under the rules, you are considered disabled if you cannot do the work you did before and it is concluded that you cannot adjust to other work because of your medical condition. It must be expected that your disability will last for at least one year or result in death. In addition, you must have worked long enough and recently enough under Social Security to qualify for disability benefits. This means that a person must have worked at least 5 of the 10 years immediately before the disability and paid FICA taxes during that time.

A high percentage of initial SSDI claims are denied by Social Security, but there are various levels of the appeals process. To win a claim at any level, an applicant must provide medical evidence of a disabling condition. The best source of this evidence is the applicant's doctor, not the applicant.

SSI

Supplemental Security Income is a program that provides monthly payments to people who have limited income and resources if they are 65 or older or if they have a disability. SSI benefits are not based on your work history or that of a family member. Depending on the state where you live, the benefits and services that come with SSI include food stamps and paid Medicare premiums (all states). In most states, SSI recipients can also get Medicaid coverage for hospital stays, doctor bills, prescription drugs, and other health costs.

The Appeals Process

Social Security, ever vigilant toward waste and fraud, does not always make it easy to get or keep benefits. If the agency decides that you are not eligible or are no longer eligible for benefits, or that the amount of your payments should be changed, you will receive a letter explaining the decision. If you don't agree, you can ask them to look at your case again. If you wish to appeal, you must make your request in writing within 60 days of the date you receive the letter. There are four levels of appeal.

- A reconsideration is a complete review of your claim by someone who didn't take part in the original decision. This person will look at all the evidence submitted when the original decision was made, plus any new evidence.

- If you disagree with the reconsideration, you may ask for a hearing. The hearing will be conducted by an administrative law judge who had no part in either the first decision or the reconsideration of your case. You and your representative, if you have one, may come to the hearing and explain your case. You may review anything in your file and provide new information.

- If you disagree with the hearing decision, you may ask for a review by the Social Security's Appeals Council. The Appeals Council looks at all requests for review, but it may deny a request if it believes the hearing decision was correct. If the Appeals Council decides to review your case, it will either decide your case itself or return it to an administrative law judge for further review.

- If you disagree with the Appeals Council's decision or if the Appeals Council decides not to review your case, your final option is to file a lawsuit in a federal district court.

Because the rules are complicated, many applicants hire lawyers who specialize in Social Security law. The National Organization of Social Security Claimants' Representatives may be able to suggest local referrals; see page 252 for contact information.

For any questions about SRI, SSDI or other disability benefit programs, contact the nearest Social Security office.

Source
Social Security Administration

OLMSTEAD CASE: NO PLACE LIKE HOME

In a historic decision known as the Olmstead case, The Supreme Court ruled that states are required to provide care for persons with disabilities in "the most integrated setting," utilizing community-based services for those who would otherwise be placed in nursing homes. In other words, home is better than a nursing home.

According to the court, "Unjustified isolation . . . is properly regarded as discrimination based on disability." The Court also noted that "institutional placement of persons who can handle and benefit from community settings perpetuates unwarranted assumptions that persons so isolated are incapable or unworthy of participating in community life," and that "confinement in an institution severely diminishes the everyday life activities of individuals, including family relations, social contacts, work options, economic independence, educational advancement, and cultural enrichment."

The Olmstead case was brought by two Georgia women who asserted that institutionalization violated their ADA rights. The effect of the case has been mixed; some states are not in any hurry to implement the court's ruling. For more on the need for in-home services and nursing home reform, see *www.adapt.org*

SOCIAL SECURITY RESOURCES

Social Security Administration (SSA) offers numerous resources to explain various benefit programs, including SSI, SSDI, Medicare, Medigap policies, etc. Social Security Administration, Office of Public Inquiries, Windsor Park Building, 6401 Security Boulevard, Baltimore, MD 21235; toll-free 1–800–772–1213; or visit the Internet site *http://www.ssa.gov/disability*

The National Organization of Social Security Claimants' Representatives (NOSSCR) provides representation and advocacy on behalf of persons seeking Social Security and Supplemental Security Income. NOSSCR, 560 Sylvan Avenue, Englewood Cliffs, NJ 07632; toll-free 1–800–431–2804; or visit the Internet site *http://www.nosscr.org*

MEDICARE AND DISABILITY

You are eligible for healthcare coverage from Medicare if you or your spouse worked and paid taxes for at least 10 years, you are at least 65 years old, and are a citizen or permanent resident of the United States. You might also qualify if you are a younger person with a disability.

Note: Medicare is not the same as Medicaid, which is a joint federal and state program that helps with medical costs for some people with low incomes and limited resources. Nearly 7 million individuals with disabilities were covered by Medicaid in 1998. Almost 80 percent were eligible because they received cash assistance through the SSI program. The remainder generally qualified for Medicaid by incurring large hospital, prescription drug, nursing home, or other medical or long-term care expenses. Medicaid is the only national program that pays for the complete range of services that enable many persons with disabilities to live in their own homes and communities. Most states, however, still spend 70 percent or more of their Medicaid funding on nursing homes and other institutions.

Medicaid is means-tested; it has extensive rules for determining an individual's income and resources. Furthermore, because it is not a uniform federal program like Medicare, Medicaid coverage and eligibility varies from state to state. In an effort to encourage more states to provide Medicaid to working individuals with disabilities, Congress permitted states to expand their Medicaid programs through a Medicaid "buy-in." This allows people with disabilities to continue to receive Medicaid services even if they return to work. Most states also allow waivers for some eligibility restrictions. Check with your state's Medicaid office (see page 258).

Medigap policies are Medicare supplement insurance policies sold by private insurance companies to fill "gaps" in what is called Original Medicare Plan coverage, such as out-of-pocket costs for Medicare co-insurance and deductibles or services not covered by Medicare. These policies can reduce out-of-pocket costs if those costs exceed the monthly Medigap premiums.

Medicare Part A (hospital insurance) is available when you turn 65. You don't have to pay premiums if you are already receiving retirement benefits from Social Security or the Railroad Retirement Board and you or your spouse had Medicare-covered government employment. Most people get Part A automatically when they become 65. If you (or your spouse) did not pay Medicare taxes while you worked and you are age 65 or older, you still may be able to buy Part A.

If you are not yet 65, you can get Part A without having to pay premiums if you have received Social Security or Railroad Retirement Board disability benefits for 24 months.

Medicare Part B (medical insurance) is an option that helps pay for doctors and related services, outpatient hospital care, and some things Part A does not cover, such as physical and occupational therapy and home healthcare when it's medically necessary.

The Part B premium is $93.50 per month in 2007. This cost might be higher for those who did not choose Part B when they first became eligible at age 65. The cost of Part B may go up 10 percent for each 12-month period that you could have had Part B but did not sign up for it, except in special cases.

It is important to know that Medicare does not cover everything; it does not pay the total cost for most services or supplies that are covered. Talk to your doctor to be sure you are getting the service or supply that best meets your healthcare needs.

The Original Medicare Plan usually pays 80 percent of the approved amount for certain approved pieces of medical equipment. Ask your supplier "Do you accept assignment?" This could save you money. Medicare pays for some home healthcare costs. Benefits are available if people meet four conditions: Their doctor says they need medical care in their home and makes a plan for that care; they need intermittent skilled nursing care, physical therapy, speech language services, or occupational therapy; they are homebound; and the home health agency caring for them is Medicare-approved.

Medicare does not pay for 24-hour a day care at home; prescription drugs; meals delivered to the home; homemaker services such as shopping, cleaning and laundry; personal care given by home health aides such as bathing, toileting or dressing when this is the only care needed.

Find a Medicare approved home health agency by asking your

doctor or hospital discharge planner, using a community referral service, or looking in the telephone directory under "home care" or "home healthcare." Some hospitals will try to steer you toward their own home health agency, but you are free to choose any agency that meets your medical needs.

If you have questions about your home healthcare benefits and you are in the Original Medicare Plan, contact Medicare (page 258) to get the number for your Regional Home Health Intermediary. If you have questions about home healthcare and you are in a Medicare managed care plan, call your plan.

Although the Original Medicare Plan does not provide prescription drug coverage, your state may offer discounted or free medications programs. Check with your state's Department of Aging or local Area Agency on Aging. For those numbers, contact Medicare. Your state also has programs that pay some or all of the Medicare premiums for people with limited incomes. Call your state's Medical Assistance Office to learn about Medicare Savings Programs (contact Medicare for telephone numbers; see page 258).

You have the right to file an appeal for any unsatisfactory decision about your Medicare services. Ask your doctor or provider for any information related to the bill that might help your case. Your appeal rights are on the back of the Explanation of Medicare Benefits or Medicare Summary Notice that is mailed to you from the company that handles bills for Medicare. The notice will also tell you why your bill was not paid and how to appeal.

If you are in a Medicare managed care plan, you can always appeal if your plan does not pay for, does not allow, or stops a service that you think should be covered. If you think having to wait for a decision could seriously harm your health, ask the plan for a fast decision. The plan must answer you within 72 hours. A Medicare managed care plan must tell you in writing how to appeal. After you file an appeal, the plan will review its decision. If your plan does not decide in your favor, the appeal is reviewed by an independent group that works for Medicare, not for the plan.

Medicare Part D: is a program that provides assistance for prescription drugs. The drug benefit, which began in January 2006, is not provided within the traditional Medicare program. Instead, beneficiaries must enroll in one of many Part D plans offered by private companies.

Medicare drug benefits are available through two types of private plans: beneficiaries can join a Prescription Drug Plan (PDP) for drug coverage only or they can join a Medicare Advantage plan (MA) that covers prescription drugs (MA-PD). There are 34 PDP regions and 26 MA regions in the U.S. The drug plans control drug costs through a system of tiered formularies; lower cost drugs are assigned to lower tiers and thus are easier to prescribe.

Those beneficiaries who are dual eligible, having both Medicare and Medicaid, are automatically enrolled into a Prescription Drug Plan (PDP) in their area. If the dual eligible person is already enrolled in an MA-only plan, he or she is automatically removed from the MA plan upon enrollment in the PDP.

Dozens of Medicare prescription drug plans are available. Plans can choose to cover different drugs, or classes of drugs, at various co-pays, or choose not to cover some drugs at all. Medicare has made available an interactive online tool called the Prescription Drug Plan Finder (see *www.medicare.gov*) that compares drug availability and costs for all plans in a geographic area.

The Annual Enrollment Period for Part D runs from November 15 – December 31. Only during this period can people with Medicare enroll in a plan or change from one plan to another. Those who are already in a plan should decide whether it will be right for them in the following year; if they do not choose to switch they will remain in their current plan.

Plans will have different costs and benefits from year to year, thus it is advisable for all beneficiaries to consider their options.

Medicare Part D will provide a full drug subsidy with lower co-payments to beneficiaries with incomes up to 135 percent of the federal poverty level. Part D will also provide a partial subsidy of premium, deductible and co-insurance to beneficiaries with incomes up to 150 percent of FPL. Unlike rules for Medicare Savings Programs, which allow for a family unit of only one or two, Part D recognizes larger family units and extends coverage.

Resources
Social Security Administration, Centers for Medicare & Medicaid Services, Medicare

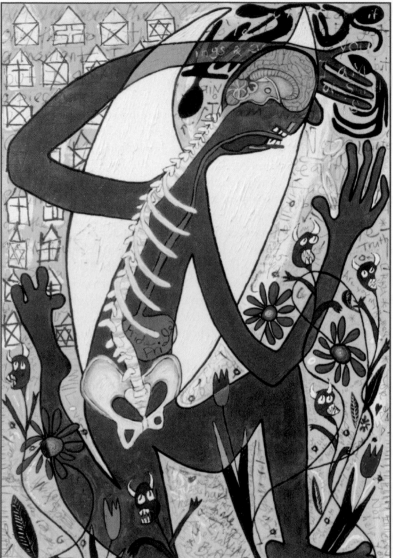

SWALLOWING MY PRIDE IN THE GARDEN OF GOOD AND EVIL
24 x 26 INCHES, OIL ON CANVAS, 2001

"REALIZING MY HUMILITY, LETTING GO OF WHETHER OR NOT I AM RIGHT OR
WRONG, IN CONTROL, OR NOT; I MUST LEARN TO ACCEPT THIS LIFE FOR
WHAT IT IS AND FIND FAITH FROM WITHIN NO MATTER HOW MY BROKEN
INSIDES REVEAL OTHERWISE. THIS PAINTING IS DEDICATED TO ALL WHO HAVE
TO MAKE KNOWN THEIR 'DISABILITY' TO OTHERS."

— CAROL ES

MEDICARE AND DISABILITY RESOURCE

Medicaid is a federally supported healthcare program administered by each state. For connections to your state's program, call toll-free 1–877–267–2323 or visit the Internet site *http://cms.hhs.gov/medicaid*

Medicare offers loads of resources, state-by-state connections and full details on federal healthcare programs, appeals, etc. Call toll-free 1–800–MEDICARE for information, connections to all Medicare and state Medicaid offices, and more. The Internet site *http://www.medicare.gov* is comprehensive and user-friendly. Click on the "Helpful Contacts" link on the home page for the list of phone numbers for your state.

The Medicare Rights Center (MRC) is a not-for-profit organization working to insure that older adults and people with disabilities get affordable healthcare. It offers helpful and reliable Medicare information for consumers and professionals, including information on State Health Insurance Assistance Programs. Medicare Rights Center, 1460 Broadway, 17th Floor, New York, NY 10036; telephone 212–869–3850; or visit *http://www.medicarerights.org*

Medigap (Medicare supplemental) is extra insurance for which you pay premiums to cover some of the costs not allowed by Medicare, such as co-insurance payments for doctor and hospital services. All states have basic Medigap plans. AARP offers a Medigap insurance program; visit *http://www.aarp.org* or call toll-free 1-800-523-5800. For comparisons of policies visit *http://www.medicare.gov* and search under "Medigap."

The Center for Medicare Advocacy, Inc. provides education, advocacy and legal assistance to help elders and people with disabilities obtain necessary healthcare. The focus is on the needs of Medicare beneficiaries, people with chronic conditions, and those in need of long-term care. The Center for Medicare Advocacy, Inc., 1101 Vermont Avenue, N.W., Washington, D.C. 20005; telephone 202–216–0028; or visit the Internet site *http://www.medicareadvocacy.org*

Centers for Medicare & Medicaid Services (CMS), formerly the Health Care Financing Administration, provides health insurance for more than 74 million Americans through Medicare, Medicaid and the State Children's Health Insurance Program (SCHIP—a state and federal partnership designed to help children without health insurance, many from families with incomes too high to qualify for Medicaid but too low to afford private health insurance; see Insure Kids Now!, below). Centers for Medicare & Medicaid Services, 7500 Security Boulevard, Baltimore, MD 21244–1850; toll-free 1–877–267–2323; or visit *http://cms.hhs.gov*

Advancing Independence: Modernizing Medicare & Medicaid (AIMMM) is an advocate for Medicare and Medicaid reforms to enhance the health, independence and productivity of Americans with disabilities. AIMMM, 1875 Eye Street, NW, 12th Floor, Washington, DC 20006; telephone 202-429-6810 or see the Internet site *http://www.aimmm.org*

Insure Kids Now! is a national campaign from the U.S. Department of Health and Human Services to link the nation's 10 million uninsured children—those from birth to age 18—to free and low-cost health insurance. In most states, uninsured children 18 years old and younger whose families earn up to $34,100 a year (for a family of four) are eligible. Call toll-free 1–877–543–7669 to get in touch with your state's program; *http://www.insurekidsnow.gov*

State Health Insurance Assistance Programs offer help with buying a Medigap policy or long-term care insurance, dealing with payment denials or appeals, Medicare rights and protections, complaints about your care or treatment, choosing a Medicare health plan, or problems with Medicare bills. To find your state's health insurance assistance program call toll-free 1–800–MEDICARE (1–800–633–4227) or visit *http://www.medicare.gov* and click on "Helpful Contacts."

Families USA acts as a watchdog over policies related to affordable health and long-term care. The group features consumer-based subgroups including The Medicaid Advocacy Network, The Children's Health Campaign, and The Medicare Action Network. Families USA, 1201 New York Avenue, NW, Suite 1100, Washington, DC 20005; telephone 202-628-3030; *http://www.familiesusa.org*

SeniorLaw offers information on Medicare, Medicaid, estate planning, trusts, legal rights, family issues. SeniorLaw, 350 Fifth Avenue, Suite 1100, New York, NY 10118; 212-387-8400; *http://www.seniorlaw.com*

GETTING WORK

Until recently, people with disabilities who received Social Security benefits were effectively penalized for taking a job. Any income above certain limits set by the government was deducted from one's benefits, thus jeopardizing the only source of health insurance available to people with long-term health conditions.

While many continue to see disincentives to working (fewer than 1 percent of the people who get Social Security and SSI disability benefits leave the rolls each year to go to work), things have improved. Below are details on two Social Security programs designed to encourage people with disabilities to enter the job force without fear of losing healthcare benefits. One is the Ticket to Work program, the other the Plan to Achieve Self-Support (PASS).

The Ticket to Work Program

The Ticket to Work and Work Incentives Improvement Act of 1999 increases the choices people with disabilities have to obtain rehabilitation and vocational services while removing barriers that require a choice between healthcare coverage and work.

Beneficiaries of Social Security and Supplemental Security Income (SSI) receive a "Ticket" to obtain vocational rehabilitation and other employment support services from an approved provider of their choice. The goal of the Ticket Program is to give disability beneficiaries the opportunity to achieve steady, long-term employment by providing them greater choices and opportunities to go to work if they choose to do so.

In 2001, the Social Security Administration (SSA) began contracting with national, state and local service providers to become Employment Networks (ENs). These providers (employment agencies, independent living centers, state vocational rehab offices, community nonprofits, churches, etc.) work with beneficiaries to provide support and employment-related assistance. Beneficiaries receiving Tickets may contact any EN of their choice to design an employment plan.

The law expands Medicaid and Medicare coverage to more working people with disabilities. States may permit working individuals with an income above 250 percent of the federal

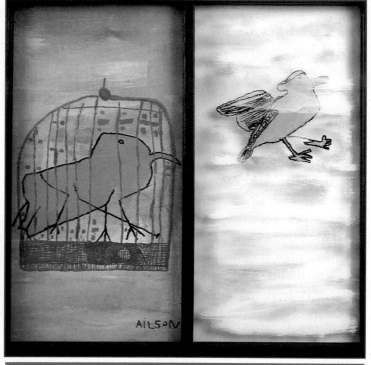

AILSON CARVALHO, WHO HAS DOWNS SYNDROME, WAS BORN AND RAISED IN BRAZIL. HE NOW LIVES IN THE WASHINGTON, D.C. AREA.

© Ailson Carvalho

FLYING FREE — AILSON CARVALHO

poverty level to purchase Medicaid coverage.

When a person's Social Security or SSI disability benefits have ended because of earnings from work, he or she may request reinstatement of benefits, including Medicare and Medicaid, without filing a new application.

An individual using a Ticket will usually not have to undergo regularly scheduled disability reviews; beneficiaries who have been receiving benefits for at least 24 months will not be asked to go through a disability review because of the work they are doing. Regularly scheduled medical reviews could still be performed and benefits could be terminated if earnings are above the limits.

The law directs Social Security to establish a community-based work incentives assistance program to disseminate accurate information about work incentives and to give beneficiaries more choices. Social Security has established a program of cooperative agreements and contracts to provide benefits planning and assistance to all Social Security disability beneficiaries. SSA also offers information about protection and advocacy services in each state.

For information on the Ticket Program call Maximus, Inc., the Ticket Program manager, toll-free 1–866–968–7842 or visit *www.yourtickettowork.com*

Preparing a PASS

The PASS (Plan to Achieve Self-Support) is a work incentive plan that allows people to work and keep Social Security health-care benefits. Under regular Supplemental Security Income rules, your SSI benefit is reduced by any other income you have. But income you set aside for a PASS does not reduce your SSI benefit: You can get a higher SSI benefit when you have a PASS.

One's plan is submitted to Social Security, usually with the help of a counselor, stating what the work goal is, what is needed to achieve it, how long that will take, and what it will cost. The work goal can be anything you realistically expect to accomplish that will generate adequate income. It can be part- or full-time, at home or not, working for wages or starting a business of your own.

The things you buy must be related to the goal—training, testing or tuition, a car or van, a computer or tools and supplies of your trade or business, daycare for a child while you work or attend school, other sorts of adaptive technology, etc.

To start, ask your local Social Security office for a copy of PASS form SSA-545-BK. This has most of the information needed to review your plan. Next, choose a work goal for a job you want to do. Figure out what steps you need to take to reach your goal and how long it will take you to complete each step. Find out how much money you'll need to set aside each month to pay for items or services you will need to reach your goal. Get several cost estimates for the things you need.

If you're planning to set aside income for your plan, your SSI benefit will usually increase to help pay your living expenses. Contact Social Security; the agency can estimate what your new SSI payment will be. Keep any money you save for your goal separate from any other money you have. The easiest way to do this is to open a separate bank account for the PASS money.

If you intend to start a business, you will also need a business plan, including: kind of business you want to start, hours of operation, location; how you will pay for your business; how you will market your product or service; who your suppliers and customers will be; your expected earnings.

It may be a good idea to get help writing your PASS from a vocational rehabilitation counselor, an organization that helps people with disabilities, or the people at your Social Security office. Some organizations charge a fee for this service. On the Internet, see *http://www.passonline.org*, for a PASS tutorial from Cornell University and the Social Security Administration.

Complete form SSA-545-BK, sign and date it. Take or mail the form to your local Social Security office.

After you submit your plan, Social Security will review it and decide if there is a good chance that you can reach your goal, if the things you plan to buy are necessary and reasonably priced, and if any changes are needed. They will discuss any changes with you. If your PASS is denied, there is an appeal process.

If your plan is approved, Social Security will contact you from time to time to make sure that you are following your plan and on the way to your goal. Make sure that you keep receipts for the items and services you buy for the plan.

Vocational Rehabilitation (VR)

Every state has a federally funded agency that administers vocational rehabilitation, supported employment, and independent living services. VR assists people in finding jobs through local searches and by promoting self-employment and telecommuting opportunities. VR services vary widely depending upon the state but typically include medical, psychological and vocational assessments; counseling and guidance; vocational and other types of training; interpreter and reader services; services to family members; rehabilitation technology; placement; post-employment services; and/or other goods and services necessary to achieve rehab objectives. In some cases VR pays for transportation and vehicle modification.

Sources

Social Security Administration, Rehabilitation Services Administration, Maximus, Inc., Cornell University

GETTING WORK RESOURCES

Social Security Administration operates the Ticket to Work and PASS programs. For information call toll-free 1–800–772–1213. Visit the Internet site *http://www.ssa.gov* for details on all SSA programs. Use the Search function on the home page and type in "Ticket" or "PASS" or other topics of interest.

The Rehabilitation Services Administration (RSA) administers grant programs and projects that serve individuals with disabilities in the areas of vocational rehabilitation, supported employment and independent living. RSA, 400 Maryland Avenue, S.W., Washington, D.C. 20202–2551; telephone 202–245–5482; on the Internet visit *http://www.ed.gov/about/offices/list/osers/rsa/index.html*

Disability and Business Technical Assistance Centers: The **National Institute on Disability and Rehabilitation Research (NIDRR)** has established 10 regional centers to provide information, training and technical assistance to employers, people with disabilities and other entities with responsibilities under the ADA. The centers act as a "one-stop" resource on ADA issues in employment, public services, public accommodations and communications. To locate the center in your region call toll-free 1–800–949–4232; or visit the Internet site *http://www.adata.or*g

Office of Disability Employment Policy (ODEP) is a federal agency that works to increase job opportunities for adults and youth with disabilities while striving to eliminate barriers to employment. Contact ODEP by way of the U.S. Department of Labor, Frances Perkins Building, 200 Constitution Avenue, NW, Washington, DC 20210; toll-free 1-866-ODEP-DOL, or visit *http://www.dol.gov/odep*

The Job Accommodation Network (JAN) is a free consulting service that provides information about job accommodations, the Americans with Disabilities Act (ADA), and the employability of people with disabilities. JAN also staffs the **Small Business and Self-Employment Service (SBSES)** of the Office of Disability Employment Policy; SBSES provides information, counseling and referrals about self-employment and entrepreneurship for people with disabilities. Call toll-free 1-800-526-7234 or visit the Internet site *http://janweb.icdi.wvu.edu*

The National Business & Disability Council is a resource for employers seeking to integrate people with disabilities into the workplace and also for companies hoping to reach them in the consumer marketplace. The National Business & Disability Council, 201 I.U. Willets Road, Albertson, NY 11507; telephone 516–465–1515; *http://www.nbdc.com*

The National Center on Workforce and Disability/Adult is funded through the U.S. Department of Labor's Office of Disability Employment Policy (ODEP) and provides training, technical assistance and information to improve access for all in the workforce. The Institute for Community Inclusion, UMass Boston, 100 Morrissey Boulevard, Boston, MA 02125; toll-free 1-888-886-9898; *http://www.onestops.info*

The National Collaborative on Workforce and Disability for Youth (NCWD/Youth) works to ensure that youth with disabilities have full access to services in order to maximize their opportunities for employment and independent living. NCWD/Youth, Institute for Educational Leadership, 4455 Connecticut Avenue, NW, Suite 310, Washington, DC 20008; toll-free 1-877-871-0744 or see *http://www.ncwd-youth.info*

PASS Tutorial: Cornell University, The Social Security Administration and the New York State Office of Vocational and Educational Services for Individuals with Disabilities have teamed up to create a useful Internet site to provide assistance for the Plan for Achieving Self-Support (PASS). Includes detailed explanation of the PASS program as well as a helpful tutorial on completing the application. Visit the Internet site *http://www.passonline.org*

Proyecto Vision: Disabled Latinos face higher rates of unemployment than other disabled Americans and non-disabled Latinos. This project connects disabled Latinos with employment services and related resources and helps Latino organizations to better serve their disabled community members. Offers bilingual services. For more call Proyecto Vision, toll-free 1–866–367–5361; or visit the Internet site *http://www.proyectovision.net*

The Abilities Fund is the first financial lending institution devoted exclusively to advancing entrepreneurial opportunities for Americans with disabilities. The Abilities Fund, 101 East Van Buren Street, Centerville, IA 52544; toll-free 1–888–222–8942; or visit *http://www.abilitiesfund.org*

GETTING WORK RESOURCES

The Consortium for Citizens with Disabilities is a coalition of about 100 national disability organizations working toward the self determination, independence, empowerment and inclusion of children and adults with disabilities in all aspects of society. CCD, 1660 L Street, NW, Suite700, Washington, DC 20036; telephone 202-783-2229; or visit the Internet site *http://www.c-c-d.org*

The Council for Disability Rights (CDR) believes that people should be encouraged and accommodated to live independently and to participate fully in community life. CDR promotes public policy and legislation, public awareness through education, and provides information and referral services. Council for Disability Rights, 30 East Adams, Suite 1130, Chicago, IL 60603; telephone 312-444-9484; or visit the Internet site *http://www.disabilityrights.org*

Disabled Businesspersons Association assists enterprising individuals with disabilities to maximize their potential in the business world, and works with vocational rehabilitation, government and business to encourage the participation and enhance the performance of the disabled in the workforce. DBA helps with business plans, setting goals and objectives, and financing. See *http://www.disabledbusiness.com*

Just One Break, founded in 1947 by Eleanor Roosevelt, Orin Lehman, and Bernard Baruch, is the nation's oldest not-for-profit, employment placement service for people with disabilities. JOB matches skilled candidates with leading corporations in all industries. Just One Break, Inc., 570 Seventh Avenue, New York, NY 10018; telephone 212-785-7300; or visit *http://www.justonebreak.com*

The AgrAbility Project assists people with disabilities employed in farming and ranching. The Project features a database of assistive technology for the agricultural industries, including adaptive tractors and other modified gear for home and workplace. Twenty-one states have developed AgrAbility programs that offer resources and referral, onsite technical assistance and training for using adaptive equipment, and peer support to keep people in agriculture on the job, even after a major disability. See Website listed below for list of state projects. If your state does not have an AgrAbility Project, contact the national project office, 460 Henry Mall, Madison, WI 53706; call toll-free 1-866-259-6280; or visit *http://www.agrabilityproject.org*

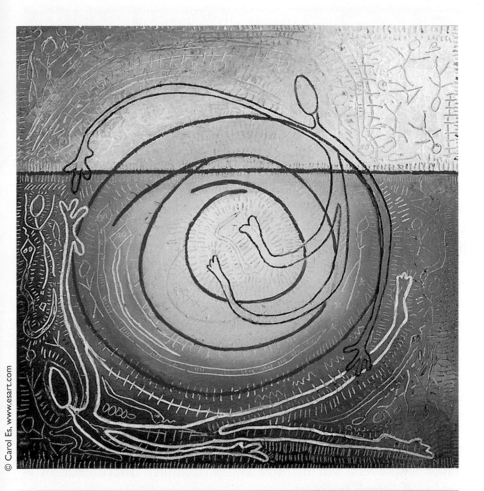

UNAFRAID OF SNAKES AND BEES
OIL ON CANVAS, 12 X 12 INCHES

"I THINK WE ALL FEAR A VARIETY OF THINGS AT DIFFERENT DEGREES AT DIFFERENT TIMES. I HAVE FEARED THINGS LIKE SNAKES, BEES, DEATH, RELATIONSHIPS, INJURY, FATE, THE UNKNOWN, AND MY CAPABILITIES. I REALIZE THESE FEARS MAKE ME HUMAN. THIS PAINTING REMINDS ME OF THIS AND HELPS ME COPE AND ACCEPT THE NATURE OF THINGS."

– CAROL ES

LEGAL BASICS: JOB HUNTING WITH A DISABILITY

BY HARRIET MCBRYDE JOHNSON, ATTORNEY AT LAW

Note: This article offers general information about law and is not intended as a substitute for individual legal advice.

Under the best of circumstances, job hunting is probably the hardest job you'll ever have. For anyone, it requires energy and dogged persistence—keeping at it in the face of rejection. A disability can make it even tougher. Functional limitations may make some jobs impossible. You may need to find a unique job that will accommodate your unique situation. Instead of merely adapting to the workplace, you may need a workplace that adapts to you.

Added to all of this is that ugly fact of life we'd like to forget: discrimination. Despite some real progress, many employers still have trouble seeing people with disabilities as part of the workforce. In your job hunt, you're likely to encounter unfounded myths, fears, and stereotypes. The good news is that the law, particularly the Americans with Disabilities Act, offers some help. It hasn't leveled the playing field. It hasn't made job hunting easy. But you can improve your chances of winning the job that's right for you by being armed with a little knowledge of how the laws work.

Q: Are all employers covered by the ADA? **A:** No, only those with 15 or more employees. Some states have comparable laws covering smaller employers, but in most states disability discrimination is legal in very small business.

Q: Does the ADA guarantee me a job? **A:** No, it only protects your right to compete. If you are qualified and able to do the job, you cannot be denied the job just because of your disability. Moreover, if you're able to do the job with an accommodation, the employer must provide "reasonable" accommodation to your disability.

Q: Do I report my disability when I apply for a job? **A:** You are under no obligation to do so. Under the ADA, employers may not inquire about disabilities until after a "conditional offer" of employment has been made. That means you should be evaluated initially the way other people are evaluated, based on your education, experience, and skills.

Q: What if I want to report my disability? It's part of who I am.

A: It's your call but disclosure does carry a lot of risk. For most employers, disability is still a definite negative. If you bring it out too early, employers may decide to avoid an uncomfortable situation simply by not selecting you for an interview.

Q: What about job interviews? A: Even in an interview, ADA employers may not ask about disabilities; they may ask about your ability to perform essential job functions. For example, if driving is part of the job, you can be asked if you have a driver's license.

Q: What is a "conditional offer of employment." A: Basically, under the ADA, the employer should first evaluate your qualifications without considering disability. Before asking medical questions, the employer must tell you that you're selected, contingent on your satisfying medical requirements. This means you should have a job offer, with all important terms like what you'll be doing, how much you'll be paid, and when you'll start. After the offer, you are subject to the same medical screening that applies to all applicants: you should not be singled out for special scrutiny because of your disability.

Q: If the employer gets my medical information anyway, what good does the ADA do me? A: It may enable you to prove that your disability was the only reason you were not hired. You've already been told you have a job; if you get un-hired after the company physical, the company can't claim some other reason. This is a tremendous boost for any possible discrimination charge. Employers know this, so the ADA gives them practical reason to evaluate you fairly.

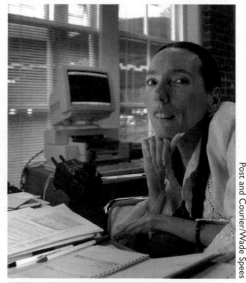

Post and Courier/Wade Spees

HARRIET MCBRYDE JOHNSON

Johnson, who died in 2008, was a writer and lawyer in Charleston, SC. Her books include Too Late to Die Young: Nearly True Tales from a Life, *and* Accidents of Nature.

FINANCIAL PLANNING

The suddenness of a stroke, spinal cord or brain injury can be devastating emotionally and physically but also financially. At first, making plans and gaining control of one's financial future is difficult for people who may be preoccupied with day-to-day survival after disability. While situations vary, there are some basic steps to take to reduce anxiety about paying bills and affording necessary equipment and care down the road.

Here are some steps to consider, as outlined in *On The Move, a Financial Guide for People With Spinal Cord Injury*. The 15-page booklet (from the Paralyzed Veterans of America and the National Endowment for Financial Education) lays out a series of questions based on three phases of injury: getting through "the first days," the acute phase of the injury; "resuming life's activities;" and "planning for the future."

Get organized: ask for help; talk to your employer about disability benefits, if any; locate important financial and legal papers; estimate as best you can your medical expenses; prioritize your bills; and keep good records.

Consider all sources of funds for medical care and equipment, including your health insurance, VA benefits, auto insurance, workers comp, lawsuits, etc. Try to keep your current insurance policy in force. If you don't have coverage for 62 days or more, you can be denied coverage for up to a year in your next group plan. A program called COBRA allows for continuation of coverage in some cases.

It is important to understand Social Security and federal health care benefits (see information earlier in this chapter). It is also important to know your rights and to advocate for them.

What do you do when there is no insurance money, no settlement, not enough coverage from Medicaid and still great need? You might turn to churches or service organizations (Kiwanis, Elks, etc.) for help. See the NATF financial option for seeking funds from your own donor base, page 271.

For a free copy of *On the Move*, contact PVA, 801 Eighteenth Street, NW, Washington, DC 20006; toll-free 1-888-860-7244; see *http://www.pva.org*, click on Publications.

TAPPING YOUR OWN NETWORK

Barely half of people with spinal cord injury have insurance at the time of trauma. Even when there is insurance it is usually quite limited. You might turn to your own community network for help. The NTAF Catastrophic Injury Program offers a step-by-step framework to raise funds locally. Because NTAF is a 501c3 non-profit and approved by the IRS, all funds raised are tax-deductible.

NTAF collects and manages funds in honor of persons with spinal cord trauma; the funds are disbursed as needed.

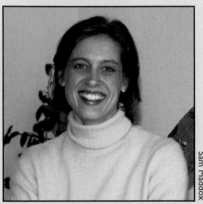

LYENA STRELKOFF

NTAF has helped numerous people. "At the time of my accident, I was very fortunate to have people in my life with the means and desire to offer significant financial support for my recovery," says Lyena Strelkoff, a T11 paraplegic from Los Angeles. "But their generosity was limited by the fact that no deduction could be taken. My relationship with NTAF allowed my donors to make sizable contributions and receive a tax deduction for their kindness."

The NTAF also helps coordinate fundraising efforts. "They gave us ideas for fundraisers, shared sample materials, created flyers, and gave valuable feedback on our fundraising materials," says Strelkoff.

Dave Denniston, a T10-11 paraplegic from Wyoming, raves about his experience with NTAF. "They sympathize with every situation and do all they can to help relieve the stress of dealing with the medical field. Anything I do from acupuncture to exercise therapy is covered by NTAF. Having them handle my donor's funds has been a huge blessing," says Denniston.

For more information contact NATF, 150 N. Radnor Chester Road, Radnor, PA 19087, toll-free 1-800-642-8399. On the Internet see *http://www.transplantfund.org*

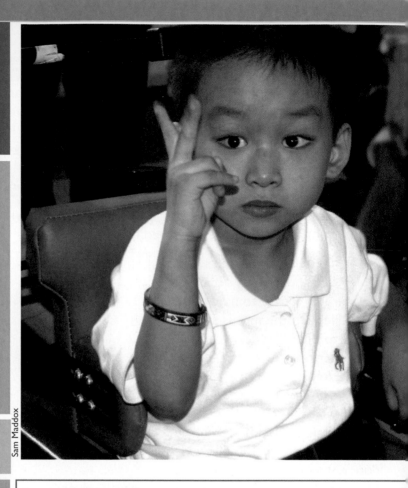

Sam Maddox

KIDS' ZONE

The most important tools for parents are other parents. There is no substitute for the advice and counsel of those who have been in similar situations.

chapter

9

Children and Paralysis

The interests of kids with disabilities are at the heart of numerous policies and programs set forth by nonprofit groups, resource centers and state and federal agencies. There are programs to ensure families have resources to live. There are programs that hope to make healthcare available. Laws have been written to guarantee that all kids, no matter what disabilities come into play, get a free public education. Of course having such policies and applying them across the land means that parents must navigate through a maze of regulation in areas of social security, healthcare, special education and even tax law.

The most important tools for parents are other parents. There is no substitute for the advice and counsel of those who have been in similar situations.

Here is a rundown of several key programs for kids (from birth to age 18) with disabilities, including numerous links to connect with other parents of kids with disabilities.

IDEA

The Individuals with Disabilities Education Act (IDEA) is a law created to ensure that all children with disabilities, regardless of the severity of their disability, have available a "free appropriate public education," including special education and related services.

IDEA makes funds available for states and cities to assist in the education of infants, toddlers, preschoolers, children and youth with disabilities. In order to remain eligible for federal funds, states must ensure that children with disabilities receive a complete individual evaluation and assessment of their specific needs. An Individualized Education Program (IEP) or an Individualized Family Services Plan (IFSP) will be drawn up for every child or youth found eligible for special education or early intervention services. An IEP is the contract between the school district and the student that lists the type and amount of services it will provide to the student. To the maximum extent appropriate, all children with disabilities are to be educated in the regular education environment.

Those receiving special education have the right to receive the related services, which may include transportation; speech pathology and audiology; psychological services; physical and occupational therapy; recreation, including therapeutic recreation; rehabilitation counseling; and medical services for diagnostic or evaluation purposes. Parents have the right to participate in all decisions related to identification, evaluation and placement of their child with a disability. Parents may appeal any decision concerning the education of their child.

IDEA was reauthorized by Congress in 2004. Among the changes in the law are provisions that all public elementary and secondary special education teachers be "highly qualified" as special education teachers, and new rules for children in private schools, For more detail see the Internet site *http://idea.ed.gov*

"Early intervention services must be provided at no cost by qualified people who work with infants and toddlers who have disabilities."

Early Intervention

Children from birth through age two may be eligible for no-cost services through The Infants and Toddlers with Disabilities Program (Part C) of IDEA. Programs for children under age three are provided by different agencies in different states: the department of education will handle some programs, or the health department or another agency may be the lead agency—it varies from state to state. Early intervention services must be provided by qualified people who work with infants and toddlers who have disabilities or who are at risk of developing disabilities. Services must be written into an Individualized Family Services Plan (IFSP) that is reviewed every six months. For information by state about how to access services for infants and toddlers, contact NICHCY; see Resources, below.

State Children's Health Insurance Program (SCHIP)

This program is administered by the state, which sets eligibility and coverage according to broad federal guidelines.

Requirements include the following: low income; ineligibility for Medicaid; must be uninsured. Programs offer inpatient and out-patient hospital services; doctors' surgical and medical services, including lab and X-ray; well-baby/child checkups and immunizations. Apply for SCHIP at public schools. In some states, one can apply through public health departments, state social service agencies, or state welfare agencies. For more contact the SCHIP office of the U.S. Department of Health and Human Services, 1–877–543–7669; or visit *http://www.insurekidsnow.gov*

Children With Special Health Care Needs (CSHCN)

Children who are eligible for Supplemental Security Income (SSI) are also eligible for CSHCN, a federal program administered via state health agencies. Most CSHCN programs help provide specialized services through arrangements with clinics, private physicians, hospital-based outpatient and inpatient treatment centers, and social services. CSHCN programs are known by a variety of names, including Children's Special Health Services, Children's Medical Services, and Handicapped Children's Program. A CSHCN program may be able to help even if a child is not eligible for SSI. The Institute for Child Health Policy at the University of Florida publishes a directory of state CSHCN programs. Institute for Child Health Policy, 5700 S.W. 34th Street Suite 323, Gainesville, FL 32608; telephone toll-free 1–888–433–1851; or visit the Internet site *http://cshcnleaders.ichp.edu/* and click on the directory link.

Special-Needs Trust

In traditional estate planning, wills and trusts generally specify what is to be paid to whom and when. Planning for people with disabilities is quite different; standard wills and trusts can leave beneficiaries liable to the government and other creditors. Parents (or other family members) of a disabled child can get around this liability issue by establishing what is called a special-needs trust. This planning tool places the disabled child's share of the estate into a special trust without threat that receipt of these funds will disqualify them from essential public benefits, including health-

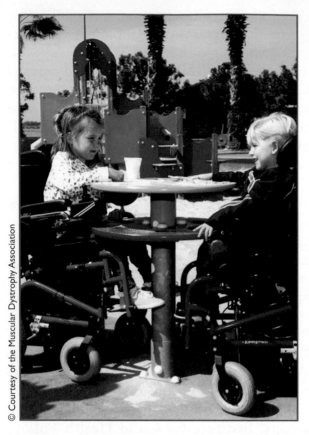

© Courtesy of the Muscular Dystrophy Association

care. Typically, when a special-needs trust is established by parents, the parents serve as the trustee until they die or become incapacitated. When that occurs a successor, or trustee, selected in advance by the parents, continues to serve according to instructions contained in the trust. The disabled person has no power or authority to direct the payment of funds; that power is turned over to the trustee, who pays for items and services beyond the bare necessities the government provides.

When setting up a special-needs trust it's a good idea to work with an expert lawyer. This is a complicated area of the law; government agencies have imposed very stringent rules and regulations upon these types of trusts. Look for an attorney who specializes in probate law, trusts and wills and estate planning. Connect with other parents or disability organizations, or contact the bar association in your area for referrals.

Sources

National Information Clearinghouse for Children and Youth with Disabilities (NICHCY); Office of Special Education Programs (OSEP); Parent Advocacy Coalition for Educational Rights (PACER)

KIDS' ZONE RESOURCES

Alliance for Parent Centers provides training and information to parents of infants, toddlers, school-aged children and young adults with disabilities, as well as the professionals who work with the families. For the regional parent center in your area, contact the Technical Assistance Alliance for Parent Centers Coordinating Office, PACER Center, 8161 Normandale Boulevard, Minneapolis, MN 55437; toll-free 1–888–248–0822; or visit *http://www.taalliance.org*

The Arc is an organization of people with mental retardation and related developmental disabilities, parents and other family members, and professionals who work with them. The Arc of the United States, 1010 Wayne Avenue Suite 650, Silver Spring, MD 20910; telephone 301–565–3842; or visit the Internet site *http://www.thearc.org*

Council for Exceptional Children (CEC) is a professional organization dedicated to improving educational outcomes for students with disabilities and/or other special exceptions. CEC advocates for appropriate governmental policies, sets professional standards, provides professional development, and advocates for underserved individuals. Council for Exceptional Children, 1110 North Glebe Road Suite 300, Arlington, VA 22201; toll-free 1-800-224-6830; or visit the Internet site *http://www.cec.sped.org*

Easter Seals has been helping individuals with disabilities and special needs and their families live better lives for more than 80 years. Primary Easter Seals services include rehabilitation, physical therapy, occupational therapy, speech and hearing therapy, job training, employment, child care, adult day services and much more. Easter Seals has dozens of local offices. Contact the national office for details. Easter Seals, 230 West Monroe Street Suite 1800, Chicago, IL 60606; toll-free 1–800–221–6827; or visit the Internet site *http://www.easterseals.com*

Educational Resources Information Center (ERIC) is an internet-based digital library of education research and information sponsored by the Institute of Education Sciences (IES) of the U.S. Department of Education. ERIC gathers and disseminates professional literature, information and resources on the education and development of individuals of all ages who have disabilities and/or

KIDS' ZONE RESOURCES

who are gifted. ERIC EC, toll-free 1–800-538-3742; or visit the Internet site *http://eric.ed.gov*

Family Center on Technology and Disability supports assistive technology organizations and programs that work with families of children and youth with disabilities. The website features a searchable database containing reviews of books, articles, research and other materials. Publishes a monthly newsletter. Family Center on Technology and Disability, 1825 Connecticut Avenue, N.W. Seventh Floor, Washington, D.C. 20009; telephone 202–884–8068; or visit the Internet site *http://www.fctd.info*

Family Voices is a national, grass roots clearinghouse for information concerning the healthcare of children with special health needs. Family Voices, 2340 Alamo SE, Suite 102, Albuquerque, NM 87106; toll-free 1–888–835–5669; or visit the Internet site *http://www.familyvoices.org*

Fathers Network is a national information resource to assist fathers involved in the lives of children with special needs. A program of the Kindering Center, funded by the Office of Children with Special Health Care Needs, Washington State Department of Health. Washington State Fathers Network, 16120 N.E. 8th Street, Bellevue, WA 98008; telephone 425–747–4004; or visit *http://www.fathersnetwork.org*

Federal Resource Center for Special Education (FRC) supports a nationwide technical assistance network to respond to the needs of students with disabilities, especially those from underrepresented populations. Federal Resource Center for Special Education, c/o Academy for Educational Development, 1825 Connecticut Avenue N.W., Washington, D.C. 20009; telephone 202–884–8215; or visit the Internet site *http://www.rrfcnetwork.org*

IDEA Partnership is a collaboration of more than 55 national organizations, technical assistance providers, state and local organizations and agencies working to improve educational results for children and youth with disabilities. The single partnership replaces four previous partnerships and is supported by the Research to Practice Division of the Office of Special Education Programs in the U.S. Department of Education. Contact the Partnership by way of the National Association of State Directors of Special Education (NASDSE), 1800 Diagonal Road, Suite 320, Alexandria, VA 22314. Toll-free call 1-877-IDEA.info. On the Internet please see *http://www.ideapartnership.org*

National Early Childhood Technical Assistance Center (NEC-TAC) supports the implementation of the early childhood provisions of the Individuals with Disabilities Education Act (IDEA). The center offers many resources and state phone contacts, hoping to strengthen service systems so children with disabilities (birth through five) and their families benefit from high-quality support and services. National Early Childhood Technical Assistance Center, Campus Box 8040, University of North Carolina, Chapel Hill, NC 27599; telephone 919–962–2001; or visit the Internet site *http://www.nectac.org*

National Information Clearinghouse for Children and Youth with Disabilities (NICHCY) is a resource for families and professionals with information about disabilities and related services. NICHCY offers details on education rights and the laws that enforce them. The clearinghouse also maintains a directory of disability related services and programs by state; to tap into the essential resources for your area contact NICHCY, P.O. Box 1492, Washington, DC 20013; toll-free 1–800–695–0285; or visit the Internet site *http://nichcy.org*. For more on early intervention, click on "Publications," then on "Parent Guides." NICHCY also offers training and curriculum modules on IDEA.

National Organization for Rare Disorders (NORD) is a federation of voluntary health organizations dedicated to helping people with rare "orphan" diseases and assisting the organizations that serve them. NORD maintains three searchable databases and an alphabetical index of over 1,000 diseases. National Organization for Rare Disorders, 55 Kenosia Avenue, Danbury, CT 06813; toll-free 1–800–999–6673; or visit the Internet site *http://www.rarediseases.org*

Office of Special Education Programs (OSEP) is part of the Office of Special Education and Rehabilitative Services in the U.S. Department of Education. OSEP's role is to improve results for infants, toddlers, children and youth with disabilities by providing leadership and financial support to assist states and local districts. OSEP administers the Individuals with Disabilities Education Act

KIDS' ZONE RESOURCES

(IDEA), which authorizes grants to states, institutions of higher education and other nonprofit organizations to support research, technical assistance, technology development and parent-training and information centers. Office of Special Education Programs, U.S. Department of Education, 400 Maryland Avenue, S.W., Washington, D.C. 20202; telephone 202–401-2000; or visit *http://www.ed.gov* search for OSEP.

Parent Advocacy Coalition for Educational Rights (PACER) was created in 1977 by parents of children and youth with disabilities to help other parents and families facing similar challenges and opportunities. PACER addresses special needs for all stages of childhood and all disabilities, and identifies resources and services available to help families learn and grow. PACER is also the coordinating office for Families and Advocates Partnership for Education (FAPE) to reach parents, administrators, service providers and policymakers with information about implementing IDEA. PACER Center, 8161 Normandale Boulevard, Minneapolis, MN 55437; telephone 952–838–9000; or visit the Internet site *http://www.pacer.org*

Parents Helping Parents (PHP) was formed to make sure children of all ages and backgrounds receive the resources, healthcare, education, and other services they need to reach their full potential. PHP offers information, training and support to families, professionals and the communities in which they live. Parents Helping Parents, 3041 Olcott Street, Santa Clara, CA 95054; telephone 408–727–5775; or visit the Internet site *http://www.php.com*

Shriners Hospitals: The Shrine of North America has established 22 pediatric hospitals in the United States, Canada and Mexico for kids with neuromusculoskeletal conditions, burn injuries and certain other special health care needs; there is no charge for any services. Three specialized rehabilitation units have been established for young people (up to age 18) with spinal cord injuries. The SCI facilities are located in Philadelphia, Chicago and Sacramento. For more information contact Shriners International Headquarters, 2900 Rocky Point Drive, Tampa, FL 33607; telephone toll-free 1–800–237–5055; or visit the Internet site *http://www.shrinershq.org* and click on "Hospital Directory."

Sibling Support Project, part of the Arc of the United States, is a peer support program dedicated to the interests of brothers and sisters of people with special health and developmental needs. The Sibling Support Project, 6512 23rd Avenue, N.W. Suite 213, Seattle, WA 98117; telephone 206–297–6368; or visit the Internet site *http://www.thearc.org/siblingsupport*

Special Needs Advocate for Parents (SNAP) features national online and print information for parents of children with disabilities. SNAP offers advocacy and resolution of medical insurance problems, referrals to educational advocates, support groups, and related organizations and professionals. Special Needs Advocate for Parents, 11835 W. Olympic Blvd. #465, Los Angeles, CA 90064; or visit *http://www.snapinfo.org*

Through the Looking Glass/National Parent-to-Parent Network connects parents with disabilities and others who may have shared similar experiences or faced common barriers related to child custody, adoption, pregnancy and birthing, specialized baby care equipment, etc. Through the Looking Glass, 2198 Sixth Street Suite 100, Berkeley, CA 94710-2204; toll-free 1–800–644–2666; or visit the Internet site *http://www.lookingglass.org/ppn.php*

United Cerebral Palsy (UCP), a partner with the Paralysis Resource Center, is a national organization with 110 affiliates in almost every state that strives to include persons with disabilities into every facet of society. UCP is the leading source of information on cerebral palsy, although 65 percent of the people served by UCP have disabilities other than CP. UCP National, 1660 L Street, N.W. Suite 700, Washington, D.C. 20036; telephone toll-free 1–800–872–5827; or on the Internet visit *http://www.ucp.org*

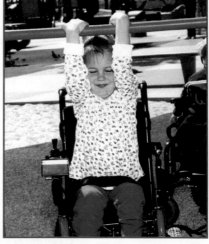

© Courtesy of the Muscular Dystrophy Association

KIDS' ZONE RESOURCES

University Of Montana Rural Institute: Center for Excellence in Disability Education, Research, and Service is part of the national network of programs funded by the Federal Administration on Developmental Disabilities (ADD). The program is committed to the independence, productivity and inclusion into the community of persons with disabilities. The University of Montana Rural Institute, 52 Corbin Hall, Missoula, MT 59812; toll-free 1–800–732–0323; or visit the Internet site *http://ruralinstitute.umt.edu*

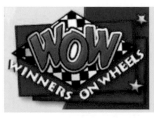

Winners On Wheels (WOW) is a national organization for children who use wheelchairs, featuring a social/recreation program that assists children in developing positive self-esteem and promoting independence and fun. WOW believes that encouraging personal achievement through creative learning and fun develops an individual's self-esteem. Winners On Wheels, 302 E. Church Street, Lewisville, TX 75057; toll-free 1–800–WOWTALK; or visit *http://www.wowusa.com*

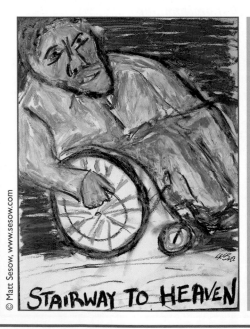

© Matt Sesow, www.sesow.com

STAIRWAY TO HEAVEN

STAIRWAY TO HEAVEN

"THIS PAINTING RELATES TO THE COMMON THEME OF PEOPLE CLIMBING A STAIRWAY TO HEAVEN. I WONDERED WHAT PEOPLE WHO COULDN'T WALK WOULD DO? AND DOES THAT IMPLY THEY DON'T GO TO HEAVEN?"

- MATT SESOW

Exceptional Parent is a media company that offers information to families and professionals involved in the care and development of people with disabilities and special healthcare needs. Publishers of Exceptional Parent magazine. Exceptional Parent, 551 Main Street, Johnstown, NJ 15901; call toll-free 1-800-372-7368; or visit *http://www.eparent.com*

Kids on Wheels is a unique book, and now also a magazine, written in two parts: one for parents; one for kids living with disabilities. The idea, says founding editor Jean Dobbs, is to respect and empower young people, "to plant the seeds of independent living, disability pride and 'the dignity of risk.'" The book is a full reference guide to pediatric physical medicine, community living, education, benefits, active living, etc. The quarterly magazine carries the theme forward with news, features and personality. From Leonard Media, which publishes *New Mobility*. P.O. Box 220, Horsham, PA 19044, toll-free call 888-850-0344. See *http://www.kidsonwheels.u*s

On the Internet
Ability OnLine is a computer friendship network for children and youth with disabilities that helps them connect to one another and to friends and family members. The site also provides a place for parents, caregivers and healthcare professionals to discuss issues of interest. The Toronto-based online connection promotes inclusion and full community participation. Traffic is monitored; access is free, registration required. Visit *http://www.abilityonline.org*

All Kids Can! is an online disabilities awareness program that helps students of all ages learn attitudes of acceptance, dignity and respect toward all people, especially those with disabilities. See *http://www.allkidscan.com*

Band-Aides and Blackboards is a Web community that sensitizes people to the reality of growing up with a medical problem. Many kids with diseases or conditions keep them secret, avoiding the stigma attached to not being physically perfect. This site, with sections for kids, teens and adults, makes the case that we're all more alike than different. *http://www.lehman.cuny.edu/faculty/jfleitas/bandaides/*

KIDS' ZONE RESOURCES

U Can Do! is an Internet community that celebrates the differences and abilities of all people, helps young people develop a positive attitude and broader perspective about themselves, and fosters a "can do" attitude to expand the possibilities for us all. The site features activities, dream sharing, etc. On the Internet see *http://www.ucando.org*

DO-IT (Disabilities, Opportunities, Internetworking, and Technology) aims to increase participation of people with disabilities in challenging academic programs and careers and to promote the use of information technology to maximize independence and productivity. DO-IT offers a mentor and pen-pal system for support and shared experience. Funding for the program is provided by the National Science Foundation, the State of Washington, and the U.S. Department of Education. DO-IT, University of Washington, Box 355670, Seattle, WA 98195; telephone 206–685–3648; or visit *http://www.washington.edu/doit*

EDLAW: Attorney S. James Rosenfeld, founding managing editor of *Education for the Handicapped Law Report*, created this legal resource to address issues related to law and education. The Child Advocate website features his webpage entitled Section 504 and IDEA. *http://www.childadvocate.net/504_and_IDEA.htm*

Education on Disability and Gender Equity (EDGE) is a Website curriculum project that offers readings, activities, resources and analysis so high school students can gain a better understanding of disability and gender and their impact on society. *http://www.disabledwomen.net/edge*

Keep S'myelin is a colorful online magazine to help kids better understand multiple sclerosis, from the National Multiple Sclerosis Society. *http://www.nmss.org*, search Keep S'myelin

Zigawhat is a Web information hub mainly for kids, maintained by the folks at the National Dissemination Center for Children with Disabilities (NICHCY). Kids a can share their story, connect with others, learn about their own health issues, play games and have fun. *http://www.nichcy.org/kids/index.htm*

Momentous Reality

Courtesy MDA

The next century, the next millennium
Is being made, now, today, each second.
We could be working towards
World peace, living as one spirit.
Or, we could be working towards
Disaster, chemical and nuclear wars.
The harmony, and existence of the future
Depends on the harmony and existence
Of each individual here, today.
We must be brave going into the future.
We must remember to play after each
          storm.
We must not live in fear of bad things
Blocking our way or overcoming our optimism.
If we can work together to face the future,
If we can unite as one,
Then our future will look, and be, very bright.
Even though the future seems far away,
It is actually beginning right now.
And while we are living in the present,
We must celebrate life everyday,
Knowing that we are becoming history
With every word, every action, every moment.
Because we, today, are the history of tomorrow,
We must ask ourselves each day
What we are doing that may have
An influence on the future.
It really won't be for many years that
The future will indicate if something we said,
Or if something we did or did not do,
Had an impact on a single individual,
Or if it trickled out to touch the whole world.

Written by Mattie Stepanek; he was ten years old at the time. Mattie, who had a form of muscular dystrophy, died in 2004; he was 14.

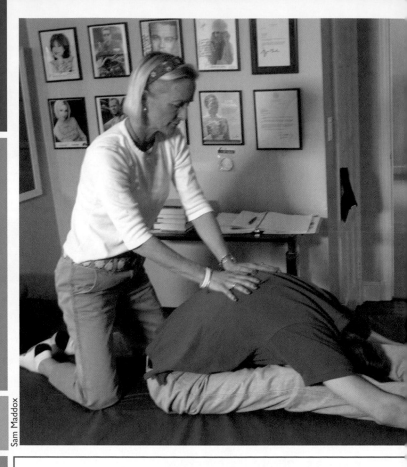

Sam Maddox

CAREGIVERS

Caregiving duties cannot be skirted and cannot always be delegated. But the job does not have to be performed in isolation. Connect to others with similar situations.

Dear Caregiver,

After my husband, Chris, was injured it became obvious that paralysis is a family issue. Taking care of our families' physical, emotional, social and economic needs can be fulfilling and rewarding. But caregiving a person who is paralyzed is a job we don't always expect to get.

We mourn our loved one's loss of mobility and independence. We also mourn our own losses: We feel isolated; we have no personal time; we feel exhausted, overwhelmed. And we feel no one else understands the demands placed upon us.

A caregiver must deal with medical concerns, hygiene, transportation, financial planning, advocacy, and end-of-life issues. Being an effective caregiver means gaining some sense of control over the situation. One way this is done is through information, and by sharing experiences or solving problems with other caregivers.

Please know that you are not alone, that you are extremely valuable, and that you and your family can lead active, fulfilling lives despite the challenges of paralysis. Don't ever be embarrassed to ask our Resource Center for assistance.

Best Wishes,
Dana Reeve

ED. NOTE: THIS MESSAGE WAS WRITTEN IN 2005, A YEAR BEFORE DANA REEVE'S DEATH.

Helping someone you care for to continue living independently in the community is valuable work. Caregiving can be a satisfying experience; it demonstrates fulfillment of a commitment to a loved one. True enough, though, caregiving is not a role anyone really chooses. It seems to choose us, emerging from events and circumstances outside our expectations, beyond our control.

Family members provide the vast majority of care for people who are chronically ill or disabled. According to the National Family Caregivers Association (NFCA), family caregivers underpin our healthcare system in a profound way. More than 50 million people provide some level of care for a loved one, which would translate into annual wages of $257 billion if it weren't done for "free." As the population ages, as medical science keeps people alive longer and as healthcare policies send people home from hospitals sicker and quicker, the number of family caregivers can only grow.

Caregiving is a job that cannot be skirted and cannot always be delegated. It is frustrating. It is physically and emotionally draining. It can steal our dreams or break our hearts. It makes us sad for our loved one's loss . . . and for our own loss. While caring for loved ones can be enormously satisfying, there are days, to be sure, that offer little reward.

The job takes its toll. Caregivers suffer far more depression, stress and anxiety than the general population. In an NFCA member survey, 61 percent of caregivers reported depression, 51 percent sleeplessness, and 41 percent back problems.

Caregivers feel isolated; they often report that their lives are not "normal" and that no one else can possibly understand what they are going through.

There is a financial impact, too. Families helping a person with a disability in daily living activities spend more than twice as much on out-of-pocket medical expenses than families without a disabled person. Frequently the caregiver must make sacrifices at work to attend to duties at home.

But this is your family, your loved one. What are your choices? You can't just walk away. You learn to deal with the frustration while learning how to best get the job done. The lessons are often learned the hard way—for the most part, caregivers learn by trial and error how to manage daily routines for food preparation, hygiene, transportation and other activities at home.

Here are a few caregiving tips compiled from the Paralysis Resource Center information collection:

- Rule number one for all caregivers is to take care of yourself. Providing care while holding down a job, running a household, or parenting can burn anyone out. A person who is exhausted or sick is more likely to make bad decisions or take out frustrations inappropriately. Stress is known to contribute to a variety of health problems. The more in balance you keep your own well-being, the more you will enhance your coping skills and stamina. By taking care of yourself, you will be better able, both physically and emotionally, to provide care for your loved one.

- Connect to the caregiving community. Share and learn and benefit from the collective wisdom of the caregiver community. It is important that caregivers connect with one another to gain strength and to know that they are not alone. For many, the isolation that comes with the job is eased by attending support-group meetings with others in similar situations. Support groups provide emotional support and caregiving tips, as well as information on community resources. Online support groups on the Internet can be very helpful. Therapeutic counseling may also facilitate better problem solving. Counseling can help one cope with feelings of anger, frustration, guilt, loss or competing personal, work and family demands.

- Know as much as possible about your loved one's condition. Be informed about medical issues and how the disease or disability can affect a person physically, psychologically, behaviorally and etc. You are an important member of your loved one's healthcare team. Chapter 1 provided an overview of the primary causes of paralysis. The Internet is another powerful tool for learning about the medical basis of disability. Doctors and other health professionals can help you understand how a loved one's condition might change, and how that change might affect the demands on the caregiver.

- Take advantage of opportunities for respite care. Refresh yourself and take an occasional break from daily duties. An extended vacation may not be realistic but it is essential for caregivers to schedule some down time. This may be a short outing, quiet time at home, a movie with a friend, etc. To get away, the caregiver may require respite care/assistance from others. See Resources at the end of this chapter for some possible connections to help you get a break.

- Be an advocate. Keep in mind you may be the only one equipped to speak out on your loved one's behalf or to ask difficult questions. Prepare your loved one's health history and take it with you to appointments. Anticipate the future as best as you can. Financial and legal planning are important considerations. Issues such as financing long-term care, protecting assets, obtaining the authority for surrogate decision making, and other matters often need attention. Make an appointment with an attorney knowledgeable in estate planning, probate, and, if possible, public benefits planning. Careful planning is often required to coordinate community services and involved friends and family. Decisions about placement in a nursing home or other care options can often be facilitated by a trained

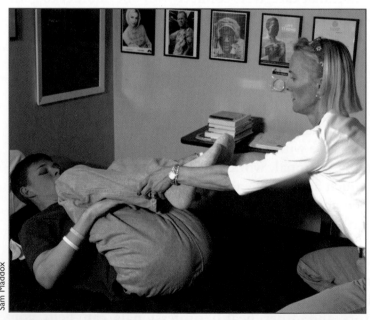

Sam Maddox

TAYLOR AND MARNIE PRICE

professional familiar with brain impairments, caregiving and community resources. In some cases, it is necessary to make end-of-life decisions regarding your loved one.

- Understand as best as you can how the system works for insurance, social security and others means of public assistance. There are experts at public agencies who can help. See Chapter 8, Working the System, pages 244 - 275.

- Ask for help. Many caregivers are so accustomed to providing help and seeing to another person's needs that they don't know how to ask for aid themselves. Your family is your first resource. Spouses, brothers and sisters, children, and other relatives can do a lot to ease your caregiving burden. Let them know what they can and should do. Look to your church for aid and counsel. Make your minister or religious leader aware of your situation. Encourage your loved one's friends and neighbors to provide what comfort they can. If you need to hire an attendant, several good resource guides are listed below.

- Know as much as you can about tools and adaptive equipment. It is essential that caregivers know about the homecare products and services that might make their jobs easier. See the Tools, chapter 7 in this book, pages 212 - 243, for ways to stay current and up-to-date on all technology has to offer.

"Rule number one for all caregivers is to take care of yourself. The more in balance you keep your own well-being, the more you will enhance your coping skills and stamina."

As you settle into the role of caregiver, you may find yourself making decisions for people who used to decide for you. It's sometimes a trick to balance competing needs for control. But it's important to respect the right of the person being cared for to make choices. Choice is good; by deciding things we have a sense of control over our lives. Allow your loved one as much choice as possible, from the food on the menu to their daily wardrobe to TV programming.

Gain confidence in your abilities and pride in your achievements. Easier said than done—how do you stand up for yourself, take care of yourself, and find a balance between your own needs and those of your loved ones? The NFCA offers the following Principles of Caregiver Empowerment – the foundation by which the association urges caregivers to try to live.

• **Choose to take charge of your life.** Don't let your loved one's illness or disability always take center stage. We fall into caregiving often because of an unexpected event, but somewhere along the line you need to step back and consciously say, "I choose to take on this caregiving role." It goes a long way toward eliminating the feeling of being a victim.

• **Honor, value and love yourself.** You're doing a very hard job and you deserve some quality time, just for yourself. Self-care isn't a luxury. It's a necessity. It is your right as a human being. Step back and recognize just how extraordinary you are. Remember, your own good health is the very best present you can give your loved one.

• **Seek, accept and, at times, demand help.** Don't be ashamed to ask for help. When people offer assistance, accept it and suggest specific things that they can do. Caregiving, especially at its most intense levels, is definitely more than a one-person job. Asking for help is a sign of your strength and an acknowledgment of your abilities and limitations.

• **Stand up and be counted.** Stand up for your rights as a caregiver and a citizen. Recognize that caregiving comes on top of being a parent, a child, a spouse. Honor your caregiving role and speak up for your well-deserved recognition and rights. Become your own advocate, both within your own immediate caregiving sphere and beyond.

Sources

National Family Caregivers Association, The Family Caregiver Alliance, Aging and Adult Services Administration/Department of Social and Health Services, State of Washington; American Stroke Association, AARP

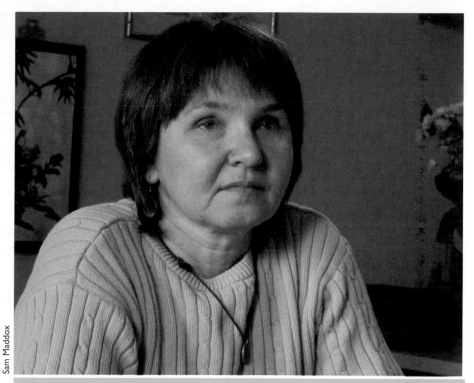

Sam Maddox

Kate Willette

Your partner gets hurt and your life is changed because of something that happened to him. That is the hard truth. I remember saying to him, "Come back. Please come back." And, he would say, "I'm trying."

A caregiver-spouse has to say to at some point, "I freely choose this," in the same way before the injury happened. And, if you don't freely choose this with your whole heart, I don't see how you can make it, because there's going to be some part of you that is always mad, that always somehow resents this other person for what they've taken away from you. Being a family care giver is relentless. You can never, ever really get away from it. It really helps to have a sense of humor; but, I think the most important thing isn't really how you communicate. It's the very basic choice and knowing that no one's making you do anything. If you can accept this, you'll find ways to work it out, whatever it is.

Willette chronicled her experiences as a caregiver in the book Some Things Are Unbreakable; *order from www.lulu.com*

CAREGIVERS RESOURCES

The National Family Caregivers Association (NFCA) educates, supports and empowers families who care for chronically ill, aged or disabled loved ones. NFCA, a partner organization of the Christopher and Dana Reeve Foundation Paralysis Resource Center, reaches across different diagnoses, relationships and life stages to address the common needs and concerns of all family caregivers. NFCA, 10400 Connecticut Avenue #500, Kensington, MD 20895–3944; toll-free 1–800–896–3650; or visit the Internet site *http://www.nfcacares.org*

National Alliance for Caregiving is a coalition or national groups that supports to family caregivers and the professionals who help them. National Alliance for Caregiving, 4720 Montgomery Lane, 5th Floor, Bethesda, MD 20814. See Website *http://www.caregiving.org*

The Caregivers Advisory Panel collects confidential information on the opinions and needs of family caregivers to help healthcare product manufacturers and service providers. Caregivers Advisory Panel, 3949 Old Post Road Suite 200C, Charlestown, RI 02813; toll-free 1–877–595–6227; or visit the Internet site *http://www.caregiversadvisorypanel.com*

Well Spouse is a national organization that gives support to wives, husbands, and partners of the chronically ill and/or disabled. Addresses issues common to family caregivers: anger, guilt, fear, isolation, grief, and financial threat. Well Spouse, 63 West Main Street Suite H, Freehold, NJ 07728; 1–800–838–0879; *http://www.wellspouse.org*

Caregiving.com is an Internet community site operated by Denise Brown for families and healthcare professionals who care for chronically ill or disabled family members. See *www.caregiving.com*

The Family Caregiver Alliance (FCA) is the lead agency in California's system of Caregiver Resource Centers and operates the National Center on Caregiving to develop support programs for family caregivers in every state. FCA champions the caregivers' cause through education, services, research and advocacy. For residents of the San Francisco Bay Area, FCA provides direct support services for caregivers of those with Alzheimer's disease, stroke, traumatic brain injury, Parkinson's, etc. FCA, 180 Montgomery Street, Suite 1100, San Francisco, CA 94104; telephone 415–434–3388; or visit the Internet site *http://www.caregiver.org*

AARP (formerly the American Association of Retired Persons) features numerous fact sheets and resources on caregiving, including legal issues, care, long distance caregiving, end of life issues. AARP, 601 E Street, NW, Washington, D.C. 20049; toll-free 1-888-OUR-AARP; or visit the Internet site *http://www.aarp.org* and search under "Caregiving."

The National Citizens' Coalition for Nursing Home Reform (NCC-NHR) was formed to represent the consumer voice at the national level regarding nursing home issues. They feature fact sheets on nursing home topics, including a guide to choosing one. They publish the book *Nursing Homes: Getting Good Care There* (by Sarah Greene Burger, Virginia Fraser, Sara Hunt and Barbara Frank), a consumer guide on achieving the best possible nursing home experience for a relative or friend. NCCNHR, 1828 L. Street, NW Suite 801, Washington, D.C. 20036; telephone 202-332-2276; or visit the Internet site *http://nursinghomeaction.org*

Caregiver Media Group provides information, support and guidance for family and professional caregivers. Publishes *Today's Caregiver* magazine and offers a Website with topic-specific newsletters, online discussion lists, chat rooms and an online store. Caregiver Media Group, 3005 Greene Street, Hollywood, FL 33020; telephone 954–893–0550; or visit the Internet site *http://www.caregiver.com*

National Respite Coalition and National Respite Locator Service helps parents, caregivers and professionals get a break using respite services in their local area. ARCH National Respite Network, 4016 Oxford Street, Annandale, VA 22003, telephone 703-256-9578. On the Internet see *http://www.archrespite.org*

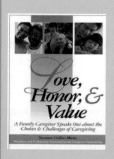

Love, Honor & Value, by Suzanne Mintz, co-founder of the National Family Caregivers Alliance, is for those who are just beginning a caregiving journey and those for whom family caregiving is an integral part of their lives. Order from NFCA, http://www.nfcacares.org. This is a book that can make a difference for those trying to find their way through the maze of caregiving.

ON THE INTERNET

FamilyCare America hopes to improve the lives of the caregivers by creating a highly accessible resource for caregivers. FamilyCare America also serves corporate needs through specialty publishing and human resource programs. See *http://www.familycareamerica.com*

Shepherd's Centers of America (SCA) is an interfaith, not-for-profit organization that coordinates nearly 100 independent Shepherd's Centers across the United States to help older adults remain independent. See *http://www.shepherdcenters.org*

Hiring and Management of Personal Care Assistants for Individuals with SCI is a downloadable, 26-page booklet in PDF format from the SCI Project at Santa Clara Valley Medical Center. Covers everything from locating and hiring, to training and paying personal assistants. Includes forms, checklists and resources. See *http://www.tbi-sci.org/pdf/pas.pdf*

Paralysis Community, a resource of *www.paralysis.org*, the homepage of the Christopher & Dana Reeve Foundation Paralysis Resource Center. This is a safe and secure online social networking site with a robust discussion area on many areas of paralysis, including caregiving. Join us: Write a blog; connect with friends. Click on Community Forums at the top of the *www.paralysis.org* home page; registration is quick and easy to access the many community features.

CareCure Forum for caregivers. Active and helpful message board for loved ones and caregivers of people with paralysis. On the Internet see *http://sci.rutgers.edu* and click on the "Caregiving" section.

Spinal Cord Injury Caregivers is a Yahoo Internet forum, a place to share information and to support other caregivers who are caring for people with SCI. See *http://groups.yahoo.com/group/scic*

Nursing Home Compare, sponsored by Medicare. Information about the past performance of most nursing homes in the U.S. Also features *A Guide to Choosing a Nursing Home* and a nursing home checklist. See *http://www.medicare.gov/NHCompare/home.asp*

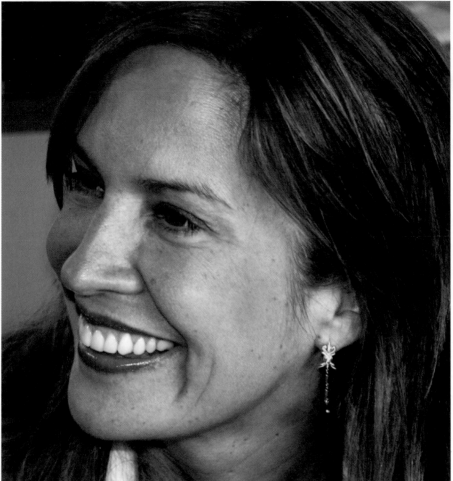

Sam Maddox

Dana Reeve

After Chris was injured we sort of operated as if it was like land-
ing on another planet. It can look very bleak and overwhelming.
There's a tremendous amount of adjustment that needs to go on
mentally. And facing the new normal, facing the adjustments, the
loss...you have to grieve for the loss. Because it's true - the only
way for grief to be alleviated is to grieve. You need to acknowl-
edge the loss. But at the same time, once you do that, you're opening up a whole new area where you can have tremendous hope.

Key resources for the paralysis community

ADVOCACY

ADAPT started as American Disabled for Accessible Public Transit, blocking buses in cities across the nation to demonstrate the need for access to public transit. The organization played a major role in gaining passage of the Americans with Disabilities Act and continues to take its message to the streets so people with disabilities can live in the community with real supports instead of being locked away in nursing homes and other institutions. ADAPT national office, 201 S Cherokee, Denver, CO 80223; 303-733-9324; on the Internet see *http://www.adapt.org*

American Association of People with Disabilities (AAPD) is the largest national cross-disability member organization in the United States, dedicated to ensuring economic self-sufficiency and political empowerment for 56 million Americans with disabilities. AAPD works with other disability organizations for the full implementation of disability nondiscrimination laws. AAPD, 1629 K Street NW, Suite 503, Washington, DC 20006; toll-free 1-800-840-8844; on the Internet *http://www.aapd.com*

Justice for All is an e-mail network formed to defend and advance disability rights and programs in Congress. For instructions on how to join this important communications link, see *http://www.jfanow.org*

National Organization on Disability: Since 1982, NOD has been working to expand the participation of people with disabilities in all aspects of American life. NOD promotes voting, housing, employment, religious access, accessible urban design, statistical surveys, marketing to the disability community, much more. National Organization on Disability, 910 Sixteenth Street, N.W., Suite 600, Washington, DC 20006; telephone 202-293-5960; on the Internet see *http://nod.org*

National Council on Disability (NCD) is an independent federal agency making recommendations to the President and Congress on issues affecting 54 million Americans with disabilities. NCD is composed of 15 members appointed by the President and confirmed by the U.S. Senate. NCD promotes policies and programs that guarantee equal opportunity and empowers people with disabilities to achieve economic self-sufficiency, independent living, and inclusion into all aspects of society. NCD was instrumental in the passage of the Americans with Disabilities Act. NCD, 1331 F Street, NW, Suite 850, Washington, DC 20004; telephone 202-272-2004; on the Internet see *http://www.ncd.gov*

CULTURE & EDUCATION

The Disability History Project is a community history project for people with disabilities to set forth and share a rich history and culture. On the Internet see *http://www.disabilityhistory.org*

The Disability Museum is a virtual collection to chronicle the disability experience and dispel lingering myths, assumptions, and stereotypes. See *http://www.disabilitymuseum.org*

Society for Disability Studies explores issues of disability and chronic illness from scholarly perspectives. SDS membership includes social scientists, health researchers, and humanities scholars, as well as those in the disability rights movement. Publishes Disability Studies Quarterly (DSQ), and hosts an annual conference. Contact Carol J. Gill, Ph.D., Executive Officer, SDS, Department of Disability and Human Development, University of Illinois at Chicago (MC 626), 1640 W. Roosevelt Road #236, Chicago, IL 60608; telephone 312-996-4664; on the Internet see *http://www.uic.edu/org/sds*

Association on Higher Education And Disability (AHEAD) is an international, organization of professionals committed to full participation in higher education for people with disabilities. AHEAD, 107 Commerce Center Drive, Suite 204, Huntersville, NC 28078; on the Internet see *http://www.ahead.org*

INDEPENDENT LIVING

National Council on Independent Living (NICL) advances the independent living philosophy of self-determination and full integration and participation of people with disabilities in society. NCIL represents over 700 organizations and individuals that advocate for the human and civil rights of people with disabilities. NCIL, 1710 Rhode Island Avenue, NW, 5th Floor, Washington DC 20036; telephone 202-207-0334; see *http://www.ncil.org*

Independent Living Research Utilization (ILRU) is a national center for information, training, research, and technical assistance in independent living. ILRU is a program of The Institute for Rehabilitation and Research and is affiliated with Baylor College of Medicine. Maintains a useful database of Independent Living Centers in the United States. ILRU, 2323 South Shepherd, Suite 1000, Houston, Texas 77019; telephone 713-520-0232; on the Internet see *http://www.ilru.org*

INTERNATIONAL

United States International Council on Disabilities (USICD) is a federation of disability-oriented agencies, associations, facilities and consumers to furthering the full integration into society of people with disabilities. USICD has taken the lead for the United States in worldwide efforts to draft a disability rights convention through the United Nations. USICD, 1710 Rhode Island Avenue, NW, 5th Floor, Washington, DC 20036; telephone 202-207-0338; on the Internet see *http://www.usicd.org*

Disabled Peoples' International advocates for the full participation of all disabled people in the mainstream of life, particularly those in developing countries. The DPI cross-disability network has approximately 120 national members. Disabled Peoples' International, 902-388 Portage Avenue, Winnipeg, Manitoba, Canada R3C 0C8; telephone: 204-287-8010; on the Internet see *http://www.dpi.org*

Rehabilitation International is a worldwide network of people with disabilities, service providers and government agencies working together to improve the quality of life for disabled people and their families. RI actively participates in the International Disability Alliance (IDA), a coalition of international organizations. Founded in 1922, it now has more than 700 member organizations in 100 nations. RI, 25 East 21 Street, New York, NY 10010; telephone 212-420-1500; on the Internet see *http://www.rehab-international.org*

MEDIA

Abilities is Canada's cross-disability lifestyle magazine. Covers health, active living, disability rights, resources, etc. Canadian Abilities Foundation, 340 College Street, Suite 401, Toronto, Ontario M5T 3A9; telephone 416-923-1885; on the Internet see *http://www.abilities.ca*

Ability Magazine crosses celebrity journalism with disability awareness. Contact the publication at 1001 W. 17th Street, Costa Mesa, CA 92627; telephone 949-854-8700; see *http://www.abilitymagazine.com*

Exceptional Parent is a magazine with support, ideas, encouragement and outreach for parents and families of children with every type of disability. Covers technology, toys, healthcare, education, advocacy, more. Exceptional Parent, 65 East Route 4, River Edge, NJ 07661; 1-800-372-7368; see *http://www.eparent.com*

Kids On Wheels is a full-color quarterly magazine that enables children with disabilities and their parents to live active, independent lives. One version is for kids, the other for parents. From the publishers of New Mobility. Kids On Wheels, P.O. Box 220, Horsham, PA 109044; toll free telephone 888-850-0344, on the Internet see *http://www.kidsonwheels.us*

Mouth is a bi-monthly magazine about disability rights and empowerment that says this about itself: "This rude little magazine demands answers from the people in charge, laughs at the lying answers, and occasionally bites down, hard, somewhere near the throbbing jugular." Mouth, 4201 SW 30th Street, Topeka, KS 66614; see *http://www.mouthmag.com*

New Mobility is a monthly lifestyle magazine for the wheelchair community. Features and news about active living, medical issues, current affairs, personalities, products and more. NM, P.O. Box 220, Horsham, PA 19044; telephone 215-675-9133; see *http://www.newmobility.com*

PN (Paraplegia News) is a magazine for service veterans with disabilities, and for anyone who uses a wheelchair. Covers healthcare, issues, news and events, sports and recreation, much more. PVA Publications, 2111 East Highland Avenue, Suite 180, Phoenix, AZ 85016; toll-free 1-888-888-2201; on the Internet see *http://www.pvamagazines.com/pnnews*

Ragged Edge, the online successor to The Disability Rag, covers the tough issues concerning disability: medical rationing, genetic discrimination, assisted suicide, long-term care, attendant services. On the Internet see *http://www.ragged-edge-mag.com*

Spinal Network: The Total Wheelchair Resource Book (which begat New Mobility) comprises 586 pages of profiles, articles, photos and resources. Founded in 1987 by Sam Maddox, this is the original survival manual for paralyzing conditions. "It's mindbendingly, breathtakingly comprehensive," says cartoonist John Callahan. New edition in 2008. Telephone 215-675-9133; see *http://www.newmobility.com*

Sports 'N Spokes is a colorful bi-monthly magazine about wheelchair athletics, competitive sports and recreation. PVA Publications, 2111 East Highland Avenue, Suite 180, Phoenix, AZ 85016; toll-free 1-888-888-2201; on the Internet see *http://www.sportsnspokes.com*

The Strength Coach Radio Show, hosted by Greg Smith, a syndicated radio talk show on life and disability. See *http://www.thestrengthcoach.com*

ON LINE COMMUNITIES

CareCure Community, the online home of Rutgers University scientist Wise Young, offers lively Internet forums with news and comment on paralysis care, caregiving, cure, funding, active living, pain treatment, sexuality, research, clinical trials and more. Must-see site for research related information. See *http://sci.rutgers.edu/*

BrainTalk Communities is a huge collection of Internet message boards covering nearly every known neurological problem and disability social issue. See *http://brain.hastypastry.net/forums/*

Dangerwood is an Internet community that offers people with paralysis insights and advice from others who have already found answers. Says founder Nick Danger, "We are infinitely stronger together than we are divided." See *http://www.survivingparalysis.com*

New Mobility online includes an active bulletin board community. See *http://www.newmobility.com*

Multiple Sclerosis Complementary and Alternative Medicine (MS-CAM) is an Internet community that shares experiences with complementary and alternative medicine (CAM) therapies. See *http://www.ms-cam.org*

The Stroke Network is a community of web sites designed to help "everyone in the stroke family." Features chats, message boards, survivor profiles, resources, etc. Link to forums via *http://www.strokenetwork.org*

Chronic Pain Support Group offers a very active and supportive online environment where people meet others who live in chronic pain. Click on Messages and chat: *http://www.chronicpainsupport.org*

Paralysis Community, a section of *www.paralysis.org*, the home of the Christopher and Dana Reeve Foundation Paralysis Resource Center, is a safe and secure online social networking site. Join the discussions and meet new people, or just hang back and learn from the sidelines. Numerous discussion areas on numerous topics related to paralysis, including active living, relationships, caregiving, cure research, clinical care and creature comforts. Join the community: connect with friends. Stay abreast of news and information that affects you; stay in touch with people you'd like to affect. It's fun and useful. Registration is required but it's free to participate. To visit the Paralysis Community click on *www.paralysis.org*, then on Community Forums at top of home page.

RELIGION

Religion and Disability Program of the National Organization on Disability is an interfaith effort that urges all faith groups, congregations and seminaries to identify and remove barriers of architecture, communications, and attitudes. Helps sponsor "That All May Worship" conferences, offers publications. See Website for list of ministers with disabilities. NOD, 910 Sixteenth Street, N.W., Suite 600, Washington, DC 20006; telephone 202-293-5960; *http://www.nod.org/religion*

Joni and Friends is a Christian ministry formed by quadriplegic Joni Eareckson Tada to evangelize people affected by disability. JAF, P.O. Box 3333, Agoura Hills, CA 91376; telephone 818-707-5664; visit Joni and Friends on the Internet at *http://www.joniandfriends.org*

National Catholic Partnership on Disability (NCPD) was established in 1982 to implement the Pastoral Statement of U.S. Catholic Bishops on People with Disabilities, a document that states that Catholics with disabilities must be able to participate in the celebrations and obligations of their faith. NCPD, 415 Michigan Avenue, NE, Suite 95, Washington, DC 20017-4501; telephone 202-529-2933; *http://www.ncpd.org*

National Jewish Council for the Disabled addresses the needs of people with disabilities within the Jewish community and enhances life opportunities and insures participation in the full spectrum of Jewish life. Telephone 212-613-8156; *http://www.ou.org/ncsy/njcd*

Christian Council on Persons with Disabilities (CCPD) provides a platform and sounding board for dialogue, communication, and interaction to promote the spiritual well-being of people with disabilities. 301 E. Pine Street, Suite 150, Orlando, FL 32801; telephone 407-210-3917; on the Internet see *http://www.ccpd.org*

The Episcopal Disability Network focuses on the physical, cultural, emotional, attitudinal, educational, and programmatic barriers that prevent all persons with disabilities from enjoying full participation in church and society. EDN, 3024 East Minnehaha Parkway, Minneapolis, MN 55406; toll-free 1-888-738-3636; on the Internet see *http://www.disability99.org*

American Atheists is a loosely organized group, and movement, concerned that the line between church and state has been badly distorted. Atheists reject the tenets of religious dogma; they accept only that which is scientifically verifiable. *http://www.atheists.org/*

Christopher and Dana Reeve Foundation Paralysis Resource Center Task Force

American Association on Health and Disability supports health promotion and wellness for people with disabilities, reduces incidence of secondary conditions and health disparities. AAHD, 110 N. Washington Street, Suite 340A, Rockville, MD 20850, 301-545-6140; *http://www.aahd.us*

American Syringomyelia Alliance Project works to improve the lives of persons affected by syringomyelia, Chiari malformation and related disorders. ASAP, PO Box 1586, Longview, TX 75606-1586; telephone 903-236-7079; see *http://www.asap.org*

Amputee Coalition of America empowers people with limb loss through education, support and advocacy. ACA, 900 East Hill Avenue, Suite 285, Knoxville, Tennessee 37915-2568; Toll-free call 1-888-AMP-KNOW; see *http://www.amputee-coalition.org*

Arizona Spinal Cord Injury Association promotes physical, intellectual, spiritual, emotional and social recovery of people with SCI. 901 E Willetta Street #2306, Phoenix, AZ 85006; telephone 602-239-5929. On the Internet see *http://www.azspinal.org*

Arkansas Spinal Cord Commission meets the lifelong needs of people with spinal cord disabilities in Arkansas. 1501 North University Ave. Suite 470, Little Rock, AR 72207; toll-free 1-800-459-1517; on the Internet see *http://www.spinalcord.ar.gov*

Association of Rehabilitation Nurses advances professional rehabilitation nursing practice through education, advocacy, collaboration, and research. ARN, 4700 W. Lake Avenue, Glenview, IL 60025-1485; toll-free call 1-800-229-7530. See *http://www.rehabnurse.org*

Brain Injury Association of America provides information, education and support to assist the 5.3 million Americans living with traumatic brain injury and their families. BIAA, 1608 Spring Hill Road, Suite 110, Vienna, VA 22182; 703-761-0750; National Brain Injury Information Center: toll-free 1-800-444-6443; *http://www.biausa.org*

Brain & Spinal Injury Trust Fund Commission of Georgia assists Georgians with SCI and TBI with expenses from their injuries. Call toll-free 1-888-233-5760; visit *http://www.ciclt.net/sn/clt/bsitf*

Centers for Disease Control and Prevention, Division of Human Development and Disability works to identify the causes of birth defects and developmental disabilities and to prevent injuries. CDC, 1600 Clifton Rd, Atlanta, GA 30333, 404-639-3534 or toll-free 800-311-3435; See *http://www.cdc.gov/ncbddd/disabilities.htm*

Cerebral Palsy International Research Foundation funds research and educational activities toward discovering the cause, cure and care for those with cerebral palsy and related developmental disabilities. CPIRF, 1025 Connecticut Avenue, Suite 701, Washington, DC 20036; see *http://www.cpirf.org*

Chiari & Syringomyelia Foundation advances knowledge about Chiari malformation, syringomyelia and related cerebrospinal fluid disorders. CSF, 333 Earle Ovington Blvd. Suite 701. Uniondale, NY 11553 *http://www.csfinfo.org*

The Cody Unser First Step Foundation raises research funds to fight paralysis and to build awareness of transverse myelitis. Post Office Box 56696, Albuquerque, NM 87187; telephone 505–890–0086; or visit *http://www.codysfirststep.org*

Craig Hospital promotes optimal health and quality of life for people affected by spinal cord injury and traumatic brain injury. Contact c/o 3425 S. Clarkson St., Englewood, CO 80113; 303-789-8000, *http://www.craighospital.org*

Department of Veterans Affairs (VA) provides health care and other benefits and services to veterans, their family members and survivors. For health care benefits: 1-877-222-8387; VA Benefits: 1-800-827-1000; *http://www.va.gov*

Easter Seals provides services to ensure that people living with disabilities have equal opportunities to live, learn, work and play. 230 West Monroe Street, Suite 1800, Chicago, IL 60606; telephone 312-726-6200; see *http://www.easterseals.com*

Kennedy Krieger International Center for Spinal Cord Injury works with children with paralysis to improve health and optimize recovery of function. 707 N. Broadway, Baltimore, MD 21205; toll free 1-888-554-2080; *http://www.kennedykrieger.org*

Kessler Medical Rehabilitation Research & Education Corporation (Northern New Jersey Spinal Cord Injury System) provides medical and rehab services. 1199 Pleasant Valley Way, West Orange, NJ 07052; *http://www.kmrrec.org/nnjscis*

Life Rolls On provides hope and advocates on behalf of young people affected by spinal cord injury. LRO, 7770 Regents Road, Suite 113-199, San Diego, CA 92122, toll-free 1-866-We Will Walk (866-939-4559); *http://www.liferollson.org*

National Alliance for Caregiving is a coalition of groups that supports family caregivers and the professionals who help them. National Alliance for Caregiving, 4720 Montgomery Lane, 5th Floor, Bethesda, MD 20814. See *http://www.caregiving.org*

National Center on Physical Activity and Disability promotes the many health benefits to be gained from regular physical activity. NCPAD, 1640 W. Roosevelt Road Chicago, IL 60608-6904; toll free call 1-800-900-8086. On the Internet see *www.ncpad.org*

National Family Caregivers Association educates, supports and empowers families who care for chronically ill, aged or disabled loved ones. 10400 Connecticut Avenue #500, Kensington, MD 20895-3944; toll-free 1-800-896-3650; *http://www.nfcacares.org*

National Institute on Disability and Rehabilitation Research provides research related to the rehabilitation of individuals with disabilities, aimed at improving lives from birth through adulthood. See *http://www.ed.gov/about/offices/list/osers/nidrr*

National Multiple Sclerosis Society (NMSS) provides information on living with MS, treatment, scientific progress, MS centers, clinical research, local chapters. NMSS, 733 Third Avenue, New York, NY 10017; 1-800-344-4867; *http://www.nationalmssociety.org*

National Organization on Disability promotes participation of America's 54 million people with disabilities in all aspects of life. NOD, 910 16th Street, N.W., Suite 600, Washington, DC 20006; 202-293-5960; *http://www.nod.org*

National Respite Coalition supports accessible, planned and crisis respite services for all families and caregivers to strengthen and stabilize families. 4016 Oxford St., Annandale, VA, 22003; telephone 703-256-9578. See *http://www.chtop.org/NRC.htm*

National Spinal Cord Injury Association features chapters and support groups. Contact NSCIA, toll-free 1-800-962-9629; or visit *http://www.spinalcord.org*

Navajoland Nurses United for Research, Service and Education is dedicated to nurturing nurses who serve the people in and around the Navajo Nation. PO Box 398, Window Rock, Arizona 86515, *http://www.n-nurse.org*

Neurotech Network of The Society to Increase Mobility, Inc. promotes access to neurotechnology devices for persons with impairments. Neurotech Network, PO Box 27386, Tampa, FL 33623; 727-321-0150; *http://www.neurotechnetwork.org*

New Jersey Division of Disability Services serves individuals and families dealing with disabilities. *http://www.state.nj.us/humanservices/dds*

Office of Special Education And Rehabilitation Services provides a wide array of supports to parents and individuals, school districts and states in three areas: special education, vocational rehabilitation and research. See *http://www.ed.gov/about/offices/list/osers/index.html*

Office on Disability, Department of Health and Human Services oversees disability programs, policies and initiatives pertaining to the over 54 million persons with disabilities in the United States, 200 Independence Avenue, S.W., Room 637D, Washington, DC 20201; 202-401-5844; *http://www.hhs.gov/od*

Paralyzed Veterans of America (PVA) works toward quality health care, rehabilitation and civil rights for veterans and all citizens with spinal cord injuries and diseases. PVA, 801 Eighteenth Street, NW, Washington, DC 20006-3517; toll-free 1-800-424-8200; or on the Internet see *http://www.pva.org*

Partners for Youth with Disabilities empowers young people with disabilities to reach their full potential for personal development. PYD: 95 Berkeley Street, Suite 109, Boston, MA 02116; 617-556-4075; *http://www.pyd.org*

Post-Polio Health International enhances the lives and independence of polio survivors and home ventilator users through education, advocacy, research and networking. PPHI and International Ventilator Users Network, 314-534-0475; *http://www.post-polio.org*

Rancho Los Amigos National Rehabilitation Center provides medical and rehabilitation services in a culturally sensitive environment. Contact toll-free 877-726-2461; 7601 E Imperial Highway, Downey, CA 90242; *http://www.rancho.org*

Sam Schmidt Paralysis Foundation funds research, treatment, rehabilitation, and programs to improve quality of life for people with spinal cord injury. SSPF, P.O. Box 24355, Speedway, IN 46224-0355; telephone 317-236-9999; *http:www.samschmidt.org*

Shepherd Center specializes in the medical treatment, research and rehabilitation for people with spinal cord injuries, acquired brain injuries and other conditions. 2020 Peachtree Road, NW, Atlanta, GA 30309; 404-352-2020; *http://www.shepherd.org*

Spina Bifida Association promotes prevention of spina bifida and works to enhance the lives of all affected. SBA, 4590 MacArthur Boulevard, NW, Suite 250, Washington, DC 20007-4226; 202-944-3285 or toll-free 1-800-621-3141; *http://www.sbaa.org*

The Institute for Rehabilitation and Research/Memorial Hermann Healthcare System provides quality health services in Southeast Texas. 1333 Moursund Street, Houston, TX 77030; 713-704-4000; *http://www.memorialhermann.org/locations/tirr*

Transverse Myelitis Association advocates for those who have transverse myelitis and related rare neuroimmunologic diseases. See *http://www.myelitis.org*

Unite 2 Fight Paralysis is dedicated to achieving a cure for spinal cord injury while empowering, educating and advocating for those living with it. Unite 2 Fight Paralysis. 5640 Alder Rd., Hood River, OR 97031; toll-free 1-888-202-1992; *http://www.unite2fightparalysis.org*

United Brachial Plexus Network informs, supports and unites families and those concerned with brachial plexus injuries. UBPN, 1610 Kent St. Kent, OH 44240; telephone 866-877-7004; *http://www.ubpn.org*

United Cerebral Palsy (UCP) offers resources on health and wellness, plus lifestyle, education and advocacy resources for all people with disabilities. 1660 L Street, NW, Suite 700, Washington, DC 20036; telephone 202-776-0406; *http://www.ucpa.org*

United Spinal Association promotes inclusion for persons with disabilities, access to health care, assistive technology, recreation, housing. USA, 75-20 Astoria Boulevard, Jackson Heights, NY 11370; 718-803-3782; *http://www.unitedspinal.org*

University of Florida Dept of Epidemiology and Biostatistics is concerned with public health, disability and health policy. USF College of Public Health, 13201 Bruce B Downs, MDC56, Tampa, FL 33612; 813-974-4860; *http://health.usf.edu/publichealth/epb*

University of Kansas Medical Center, Health Policy and Management studies public health, disability and health policy. Mail Stop 3044, 3901 Rainbow Boulevard, Kansas City, KS 66160; 913-588-3763; *http://www.kumc.edu/hpm*

University of Kansas Research & Training Center for Independent Living furthers independent living for people with productive research and innovative knowledge distribution, c/o Lawrence, KS 66045 -7555; 785-864-4095; *http://www.rtcil.org*

University of New Mexico School of Medicine, Center for Development and Disability promotes full inclusion of people with disabilities. c/o 2300 Menaul Blvd. NE, Albuquerque, NM 87107; 505-272-3000; *http://cdd.unm.edu*

University of South Carolina School of Medicine focuses on areas of public health, disability and health policy. 6311 Garners Ferry Rd. (Next to VA Hospital Complex) Columbia, SC 29209; 803-733-3200; *http://www.med.sc.edu*

Utah State University, Center for Persons with Disabilities promotes self-determination, independence. 6800 Old Main Hill, Logan, UT 84322-6800; 435-797-1981; toll-free 1-866-284-2821; *http://www.cpd.usu.edu*

Visiting Nurse Associations of America advances the nation's network of nurses who provide cost-effective and compassionate home healthcare to vulnerable individuals, particularly the elderly and individuals with disabilities. 900 19th St, NW, Suite 200, Washington, DC 20006; 202-384-1420. See *http://vnaa.org*

Volunteers for Medical Engineering applies technology to solve problems faced by people with disabilities. VME, 2301 Argonne Drive, Baltimore, MD 21218; 410-554-9134. *http://www.toad.net/~vme*

4-AMINOPYRIDINE (4-AP): A drug that improves conduction of nerve impulses in some people, leading to functional gains and reduced spasticity; may cause seizures, convulsions or dizziness. Branded as Fampridine, awaiting FDA nod.

ABDOMINAL BINDER: A wide elastic binder used to help prevent hypotension (drop in blood pressure). It is also used for cosmetic purposes, e.g., holding in the abdomen.

ACTIVITY DEPENDENT PLASTICITY: The theory that physical activity triggers nervous system recovery.

ACUTE: A stage of injury or stroke starting at the onset of symptoms. The opposite of chronic.

ADL: Rehab shorthand for "activities of daily living," e.g., dressing, eating, cooking.

AMBULATION: A "walking" motion, often aided by braces and/or crutches. Using functional electrical stimulation (FES) to fire their leg muscles, people with paralysis can ambulate short distances.

AMYOTROPHIC LATERAL SCLEROSIS (ALS) A disorder involving the loss of use of muscles. The nerves controlling these muscles are destroyed. Also known as Lou Gehrig's disease.

ANKYLOSIS: Loss of mobility in a joint caused by bony calcium deposits.

ANOXIA: A state of almost no oxygen delivery to a cell, resulting in low energy production and possible death of the cell.

ANTEGRADE CONTINENCE ENEMA: Facilitates movement of bowel by introducing an enema above the rectum by way of a stoma (opening) in the abdomen.

ANTICHOLINERGIC: A type of drug prescribed to reduce spasms of smooth muscle, especially the bladder.

ANTICOAGULANTS: A drug therapy used to prevent the formation of blood clots that can become lodged in cerebral arteries and cause strokes.

ANTIPLATELET AGENTS: A type of anticoagulant drug therapy that prevents the formation of blood clots by preventing the accumulation of platelets that form the basis of blood clots; some common antiplatelets include aspirin and ticlopidine.

APHASIA: The inability to understand or create speech, writing or language; generally due to damage to the speech centers of the brain.

APOPTOSIS: A form of cell suicide; often called programmed cell death because it is triggered by a genetic signal, involves specific cell mechanisms, and is irreversible once initiated.

ARACHNOIDITIS: Burning back pain caused by an inflamed arachnoid membrane (surrounding the spinal cord) due to disease or trauma, or to the injection of contrast dye for radiologic exams.

ARACHNOID MEMBRANE: The middle of the three membranes that surround the spinal cord and brain.

ARTERIOVENOUS MALFORMATION (AVM): A congenital disorder characterized by a complex tangled web of arteries and veins.

ASIA SCORE: A measure of function after spinal cord injury; used by physicians. "A" means complete injury; "E" means complete recovery.

ASTROCYTE: A star-shaped glial support cell that helps provide the chemical environment for nerve regeneration.

ATAXIA: A problem of muscle coordination due not to weakness, rigidity, spasticity or sensory loss, but to uncoordinated of movement.

ATELECTASIS: The collapse of part or all of a lung by blockage of the air passages or shallow breathing.

ATHEROSCLEROSIS: A blood vessel disease characterized by deposits of lipid (fat) material on the inside of the walls of large- to medium-sized arteries that make the artery walls thick, hard, brittle and prone to breaking.

ATROPHY: The loss of bulk in a muscle, nerve or organ from less than normal usage or from previous damage.

AUTOIMMUNE RESPONSE: The body's defense system against foreign substances turns on itself. Multiple sclerosis is believed to be an autoimmune disease.

AUTONOMIC DYSREFLEXIA (AD): A potentially dangerous reaction (sweating, chills, high blood pressure) to a stimulus below the level of lesion in people with injuries to the spinal cord above T6. Untreated, AD can lead to stroke.

AUTONOMIC NERVOUS SYSTEM: The part of the nervous system responsible for regulating the activity of internal organs. It includes the sympathetic and parasympathetic nervous systems.

AXON: The nerve fiber or process that carries a nerve impulse from the nerve terminals in the body back to the nerve cell.

BIOFEEDBACK: A process that uses sensory information (sight or sound) about blood pressure, muscle tension and other body functions and then enables people to control these functions.

BIPAP: Bilevel positive airway pressure, a noninvasive means of assisted breathing using a mask.

BLADDER AUGMENTATION: A surgical procedure using a portion of the intestine to expand bladder capacity in people who are incontinent;

makes possible the use of intermittent catheterization.

BLOOD-BRAIN BARRIER: An elaborate network of supportive brain cells that surround blood vessels and protect neurons from the possibly toxic effects of direct exposure to blood.

BROWN-SÉQUARD SYNDROME: An incomplete spinal cord injury wherein half of the cord has been damaged. There is spastic paralysis on the same side as the lesion and loss of sensation on the opposite side of the lesion.

CASE MANAGER: A person on the rehab team who handles discharge plans, works with insurance carriers and helps with equipment and/or home modifications as needed.

CATHETER: A rubber or plastic tube inserted in the urethra to withdraw urine from the bladder.

CAUDA EQUINA: The spinal roots descending from the tail bone area of the spinal cord.

CENTRAL CORD SYNDROME: Trauma to the center part of the cord only; may affect arms but not leg movement.

CENTRAL STROKE PAIN: Pain that is a mixture of sensations, which may include heat and cold, burning, tingling, numbness, sharp stabbing and underlying aching pain.

CENTRAL NERVOUS SYSTEM: Nerve tissue within the brain and spinal cord.

CEREBROSPINAL FLUID (CSF): The circulating clear fluid that bathes the brain and spinal cord, protecting them from shock.

CERVICAL: The portion of the spinal cord in the neck area.

CHRONIC: A condition that is continuous or persistent over an extended period of time; not easily or quickly resolved.

CLONUS: Involuntary movement of rapidly alternating contraction and relaxation of a muscle.

COLOSTOMY: A surgical procedure to facilitate emptying the bowel through the wall of the abdomen.

COMA: A sleep-like state in which an injured person does not open his/her eyes, speak, or obey simple commands.

COMPLETE INJURY: Generally, a spinal cord injury that cuts off all sensory and motor function below the lesion site.

COMPUTED TOMOGRAPHY (CT) SCAN: A series of X-rays of the brain and head; also called computerized axial tomography or CAT scan.

CONCUSSION: Reversible paralysis following brain trauma, usually involving loss of consciousness and/or a transient state of confusion.

CONGENITAL: A condition present at birth.

CONSTRAINT-INDUCED THERAPY: It restricts the use of a less affected extremity. Repetitive use of the more affected extremity improves function; has helped people with stroke and may be beneficial in CP, MS, incomplete spinal cord injuries.

CONTRACTURE: A joint that has stiffened to the point that it cannot be moved through its normal range.

CONTUSION: A type of injury due to mechanical or physical force; similar to bruising in that tissue is not lacerated or transected.

CPAP: Short for continuous positive airway pressure, a means of noninvasive breathing assistance using a mask.

CYCLIC AMP— an important intracellular signaling molecule that has many functions and enhances axon regeneration.

CREDÉ: Using the hands to push on the lower abdomen to express urine.

CYST: A cavity in the spinal cord that fills with fluid and can lead to loss of function, pain. Same as syrinx. See syringomyelia.

CYSTOGRAM: An X-ray of the bladder to show reflux (backward flow of urine back to the kidneys).

CYSTOSCOPY: A direct examination of the bladder using a cystoscope inserted in the urethra.

CYTOKINES: Small, hormone-like proteins that promote an inflammatory immune response to an injury.

CYTOTOXIC EDEMA: An influx of fluids and toxic chemicals into a cell causing swelling of the cell.

DECOMPRESSION: A surgical procedure that reduces pressure on the spinal cord by bone or disc material. Sometimes performed soon after the injury.

DECUBITUS: A skin sore caused by unrelieved pressure. deep vein thrombosis: Reduced blood flow in the lower extremities after spinal cord injury; can lead to blood clots that can, in turn, lead to pulmonary embolism (blocked blood vessels that can be fatal). Treated with anticoagulant drugs and compression hosiery.

DEMYELINATION: The loss of nerve function due to loss of nerve insulation called myelin. Common in multiple sclerosis and spinal cord injury.

DERMATOME: A schematic of the body that shows the expected functional abilities for various levels of spinal cord injury.

DME: Short for durable medical equipment, such as wheelchairs, walkers, respirators, etc.

DREZ: Short for dorsal root entry zone procedure, a surgical method of pain treatment that precisely cuts nerves in the dorsal root of the spinal cord.

DURA MATER: The tough, outermost membrane surrounding the spinal cord and brain.

DYSPHAGIA: Trouble eating and swallowing.

ECU (environmental control unit): Basically, a remote control unit to operate anything in a person's environment, such as computer, lights, television, bed, etc.

EDEMA: The swelling of a cell from large amounts of water or fluid that have entered the cell.

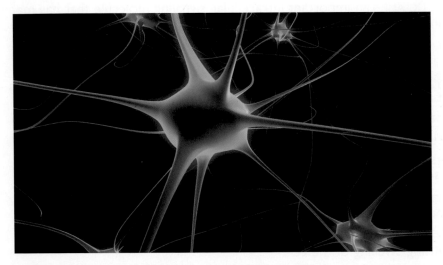

ELECTRO-EJACULATION: A method of obtaining viable sperm from men who are unable to produce a sample by other means; this involves an electrical probe in the rectum.

EMBOLIC STROKE: A stroke caused by an embolus, a free-roaming clot that usually forms in the heart and settles in the brain.

EMOTIONAL LABILITY: Uncontrolled laughing or crying; sometimes a symptom of multiple sclerosis.

EXACERBATION: In certain diseases (e.g., multiple sclerosis), a recurrence or worsening of symptoms.

EXCITATORY AMINO ACIDS: A type of neurotransmitter; proteins released by one neuron to promote an excitatory state in the other neuron.

EXCITOTOXICITY: Excessive release of neurotransmitters, causing damage to nerve and glia cells.

FUNCTIONAL ELECTRICAL STIMULATION (FES): Application of low-voltage currents to enhance the function of paralyzed muscles. Facilitates aerobic exercise, ambulation, handgrip, bladder control, etc.

FOLEY CATHETER: A type of bladder drainage system that remains inserted in the bladder and drains to a storage bag.

FRIEDREICH'S ATAXIA: An inherited, progressive dysfunction of the cerebellum, spinal cord and peripheral nerves.

GAMMA-AMINOBUTYRIC ACID (GABA): a neurotransmitter that inhibits the firing of neurons. Its activity is increased by benzodiazepine (Valium) and by anticonvulsant drugs.

GLASGOW COMA SCALE: A rating scale devised to assess the level of consciousness following brain damage. The scale assesses eye, verbal and motor responses. The GCS grades on a scale of 1–15, the lower score indicating the greater neurologic impairment.

GLIA: Also called neuroglia (derived from the Greek for glue); supportive cells of the nervous system that make up the blood-brain barrier, provide nutrients and oxygen to the vital neurons, and protect the neurons from infection, toxicity and trauma. There are three kinds: oligodendroglia, astrocytes and microglia.

GLOSSOPHARYNGEAL BREATHING: A method of "gulping" six to nine short breaths; can be used to prolong time off the ventilator or to facilitate cough. Also known as frog breathing.

GLUTAMATE: A neurotransmitter in the brain and spinal cord that excites neurons; an amino acid, also called glutamic acid. growth factors: Small proteins in the brain and spinal cord that are necessary for the development, function and survival of specific types of nerve cells.

GUILLAIN-BARRÉ syndrome: An acute nerve inflammation that damages portions of the nerve cell, resulting in muscle weakness or paralysis.

HARRINGTON RODS: Metal rods sometimes placed under the skin along the spinal column for support after spinal cord injury. hemiparesis: Weakness on one side of the body.

HEMIPLEGIA: Paralysis on one side of the body. hemorrhagic stroke: Sudden bleeding into or around the brain.

HETEROTOPIC OSSIFICATION: Bone deposits around the hips and knees and other connective tissue, generally related to inactivity.

HIPPOCAMPUS: The portion of the brain implicated in memory, learning.

HYDROCEPHALUS: A disorder associated with excessive cerebrospinal fluid in the brain; accompanies certain types of spina bifida.

HYDRONEPHROSIS: The kidney is so full of urine that it is impaired.

HYDROPHYLLIC CATHETER: Designed to be very slippery and therefore eases friction on urethra.

HYPERBARIC OXYGEN THERAPY: A system of delivering pressurized oxygen to help treat decompression sickness (the bends), smoke inhalation, air embolism and other conditions.

HYPERHYDROSIS: Excessive sweating, often seen in quadriplegics. May be caused by an overreaction of the sympathetic nervous system to an irritation below the level of injury.

HYPOTHERMIA: A technique to cool the spinal cord or brain after trauma. May reduce swelling and reduce the metabolic requirements of damaged tissue.

HYPOXIA: Lack of oxygen delivery to a cell.

ILEOSTOMY: A surgical procedure that opens the ileum (small intestine) to facilitate removal of fecal material through the abdomen.

IMMUNE RESPONSE: The body's defense mechanism to attack and eliminate microorganisms, viruses and substances recognized as foreign and potentially harmful.

INCOMPLETE INJURY: Generally, a spinal cord injury with preserved sensory or motor function below the lesion level.

INCONTINENCE: Loss of control of bowel or bladder.

INDWELLING CATHETER: A flexible tube that remains in the bladder for continuous draining.

INFARCT: An area of the brain or spinal cord tissue that is dead or dying because of a loss of blood supply.

INFORMED CONSENT: The requirement that volunteers in clinical experiments understand fully the risks and potential benefits of treatments.

INTERLEUKINS: A group of cytokine-related proteins involved in the inflammatory immune response of the ischemic cascade.

INTERMITTENT CATHETER: A flexible tube that is used to empty the bladder on a regular schedule; used for self-catheterization.

INTRACEREBRAL HEMORRHAGE: When a vessel within the brain leaks blood into the brain.

INTRATHECAL: Delivery of drugs (e.g., the spasm-control drug baclofen, or the painkiller morphine) by way of a small, implanted pump, allowing for higher dosage with fewer side effects.

ISCHEMIA: A loss of blood flow to tissue, caused by an obstruction of the blood vessel.

ISCHEMIC CASCADE: A series of events lasting for several hours to several

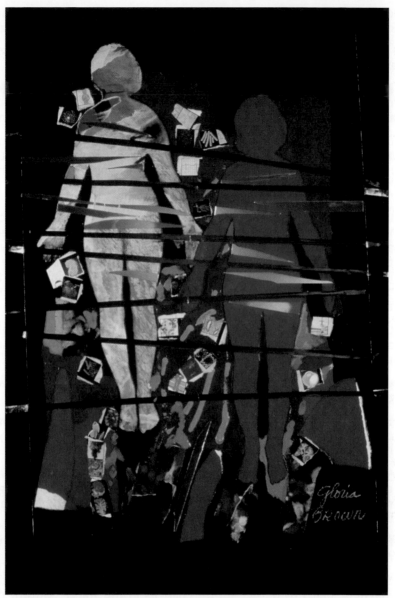

©Gloria Brown

ENTRAPMENT
24 x 36 INCHES, ACRYLIC ON CANVAS

GLORIA BROWN PAINTS TO CONVEY THE SHARED EXPERIENCE AND THE HEALING POWER OR ART, "TO TELL THE STORY AND TO MOTIVATE WOMEN TO HELP THEMSELVES BY BEING AWARE." SHE IS A CANCER SURVIVOR WHO ALSO LOST AN EYE TO GLAUCOMA.

days following initial ischemia in brain or spinal cord tissue; results in extensive cell death and tissue damage beyond the area originally affected by the lack of blood flow.

ISCHEMIC STROKE: Ischemia in the tissues of the brain.

IVP (INTRAVENOUS PYELOGRAM): A type of X-ray that examines the kidneys, bladder and ureters (the tubes that carry urine from the kidneys to the bladder).

LAMINECTOMY: An operation to relieve pressure on the spinal cord.
lesion: The site of injury or wound to the spinal cord.

LEUKOCYTES: Blood proteins involved in the inflammatory immune response of the ischemic cascade.

LOCOMOTOR TRAINING: A rehabilitation method whereby a person who is paralyzed is suspended in a harness so the legs can be moved along a treadmill to initiate patterned stepping movements. In theory, the training may unmask sensory and motor function. In fact, many people in Europe (mainly those with incomplete spinal cord injuries) have gotten functional return using treadmill training. Also called treadmill training.

LOWER MOTOR NEURONS: Nerve fibers that originate in the spinal cord and travel out of the central nervous system to the muscles. An injury to these nerves can affect bowel, bladder and sexual functions.

LUMBAR: The thickest section of the spine; the lower back below the thoracic area.

METHYLPREDNISOLONE: A steroid given to people with acute spinal cord trauma within eight hours of injury; a neuroprotective that may increase the chances for functional recovery.

MITROFANOFF PROCEDURE: This operation creates a conduit in the navel or lower abdomen connecting the bladder to a stoma, allowing intermittent catheterization for quadriplegics and women who have trouble accessing their urethra.

MOTOR NEURON: A nerve cell that carries information from the central nervous system to the muscles.

MRI (MAGNETIC RESONANCE IMAGING) scan: A type of imaging that uses magnetic fields to detect subtle changes in the water content of tissues.

MS (MULTIPLE SCLEROSIS): A chronic disease of the central nervous system. MS is believed to be an autoimmune disease, that is, the body attacks its own myelin.

MYELIN: White, fatty insulating material on nerve cells that helps rapid conduction of nerve impulses. Loss of myelin accompanies MS, spinal cord injury and other neurological conditions.

MYELOMENINGOCELE: A neural tube birth defect; a form of spina bifida usually accompanied by paralysis, wherein a portion of the spinal cord protrudes from the spinal column.

NECROSIS: A form of cell death resulting from anoxia, trauma or any other form of irreversible damage to the cell; involves the release of toxic cellular material into the intercellular space, poisoning surrounding cells.

NEUROGENIC BLADDER: A bladder with any disturbance due to an injury of the nervous system.

NEUROLOGIST: A physician who specializes in the medical treatment of diseases and disorders of the brain, spinal cord, nerves and muscles.

NEURON: The main cell of the brain and nervous system, consisting of a cell body, an axon and dendrites.

NEUROPROSTHESIS: A functional electrical stimulation device that allows paralyzed persons to do things such as breathe off a ventilator, grasp a key, stand for a transfer, empty the bladder.

NEUROPROTECTIVE AGENTS: Medications that protect the brain from secondary injury caused by stroke or trauma.

NOGO: a myelin-related molecule now the focus of clinical trials; inhibits growth of axons; can itself be blocked, allowing regenerative response.

NONSTEROIDAL ANTI-INFLAMMATORY DRUGS (NSAIDs): Medications such as aspirin and acetaminophen that reduce fever and pain; also have anti-inflammatory effects.

OCCUPATIONAL THERAPY: The process by which people with paralysis are taught to maximize their independence in the real world by use of assistive technology, management of daily living activities and maintenance of health.

OLIGODENDROCYTE: A support cell in the central nervous system.

OMENTAL TRANSPOSITION: A controversial surgical procedure that takes the tissue surrounding the lower abdomen area and places it over an area of injury. There are claims that the procedure has helped people with various types of neurological problems.

ORTHOSIS: An external device that supports the body and limbs or assists motion.

ORTHOSTATIC HYPOTENSION: Pooling of blood in the lower extremities; combined with lowered blood pressure in people with spinal cord injury, results in lightheadedness, numbness and/or pallor. Treated with elastic binders for the waist and elastic hose to prevent pooling.

OSTEOMYELITIS: infection of bone material, often related to decubitus ulcers.

OSTEOPOROSIS: Loss of bone density, common after paralysis, inactivity.

OSTOMY: An opening in the body to drain the bladder (cystostomy), to remove solid waste (colostomy or ileostomy) or allow passage of air (tracheostomy).

OXYGEN-FREE RADICALS: Toxic chemicals released in excessive amounts during necrosis of a cell; involved in secondary cell death associated with the ischemic cascade.

PARALYSIS: Injury or disease to a person's nervous system can affect the ability to move or feel.

PARAPLEGIA: Loss of function and paralysis below the cervical area of the neck; generally, the upper body retains motor and sensory function.

PARESTHESIAS: Transitory abnormal feelings such as numbness, prickling, or "pins and needles;" common in people with multiple sclerosis.

PASSIVE STANDING: Use of a frame or device to help a person stand who cannot do so otherwise; may have benefits for bone strength.

PATTERN GENERATION: There is evidence that the spinal cord itself, in the lumbar area, is able to process complex information necessary for stepping. Independent of brain input, this process is called central pattern generation. See locomotor training.

PCA: Personal care attendant.

PERCUSSION: Forceful tapping of the chest to dislodge and mobilize secretions.

PERIPHERAL NERVOUS SYSTEM: Nerves in the body away from the brain and SPINAL CORD; they have ability for self-repair that the central nervous system nerves do not.

PHRENIC NERVE STIMULATION: Application of an electrical signal to the phrenic nerve in the neck, which controls the diaphragm and, therefore, breathing.

PHYSIATRIST: A medical doctor who specializes in physical medicine and rehabilitation.

PHYSICAL THERAPY: The process of regaining maximum body function and physical abilities.

PLASMAPHERESIS: A treatment for certain immune-related diseases, including Guillain-Barré and in experiments, MS, whereby blood plasma is removed, filtered for certain antibodies and returned to the body.

PLASTICITY: The ability to be formed or molded; in reference to the brain or spinal cord, the ability for nerve cells to adapt to deficits and injury.

PNEUMOBELT: A type of noninvasive positive pressure ventilator that fits on the body like a corset. A pump fills the belt with air, which pushes the diaphragm to rise and produces an exhale. When the belt is then deflated, the diaphragm falls and air flows into the lungs.

POLIO: A disease of the central nervous system that attacks the motor nerves. Poliomyelitis, transmitted only by humans, leaves the body within a few months of infection, but often leaves people with weakened limbs or paralysis. No wild polio has been found in the United States for more than 20 years, but polio still exists in some parts of the world.

POST-POLIO SYNDROME: Accelerated aging process characterized by fatigue, pain and/or loss of function in people who had polio years ago.

POSTURAL HYPOTENSION: Reduced muscle and blood vessel activity in the lower extremities, which causes blood to pool in the legs of people who are paralyzed. Reduced blood pressure can cause lightheadedness. Wearing elastic hose is recommended.

PRESSURE SORE: A skin breakdown due to unrelieved pressure.

PRIAPISM: An erection that lasts for several hours or more; a dangerous side effect of certain drugs that improve erectile dysfunction.

QUADRIPLEGIA: Scientifically known as tetraplegia; paralysis affecting all four limbs.

RANGE OF MOTION: Normal movement of a joint, typically restricted by injury.

RECIPROCATING GAIT ORTHOSIS: This is a brace system that allows paraplegics to stand hands-free and to swing legs in a gait pattern; requires less energy than other types of braces.

REFLUX: The flow of urine backward into the kidneys; can lead to kidney breakdown.

REGENERATION: The regrowth and reconnection of damaged nerves. The process of repair occurs routinely in the peripheral nervous system, but not in the central nervous system (brain or spinal cord). In experiments, scientists have regrown nerve fibers in the spinal cord and brain by adding conditioning molecules and removing inhibitory factors. While there is hope where there was once only the dogma of doubt, functional regeneration remains a difficult problem.

REHABILITATION: A set of services intended to restore maximum function — physical, psychological, vocational and social — to a person with a disability.

RHO – An enzyme that is part of the intracellular signaling involved in the regeneration-blocking effect of Nogo and other growth cone collapsing molecules.

RP (RETROGRADE PYELOGRAM): A tool to diagnose kidney function using contrast material.

RHIZOTOMY: The cutting of nerves to interrupt spasticity or pain signals

SECONDARY CONDITIONS: A primary condition is a medical diagnosis: spina bifida, spinal cord injury, etc. A secondary condition is any medical, social, emotional, mental, family or community problem that a person with a primary condition may experience, such as pressure sores, pain, depression, reduced social life, lack of gainful work, etc.

SECONDARY INJURY: A cascade of chemical activities following trauma to the brain or spinal cord that contribute to the damage. Included are swelling, loss of blood flow, release of free radicals, excitotoxic amino acid release, etc. Experimental strategies counter these effects.

SIALORRHEA: The term for excess salivation and drooling. sheer: the friction on tissues caused by dragging across a surface; can cause skin to break down.

SHUNT: A small tube to drain a cavity or syrinx; in spina bifida it is used to reduce hydrocephalus.

SLEEP APNEA: Irregular breathing or snoring, can lead to fatigue, loss of memory, poor concentration. Increased incidence among people with respiratory weakness. Treated with BiPAP.

SPASTICITY: Uncontrolled muscle activity. This condition can be beneficial for muscle tone but can also interfere with daily activities. Known medically as spastic hypertonia. sphincter: The muscle that opens or closes the urethra or rectum.

SPHINCTEROTOMY: A surgical procedure to relax the urethral sphincter, thus improving bladder function. An alternative is the placement of a stent, which is reversible. Botulinium toxin (Botox) has also been used to relax the sphincter.

SPINA BIFIDA: Congenital spinal cord dysfunction due to malformed neural tube during prenatal development.

SPINAL SHOCK: After the initial spinal trauma, this condition, similar to a coma from a brain concussion, occurs; the nervous system shuts down and the body becomes flaccid. Can last for three or four weeks.

STROKE: A "brain attack" leading to loss of brain tissue; caused by bursting or blocked blood vessels in the brain. subarachnoid hemorrhage: Bleeding onto the surface of the brain, caused by trauma or a break in a blood vessel (aneurysm) at the base of the brain. Blood is mixed with cerebrospinal fluid, which surrounds the brain and spinal cord.

SUPRAPUBIC CYSTOSTOMY: An opening through the abdomen to drain the bladder with a catheter, known as a "super tube."

MPATHETIC NERVOUS SYSTEM: A subset of the autonomic (involuntary) ervous system that accelerates heart rate, constricts blood vessels d boosts blood pressure.

RINGOMYELIA: A disorder caused by formation of a fluid-filled cavity yrinx) within the spinal cord.

RINX: A fluid filled cavity in the spinal cord; can create pressure related functional loss and pain.

NDON TRANSFER: A type of hand surgery that offers qualified quadriple-:s significant increase in hand function. Takes advantage of functioning uscles in the arms by moving the tendons that control the hands.

NODESIS: A hand splint made of metal or plastic that is used to crease hand function.

THERED CORD: Occurs when scar tissue develops between the cord d the dura mater or arachnoid, two of the membranes covering the inal cord and brain. Tethering is believed to create and/or worsen mptoms of an existing syrinx.

TRAPLEGIA: The linguistically accurate term for paralysis affecting all ur limbs. More commonly known as quadriplegia.

ORACIC: The portion of the spinal column in the chest, between the rvical and lumbar areas.

ROMBOLYTICS: Drugs used to treat an ongoing, acute ischemic stroke ' dissolving the blood clot causing the stroke and thereby restoring ood flow through the artery.

ACHEOSTOMY: An opening in the windpipe to facilitate breathing.

ANSVERSE MYELITIS: Inflammation in the spinal cord interfering with :rve function below the level of the inflammation. An acute attack of lammatory demyelination.

EADMILL TRAINING: see locomotor training

PER MOTOR NEURONS: These are the long nerve cells that originate in e brain and travel through the spinal cord. Disruption of these cells ads to paralysis, although some reflex activity is still possible.

(VOCATIONAL REHABILITATION): A program in all states to assist people th disabilities with assessment, tools and training to find employment.

ARFARIN: A commonly used anticoagulant, also known as Coumadin.

EANING: The gradual removal of mechanical ventilation as a person's gs gain strength.

HITE MATTER: The portion of the spinal cord containing nerve tracts at are covered by myelin.

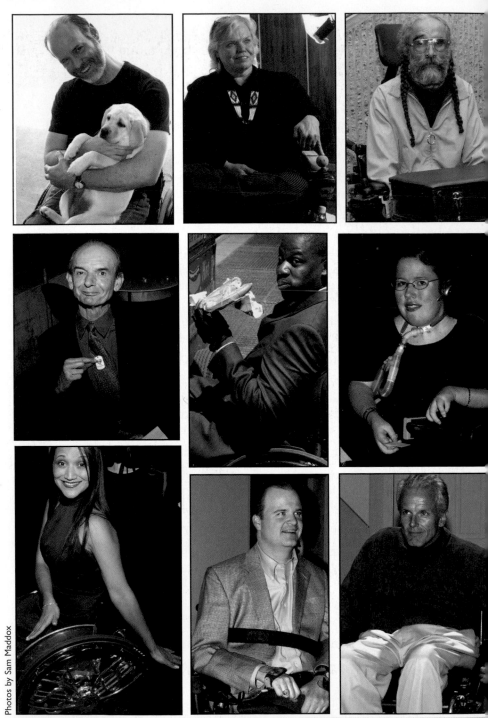

"Either you decide to stay in the shallow end of the pool or you go out in the ocean." - Christopher Reeve

INDEX

ABOUT THE AUTHOR

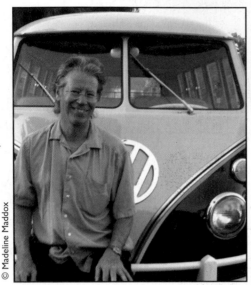

© Madeline Maddox

Sam Maddox is Knowledge Manager for the Christopher & Dana Reeve Foundation Paralysis Resource Center. He is a journalist, educator and director who oversees *www.paralysis.org* and produces the PRC multimedia catalog. In 1988 Mr. Maddox wrote and published *Spinal Network, the Total Resource for the Wheelchair Community*. Soon after he created *New Mobility*, a full service magazine for the wheelchair community. He lives in Southern California with his children Max and Madeline.

ABOUT THE PRC

The Christopher & Dana Reeve Foundation Paralysis Resource Center (PRC) was created in 2002 to provide a comprehensive information source for people living with paralysis and their caregivers to promote health, community involvement and quality of life.

The PRC, formed through a cooperative agreement with the Centers for Disease Control and Prevention, is staffed by a team highly trained Information Specialists (in English and Spanish) who research and answer queries across a wide range of issues. People may email their questions (c/o *info@paralysis.org*) or call the Center's toll-free number (1-800-539-7309) to contact an Information Specialist. The PRC website (*www.paralysis.org*) is a clearinghouse of information, with news, interactive features, multimedia productions and links to deeper resources.

The PRC is located in Short Hills, New Jersey, with a branch office in Westlake Village, California (north of Los Angeles). The fully accessible Center welcomes visitors. The PRC houses a large lending library covering all topics related to paralysis. These materials, cataloged by title, author and subject on *www.paralysis.org*, are available at no cost through interlibrary loan from local libraries.